MEDICINAL PLANTS:
Conservation, Cultivation and Utilization

MEDICINAL PLANTS:
Conservation, Cultivation and Utilization

Editors
Prof. A.K. Chopra
Dr. D.R. Khanna
Dr. G. Prasad
Dr. D.S. Malik
Dr. R. Bhutiani

2007
DAYA PUBLISHING HOUSE
Delhi - 110 035

ISBN 81-7035-486-2

Published by : **Daya Publishing House**
1123/74, Deva Ram Park
Tri Nagar, Delhi - 110 035
Phone: 27383999
Fax: (011) 23244987
e-mail : dayabooks@vsnl.com
website : www.dayabooks.com

Showroom : 4760-61/23, Ansari Road, Darya Ganj,
New Delhi - 110 002
Phone: 23245578, 23244987

Laser Typesetting : **Classic Computer Services**
Delhi - 110 035

Printed at : **Chawla Offset Printers**
Delhi - 110 052

PRINTED IN INDIA

Preface

The knowledge of medicinal plants came from our ancient literature i.e. Vedas. The literature describes plants for the cure of human ailments and diseases. The word medicinal plant often leads to the thought of some miraculous and supernatural cures. In India, medicinal plants have played a significant role in the development of our ancient Materia Medica.

With the changing times and fast developmental changes, the importance of medicinal plants i.e. conservation, cultivation and utilization of medicinal plants has declined at an alarming rate despite of their golden past for which the rapid extension of the allopathic system of medicinal treatment is the main impediment

Medicinal plants are our local heritage with global importance. An estimate measures that about 72,000 plant species including lichens to larger trees, have medicinal values. In Ayurveda about 2000 plant species are considered as medicinal.

Medicinal and aromatic plants are found throughout South Asia in forest areas from plains to Himalayas, with greatest concentration in the tropical and subtropical belts and arid region of Thar Desert. India recognizes more than 2,500 plant species with medicinal values.

India is endowed with a rich wealth of medicinal plants, placing our country as one of the top producers of herbal medicines. But today due to urbanization, industrialization and other anthropogenic activities the total forest area is reducing at an alarming rate and hence the total cultivation/collection of medicinal plants is reducing in India. If this trend of deforestation, urbanization etc. continues, we may lose the wealth of medicinal plants, which may ultimately affect the economy of our country.

The present book is aimed to fulfill the lacuna regarding awareness, importance, benefits, current status, conservation, cultivation and utilization of medicinal plants, for those who are working in this field and also the general public.

Through this book we attempt to determine and analyze the conservation, cultivation and utilization measures of medicinal plants. All eminent scientists of India have enthusiastically contributed in this book.

We are grateful to the contributors, who have impaired benefits of their research work and without their support the outcome of this book simply would not have been possible. We are confident that this book will serve its purpose. We also thank our publishers M/s Daya Publishing House, New Delhi for bringing up the book in a fantastic way.

Editors

Contents

List of Contributors

A.K. Chopra

Department of Zoology and Environmental Science, Gurukula Kangri University, Haridwar, India

A.K. Dobriyal

Department of Zoology, H.N.B. Garhwal University Campus, Pauri Garhwal – 246 001, Uttaranchal

A.K. Singh

Department of Botany, R.B.S. College, Agra

Ajay Kumar Sharma

Professor and Head, P.G. Department of Kayachikitsa, National Institute of Ayurveda, Jaipur

Ajay Singh

Department of Chemistry, Dolphin (P.G.) Institute of Biomedical and Natural Science, V.P.O. Manduwala, Near to Suddhowala, Chakrata Road, Dehradun – 248 007 (U.A.)

Alok Gupta

Research Division, Chemistry Department, Sahu Jain College, Najibabad (U.P)

Amit Agarwal

Assistant Professor, Department of Computer Science and Information Technology Graphic Era Institute of Technology, Dehradun – 248 002 (UA)

Amit Kumar

Department of Chemistry, Gurukula Kangri University, Hardwar – 249 404, Uttaranchal, India

Amit Raghuwanshi

Paharsinghpura, Haweli Path, Khargone – 451 001 (M.P.)

Anika Rana

Department of Botany and Microbiology, Gurukul Kangri University, Hardwar – 249404

Anil Kumar Dhiman

Information Scientist, Gurukul Kangri University, Haridwar – 249 404, Uttaranchal

Anjma Bhanti

Department of Botany, Raja Balwant Singh College, Agra – 282 002, India

Anupama Gautam

Department of Botany and Microbiology, Gurukul kangri University, Haridwar

Arun Arya

Department of Botany, Faculty of Science, The Maharaja Sayajirao University of Baroda, Vadodara

Arun Chugh

Navoday Ayurved and Panchkarm, A-29, Sri Ram Nagar Colony, Opposite Railway Station, Jwalapur – 249 407, Haridwar, U.A.

Arun Gupta

Ecology Research Laboratory, Department of Botany, D.A.V. (PG) College, Dehra Dun – 248 007, Uttaranchal

Arun Pratap Singh

Department of Microbiology, Dolphin (P.G.) Institute of Biomedical and Natural Science, V.P.O. Manduwala, Near to Suddhowala, Chakrata Road, Dehradun – 248 007 (U.A.)

Asha Dobhal

Department of Botany, Government Post Graduate College, New Tehri, Tehri Garhwal – 249 001

Ashish Panwar

K.V. College, Machhra, Meerut (U.P.)

Ashuthosh Sharma

Research Division, Chemistry Department, Sahu Jain College, Najibabad (U.P)

C. Shekhar

Research Division, Chemistry Department, Sahu Jain College, Najibabad (U.P)

C.J. Khune

Department of Zoology, M.B. Patel College, Sakoli

C.L. Dulkar

Botany Department, Government P.G. College, Khargone – 451 001 (M.P.)

C.M. Sharma

Associate Professor, P.G. Department of Neurology, SMS Medical College, Jaipur

C.P. Singh

Research Division, Chemistry Department, Sahu Jain College, Najibabad (U.P)

Chandra P. Kuniyal

Herbal Research and Development Institute, Gopeshwar-Chamoli – 246 401, Uttaranchal, India

Chetna Sawale

Research Student, 7, Kunda Nagar, Khargone – 451 001 (M.P.)

D.K. Bhatia

PG Department of Zoology, DBS (PG) College, Dehradun

D.R. Khanna

Department of Zoology and Environmental Science, Gurukul Kangri Vishwavidyalaya, Haridwar – 249 404, U.A.

Deepak D. Ramteke

Department of Botany, M.B. Patel College, Sakoli

Deepak Kholiya

Forest Ecology and Environment Division, Forest Research Institute, Dehradun, Uttaranchal, India

Deepika Chauhan

Department of Botany and Microbiology, Gurukula Kangri University, Haridwar – 249 404, India

Dinesh Kumar Bhardwaj

Department of Biotechnology, Shri Ram College, Muzaffarnagar – 251 001

Divya Goyal

Department of Botany, Raja Balwant Singh College, Agra – 282 002, India

G.R.S. Bisht

Sardar Bhagwan Singh (P.G) Institute of Biomedical Sciences and Research, Balawala, Dehradun

(Late) G.S. Negi

Department of Chemistry, H.N.B. Garhwal University Campus, Pauri Garhwal – 246 001, Uttaranchal

G.S. Rajwar

Department of Botany, Govt. P.G. College, Rishikesh, Dehradun – 249 201

Gyanendra Awasthi

Department of Biochemistry, Dolphin (P.G.) Institute of Biomedical and Natural Science, V.P.O. Manduwala, Near to Suddhowala, Chakrata Road, Dehradun – 248 007 (U.A.)

H.B. Vashistha

Forest Ecology and Environment Division, Forest Research Institute, Dehradun, Uttaranchal, India

H.K. Joshi

Department of Zoology, H.N.B. Garhwal University Campus, Pauri Garhwal – 246 001, Uttaranchal

Harish Chander Dutt

Department of Botany, University of Jammu, Jammu

Harish Chandra

Department of Microbiology, Dolphin (P.G.) Institute of Biomedical and Natural Science, V.P.O. Manduwala, Near to Suddhowala, Chakrata Road, Dehradun – 248 007 (U.A.)

Harish Chauhan

Ashtavaidyaratnam Vaidyasala Hospital and Research Centre, Shyampur Kangri, Haridwar

Hemlata

Herbal Research and Development Institute, Gopeshwar-Chamoli – 246 401, Uttaranchal, India

J.S. Jagwan

School of Natural Product, Department of Chemistry, HNB Garhwal University, SRT Campus, Badshahi Thaul – 249 199, Tehri Garhwal (U.A.) India

J.S. Kathait

School of Natural Product, Department of Chemistry, HNB Garhwal University, SRT Campus, Badshahi Thaul – 249 199, Tehri Garhwal (U.A.) India

Jatin Kumar Srivastava

Department of Environmental Sciences Institute of Biosciences and Biotechnology, Chatrapati Shahu Ji Maharaj University, Kalyanpur, Kanpur, India

Jinesh Shah

Department of Botany, Faculty of Science, The Maharaja Sayajirao University of Baroda, Vadodara – 390 002

Jyotsana Bhoraskar

Holkar Science College, Indore

Kajal Srivastava

P.G. Environmental Management, Department of Botany, Bareilly College, Bareilly – 243 005, (U.P.)

L.P. Awasthi

Department of Plant Pathology, N.D. University of Agriculture and Technology, Kumarganj, Faizabad – 224 229 (U.P.)

Laxmi Rawat

Forest Ecology and Environment Division, Forest Research Institute, Dehradun, Uttaranchal, India

M.F. Alam

Department of Zoology and Environmental Science, Gurukula Kangri University, Haridwar, India

M.M. Keshare

Botany Department, Government P.G. College, Khargone – 451 001 (M.P.)

Manisha Dhasmana

Department of Botany, Raja Balwant Singh College, Agra – 282 002, India

Manisha Dobhal

Department of Chemistry, H.N.B. Garhwal University Campus, Badhshaithaul Tehri, Garhwal

Manisha

Department of Botany, Raja Balwant Singh College, Agra – 282 002, India

Manjari Kumari

Department of Botany, R.B.S. College, Agra

Maya Ram Uniyal

Director, Farm, Maharishi Ayurvedic (NEPZ) Products, Noida – 201 305, U.P.

Mitesh B. Panchal

Department of Botany, Faculty of Science, The Maharaja Sayajirao University of Baroda, Vadodara – 390 002

Miti Rani

Department of Botany, RBS College, Agra

Murali Manohar

Faculty of Engineering and Technology, Gurukul Kangri Vishwavidyalaya, Haridwar – 249 404

N.K. Agarwal

Department of Zoology, HNB Garhwal University, SRT Campus, Badshahi Thaul – 249 199, Tehri Garhwal (U.A.) India

Navneet

Department of Botany and Microbiology Gurukula Kangri University, Hardwar – 249 404, Uttaranchal

Neetu Saxena

Department of Zoology and Environmental Sciences, Gurukul Kangri University, Hardwar, India

Niraj N. Upadhyay

Department of Botany, Faculty of Science, The Maharaja Sayajirao University of Baroda, Vadodara – 390 002

Nitin Dongarwar

P.G. Department of Botany, Nagpur University Nagpur

P.K. Bahuguna

Department of Zoology, H.N.B. Garhwal University Campus, Pauri Garhwal – 246 001, Uttaranchal

P.P. Badoni

Department of Chemistry, H.N.B. Garhwal University Campus, Pauri Garhwal – 246 001, Uttaranchal

Pardeep Kumar

Department of Plant Pathology, N.D. University of Agriculture and Technology, Kumarganj, Faizabad – 224 229 (U.P.)

Pawan Kumar Sagar

State Drug Testing Laboratory, Rishikul Government Ayurvedic Pharmacy, Haridwar, Uttaranchal

Prabhat

Department of Botany and Microbiology, Gurukul Kangri University, Hardwar – 249 404

Pradeep Sharma

Department of Zoology and Environmental Science Gurukul Kangri Vishwavidyalaya, Haridwar – 249 404, U.A.

Pramod Kumar

Department of Botany HNB Garhwal University Campus, B. Thaul, Tehri Garhwal – 249 199

Pramod Uniyal

Government (PG) College, Rishikesh, Uttaranchal

Premendra Singh

Department of Botany, Faculty of Science, The Maharaja Sayajirao University of Baroda, Vadodara – 390 002

Pushpa Singh

Department of Animal Science, Faculty of Applied Sciences, M.J.P. Rohilkhand University, Bareilly – 243 006, U.P. India

R. Bhutiani

Department of Zoology and Environment Science, Gurukul Kangri University, Haridwar

R.C. Dubey

Department of Botany and Microbiology, Gurukul Kangri University, Hardwar – 249404

R.K. Pande

PG Department of Zoology, DBS (PG) College, Dehradun

R.K.S. Rathore

Department of Botany, Raja Balwant Singh College, Agra – 282 002, India

R.V. Singh

Department of Plant Pathology, N.D. University of Agriculture and Technology, Kumarganj, Faizabad – 224 229 (U.P.)

Reena Pandey

Lecturer, CDM College of Ayurveda, Jagadhari, Distt. Yamuna Nagar (HR)

Rekha Sharma

Assistant Professor, Government P.G. College, Mhow

S. Sisodia

Department of Botany, Faculty of Science, The Maharaja Sayajirao University of Baroda, Vadodara – 390 002

S.B. Zade

Department of Zoology, M.B. Patel College, Sakoli

S.C. Sati

Department of Chemistry, H.N.B. Garhwal University Campus, Srinagar, Garhwal

S.K. Kamboj

Forest Ecology and Environment Division, Forest Research Institute, Dehradun, Uttaranchal, India

S.K. Mahajan

Post Graduate Department of Botany, Government College, Khargone – 451 001 (M.P.)

S.K. Pathak

Department of Zoology, Government P.G. College, Mhow

S.P. Bhatnagar

Department of Pharmaceutical Sciences, Birla Institute of Technology, Ranchi – 835 215

S.P. Joshi

Ecology Research Laboratory, Department of Botany, D.A.V. (PG) College, Dehra Dun – 248 007, Uttaranchal

Sachin Srivastava

Department of Animal Science, Faculty of Applied Sciences, M.J.P. Rohilkhand University, Bareilly – 243 006, U.P. India

Sanjay

Department of Botany and Microbiology, Gurukul Kangri Vishwavidyalaya, Haridwar – 249 404

Seema Bhadauria

Department of Botany, Raja Balwant Singh College, Agra – 282 002, India

Shailu Dalal

Department of Biotechnology, IIT, Roorkee

Shikha Singhal

S-69, Shivalik Nagar, BHEL, Haridwar – 249 403 (UA)

Shivom Singh

P.G. Environmental Management, Department of Botany, Bareilly College, Bareilly – 243 005, (U.P.)

Shri Krishna

Department of Chemistry, Gurukula Kangri University, Hardwar – 249 404, Uttaranchal, India

Shyam Singh

Department of Plant Pathology, N.D. University of Agriculture and Technology, Kumarganj, Faizabad – 224 229 (U.P.)

Sudha Dubey

Holkar Science College, Indore

Suman Bisht

Department of Botany, HNB Garhwal University Campus, Tehri Garhwal

Sunita Pathak

Department of Economics Government P.G. College, Mhow

U.S. Patil

Department of Botany, Bharatiya Mahvidyalaya, Amravati

Uttam Kumar Sharma

Reader, Department of Kayachikitsa, State Ayurvedic College, Gurukul Kangri, Hardwar

V. Kaushik

Department of Pharmaceutical Sciences, S.B.S.PG.I of Biomedical Sciences and Research, Balawala, Dehradun – 248 161 (UA)

V.K. Dua

National Institute of Malaria Research (ICMR) F/S, BHEL, Haridwar, India

V.K. Pandey

Reader, Sharir Kriya, Government Ayurveda College and Hospital, Gurukul Kangri Haridwar (U.A.)

Veena Joshi

School of Natural Product, Department of Chemistry, HNB Garhwal University, SRT Campus, Badshahi Thaul – 249 199, Tehri Garhwal (U.A.) India

Vinod Upadhyay

Hon. Advisor, Himalik Herbs India, Jwalapur, Haridwar – 249 407, India

Virendra Mandloi

Kunda Nagar (Near Canal), Khargone – 451 001 (M.P.)

Vishal K. Muliya

Department of Botany, Faculty of Science, The Maharaja Sayajirao University of Baroda, Vadodara – 390 002

Y.P.S. Pangtey

Department of Botany, DSB Campus Kumaun University, Nainital – 263 002, Uttaranchal

Introduction

The history of medicine and surgery dates back perhaps to the origin of the human race. In India, the Vedas are the epic poems, which contains rich material on the herbal medicines of that time. The Charaka Samhita, written by the physician Charaka, followed the Vedas. Charaka known as the father of medicinė in India provide medicinal treatise, which includes details of around 350 herbal medicines most of these continue to be gathered from wild plants to meet the demand of the medical profession. Thus, despite the rich heritage of knowledge on the use of plant drugs, little attention had been paid to grow them as field crops in the country till the latter part of the nineteenth century.

The book, *Yellow Emperor's Classic of Internal Medicine* is the earliest Chinese medical text written in 1st century BC and listed dozens of medicinal plants, their uses and related spells and incantations.

India is endowed with a rich wealth of medicinal plants. These plants have made a good contribution to the development of ancient Indian Materia medica. India one of the 12 mega biodiversity centers of the world is one of the richest country in plant wealth and medicinal plant heritage. Human beings have been utilizing plants for basic preventive and curative health care since time immemorial. Recent estimates suggest that over 9,000 plants have known medicinal applications in various cultures and countries, and this is without having conducted comprehensive research amongst several indigenous and other communities (Farnsworth and Soejarto 1991).

The Foundation for Revitalization of Local Health Traditions, a nongovernmental organization (NGO) dedicated to conservation of medicinal plants and a renewed appreciation of India's traditional health systems, describes India's rich plant-based medical heritage in these words:

"India's traditional medical systems are part of a time-honoured and time-tested culture that still intrigues people today. A culture that has successfully used nature to treat primary and complex ailments for over 3,000 years obviously has a contemporary relevance. In an age when toxic drugs are increasingly unwelcome and when thinking people are using viable alternatives, India's medical heritage must be documented, saved and used"

Medicinal and aromatic plants are important products found in forest areas throughout India, from the plains to the Himalayas, with the greatest concentration in the tropical and subtropical belts. About 2,500 plant species found in India, 1400 in Sri lanka, 700 in Nepal are known for having medicinal value. Some of these, found at high altitudes in particularly stressful environments, grow very slowly and cannot live elsewhere. Others are more broadly distributed and adapt more easily to different ecological conditions.

During the past decade, a dramatic increase in exports of medicinal plants attests to worldwide interest in these products as well as in traditional health systems. In the last 10 years, for example, India's export of medicinal plants has trebled. But with most of these plants being taken from the wild, hundreds of species are now threatened with extinction because of over harvesting, destructive collection techniques, and conversion of habitats to crop-based agriculture. Hence it becomes necessary to conserve, cultivate and properly utilize the medicinal plants for sustainable development of the country.

The rich knowledge base of countries like India in medicinal plants and health care has led to a keen interest by pharmaceutical companies to use this knowledge as a resource for research and development programs in the hope of discovering and producing new drugs.

The scientific studies of such plants are carried out all over in India since vedic times (i.e. more than 6000 years B.C.). This science is known as Ayurveda i.e. Ayu means life and veda means knowledge. In Sanskrit knowledge of life is called "Ayurveda". The system of Ayurveda in its diagnostic part differs very much from the Allopathic system and hence the property ascribed to medicinal plants also differs. The plants are the basic source of knowledge of Modern Medicine and still continue the same position.

Traditional medicines are used by about 60 per cent of the world's population. These are not only used for primary health care not just in rural areas in developing countries, but also in developed countries as well where modern medicines are predominantly used. While the traditional medicines are derived from medicinal plants, minerals, and organic matter, the herbal drugs are prepared from medicinal plants only.

Use of plants as a source of medicine has been inherited and is an important component of the health care system in India. In the Indian systems of medicine, most practitioners formulate and dispense their own recipes, hence this requires proper documentation and research. Public, academic and government interest in traditional medicines is growing exponentially due to the increased incidence of the adverse drug reactions and economic burden of the modern system of medicine. There are about 45,000 plant species in India, with concentrated hotspots in the region of Eastern Himalayas, Western Ghats and Andaman & Nicobar Island. The officially documented plants with medicinal potential are 3000 but traditional practitioners use more than 6000.

India is the largest producer of medicinal herbs and is appropriately called the botanical garden of the world. There are currently about 250,000 registered medical practitioners of the Ayurvedic system (total for all traditional systems: approximately 291,000), as compared to about 700,000 of the modern medicine system. In rural India, 70 per cent of the population is dependent on the traditional system of medicine, the Ayurveda.

The major hindrance in the amalgamation of herbal medicines into modern medical practices is the lack of scientific and clinical data, and better understanding of efficacy and safety of the herbal products. To ensure the quality and safety of its products and practices standardization is of vital importance.

Keeping in view the above mentioned problems related to medicinal plants an attempt has been made to pool together the expertise ideas in this book for proper conservation, cultivation and utilization of medicinal plants through advanced technologies, along with the help of science and knowledge given by Vedas and finally for sustainable and economic development of the Nation.

D.R. Khanna

R. Bhutiani

Medicinal Plants: Conservation, Cultivation and Utilization (2007) *Pages 1–10*
Editors: A.K. Chopra, D.R. Khanna, G. Prasad, D.S. Malik and R. Bhutiani
Published by: DAYA PUBLISHING HOUSE

Chapter 1

Traditional Health Care in a Remote Area of District Chamoli (Garhwal), Uttaranchal: What Could Do With?

Hemlata[1], Chandra P. Kuniyal[1*] and Y.P.S. Pangtey[2]
[1]Herbal Research and Development Institute, Gopeshwar-Chamoli – 246 401, Uttaranchal, India
[2]Department of Botany, DSB Campus Kumaun University, Nainital – 263 002, Uttaranchal

ABSTRACT

Ethnomedicobotanical surveys were conducted in a remote area namely Ghat block of district Chamoli, Uttaranchal. A total 191 plants were recorded to be used in the traditional health care system. Of the total plants used in curing various ailments, 50.26 per cent were herbs; 20.42 per cent were trees and remaining were either herbs or under shrubs, shrubs, climbers, shrubs or small trees and grasses. All the plants used traditionally in various remedies were belonging to 83 families of angiosperms and a single family of pteridophyte namely Equisitaceae. More than 53.00 per cent plants used in traditional remedies were belonging to 16 families namely; Ranunculaceae, Lamiaceae, Asteraceae, Apiaceae, Rosaceae, Fabaceae, Solanaceae, Zingiberaceae, Rutaceae, Liliaceae, Orchidaceae, Caesalpiniaceae, Polygonaceae, Euphorbiaceae, Araceae and Ericaceae. It was interesting to note that 69 diseases and other health problems are traditionally cured in this area. Root part (21.65 per cent) was predominantly used plant part in the indigenous medicinal preparations, followed by leaves (16.23 per cent), whole plant (12.04 per cent), seeds (9.42 per cent) and fruits (8.90 per cent). Other plant parts or by products used were rhizomes, stem/shoot, tuberous roots or tubers, flowers, bulbs, bark, fruit kernels, root

* Phone +91-1372-253854, 252572, Fax: +91-1372-253855. Email: cpkuniyal@rediffmail.com

bark, wood, latex, gum, resin and insect galls of different plants. Finding of this study revealed that, some of the serious diseases are successfully treated through indigenous remedies, as well; traditional health care is still alive in the remote areas, probably owing to the least modern health care facilities. Application of plants as an insecticide, anthelmentic, in sciatica pain, scabies, anemia, spermatorhoea, leprosy, jaundice, arthritis, piles and chronic bronchitis were some of the useful findings. However, it was also noticed that, in the majority of cases plants used in traditional health care are harvested in destructive and unsustainable ways. Some of the plants enlisted for priority conservation under *in situ* and *ex situ* conditions and CITES are used by native folk. These plants were *Aconitum heterophyllum*, *A. atrox*, *Angelica glauca*, *Arnebia benthamii*, *Betula utilis*, *Cinnamomum tamala*, *Dactylorhiza hatagirea*, *Ephedra gerardiana*, *Gloriosa superba*, *Nardostachys jatamansi*, *Podophyllum hexandrum*, *Polygonatum verticillatum*, *Roylea cinerea*, *Saussurea lappa*, *S. obvallata*, *Swertia chirayita*, *Symplocos paniculata*, *Taraxacum officinale*, *Valeriana jatamansi* and *Xanthoxyllum armatum*. A number of high altitude plant species such as *Aconitum heterophyllum*, *Aconitum atrox*, *Angelica glauca*, *Arnebia benthamii*, *Caltha palustris*, *Dactylorhiza hatagirea*, *Delphinium denudatum*, *Jurinea macrocephala*, *Malaxis muscifera*, *Morina longifolia*, *Nardostachys jatamansi*, *Picrorhiza kurrooa*, *Pleurospermum angelecoides*, *P. brunonis*, *Podophyllum hexandrum*, *Rheum australe*, *R. emodi*, *Saussurea lappa* and *S. obvallata* are mostly valued for their belowground parts.

During the course of this study, it was also noticed that, natives were quite dubious to express and share their trial and error based but time tested and effective knowledge. The advantage of this knowledge may be in the screening of pharmaceutically important compounds, clinical trials and development of potential drugs. As well, it was also perceived that traditional knowledge requires financial support for promotion and protection of the intellectual's property. Present investigation is aimed to suggest the strategies for utilization of ethnomedicobotanical knowledge in the remote areas in relation to its revitalization.

Introduction

It has been estimated that, worlds 70 to 80 per cent population rely on traditional health care. In addition acceptance of traditional medicines in developed world is sharply increasing (Farnsworth and Soejarto, 1991; Subrat, 2002). Herbal remedies are more acceptable prescriptions as compared to synthetic medicines. The growth of the herbal medicines in Europe and North America is ~10–20 per cent per annum (ten Kate and Laird, 1999). Mode of prescription and number of plants used in traditional medicines is variable in the parts of the world; however Farnsworth and Soejarto (1991) have estimated that worldwide ~50,000 plants are used in traditional medicines. It is interesting to note that in India only; approximately 7500 plants are traditionally used for curing various ailments (Shiva, 1996).

The significance of the medicinal plants is related to something else than the food value having miraculous property for curing ailments. Symbolically medicinal plants are held in religions, nationalistic and ideological esteem. This interrelationship is an advantage for conservation, sustainable utilization and in the development of new therapeutic agents. Knowledge of folk world is typically very important and endeavors to document, to promote and to revitalize this knowledge is quite important. Studies on indigenous knowledge with special reference to ethnomedicobotanical surveys may be useful for conservation of valuable plant resources, sustainable development and socio-economic upliftment of the marginal communities in the inaccessible areas.

Study Area

Ghat, a remote and poorly developed administrative block in district Chamoli was selected for this study. This block is located in between 79°–29′ to 79°–30′ E and 30° -10′ to 30°-29′ N in the central part of Western Himalaya. The altitude within study area varies 1000 m a. s. l. in the river valley bases to 5800 m. a. s. l. in the alpine moraines. Geographically this area is comprised of Georges, valleys, steep slopes and hills. This area is remote, inaccessible and rugged terrain makes human survival quite difficult.

42 villages namely, Bairaskund, Matai, Sakand, Mankhi, Motha, Khaltara, Sema, Sankari, Gandasu, Kameda, Banala, Bijar, Jakhni, Mokh, Kundi, Kunbagar, Kurur, Farkhet, Kumjug, Narangi, Sainti, Phali, Sarpani, Ustoli, Bheti, Tilan, Bangali, Lankhi, Moling, Luntara, Sung, Ghooni, Ramni, Boora, Padergaon, Vaduk, Pranmati, Guladi, Sitel, Sutol, Kanol and Bhuna were surveyed in this study.

Methodology

Frequent field surveys were conducted in the study area through March 2004 to December 2005. Voucher specimens were collected at flowering/fruiting stages. Field data *i.e.* place, habitats, distribution, altitude, botanical descriptions, date and herbarium number was noted in a field book. Taxonomical identity of the voucher specimens was confirmed with the help of Flora of British India Vol. 1-7 (Hooker, 1872-1897), A Forest Flora for Kumaun (Osmaston, 1927), Flora of Mussoorie (Raizada and Saxena, 1978) Flora of Chamoli Vol. 1-2 (Naithani, 1984-1985), and Flora of the District Garhwal North West Himalaya (with ethno botanical notes) (Gaur, 1999). All the specimens were collected in triplicates. During voucher specimen collection each specimen was shown to the native peoples. Whatsoever plant is used in traditional household remedies was marked and its relevant application was verified through repeated queries. Methods suggested by Jain and Rao (1977) for field and herbarium techniques were followed. All specimens were deposited in the herbarium of Herbal Research and Development Institute (HDH) Gopeshwar-Chamoli.

Results and Discussion

Ethnomedicobotanical survey in the Ghat block of district Chamoli indicates that still traditional phytoremedies are preferential first aid and mode of cure. Also, modern health care facilities are far away from remote villages. Some of the plants from other areas like high altitude regions are also collected during favorable seasons and stored for when needed. A total 191 plant species belonging to 83 families of angiosperms and 1 family of pteridophyte (Equisiteceae) were being used by native folk for curing various health problems. Out of these, 96 plants were herbs, 39 (20.42 per cent) were trees, 19 (9.95 per cent) were herbs or under shrubs or shrubs in habit, 16 (8.38 per cent) plants were shrubs, 15 (7.85 per cent) climbers, 5 shrubs or small trees and 1 was (0.52 per cent) grass namely *Cynodon dactylon*.

Important herbs used as phytoremedies in this area were *Aconitum heterophyllum*, *Angelica glauca*, *Corydalis govaniana*, *Galinsoga parviflora*, *Curculigo orchioides*, *Calanthe tricarinata*, *Delphinium denudatum*, *Aconitum atrox*, *Picrorhiza kurrooa*, *Dactylorhiza hatagirea* and *Valeriana wallichii*. Ethonomedicobotanically important tree species were *Bombax cieba*, *Aesculus indica*, *Buxus wallichiana*, *Carpinus viminea*, *Cassia fistula*, *Emblica officinalis*, *Terminalia bellerica*, *T. chebula*, *Juglans regia*, *Cedrus deodara*, *Symplocos paniculata*, and *Taxus wallichiana*. Climbers used by native communities for curing various problems were *Abrus precatorius*, *Mucuna nigricans*, *Gloriosa superba* and *Cuscuta reflexa*. *Calotropis procera*, *Adhatoda vasica*, *Indigofera atropurpuria*, *Skimmia laureola* and *Daphne papyracea* were important shrubs used by native peoples.

All the plants used in the traditional household remedies were belonging to 84 families. However, 53.92 per cent plants were belonging to 16 families only, namely Ranunculaceae, Lamiaceae, Asteraceae,

Apiaceae, Rosaceae, Fabaceae, Solanaceae, Zingiberaceae, Rutaceae, Liliaceae, Orchidaceae, Caesalpiniaceae, Polygonaceae, Euphorbiaceae, Araceae and Ericaceae.

Root parts (21.65 per cent) were predominantly used plant parts in indigenous remedies. Roots of important plant species used in indigenous system were *Aconitum atrox* (for rheumatism), *A. heterophyllum* (for fever and stomach ache), *Arnebia benthamii* (as a hair tonic), *Dactylorhiza hatagirea* (for curing cuts and wounds and as a tonic), *Picrorhiza kurrooa* (as an antipyretic), *Polygonatum verticillatum* (for treating piles) and *Saussurea lappa* for skin diseases.

Leaves of various plants used for treating different health problems were *Adhatoda vasica* (in cough), *Boenninghausenia albiflora* (as bed bug repellents), *Centella asiatica* for enhancing memory, *Equisetum arvense* for curing stomach ache and muscular pain in abdomen, *Micromeria biflora* in cuts and wounds, *Origanum vulgare* for relieving cough and cold, *Thymus linearis* as a digestive and against constipation and *Swertia chirayita* for fever.

Seeds and fruits of different plant species including *Abrus precatorius* as an abortificieant, *Gaultheria trichophylla* for relieving cold and headache, *Hippophae rhamnoides* ssp. *salicifolia* as purgative, *Mucuna nigricans* for overcoming physical weakness and fatigue, *Solanum viarum* for curing jaundice, *Terminalia chebula* for digestive disorders and *Zanthoxyllum armatum* for preventing tooth decay are extensively used.

Some of the findings were interesting, such as application of *Vitex negundo* in gout and arthritis, *Polygonatum verticillatum* for the treating piles, *Onosona emodi* for curing leprosy. Fruits of *Solanum viarum* are used as a garlet to be hanged around the neck during jaundice. Using leaves extract of *Skimmia laureola* for treating scabies and chewing leaves of *Adhatoda vasica* with honey for curing chronic bronchitis and cough were very important. Some other useful application of the plants *viz Boenninghausenia albiflora* as a natural insecticide and lice repellent, application of *Acorus calamus* and *Chenopodium ambroisoides* as an insecticide/anthelmentic for humans and animals, and application of *Ranunculus pulchellus* for curing sciatica was interesting.

Present investigation revealed that a total 23 plants are used in various skin diseases, including eczema, 14 plants are used in cough and cold, 12 in fever, 11 for checking bleeding from cuts and wounds and for wounds healing, 10 as tonic, 8 plants in diarrhoea, 8 in tooth ache, 7 in stomach ache, 6 in bone fracture, 6 plants as psycho medicines, 6 plants as digestive and purgative and 6 for curing dysentery. 5 plants to cure rheumatism, 5 during snake bite, 5 in relieving muscular pain and 5 were in use for curing diarrhoea. 4 plants in each diagnosis *viz.* urinary complaints, anthelmintic, jaundice, sores and blisters of mouth and as hair tonic are used in the study area. Similarly in treatment of blood related problems like blood sugar, blood pressure and as a blood purifier, treatment of gall stone, various eye problems and constipation, 3 plants in each ailment are used. Three plants were being used as insect repellent. To relieve gastric (2 plants), body pain and swelling (2 plants), as an antiseptic (2 plants), to relieve labor pain during delivery (2 plants) and 2 plants are used as sedative and narcotic. 2 plants were in use as biological insect repellents and fruits of two plants are used due to their cooling properties. One plant in each health problem of humans and cattle was used in colic, whoop and mouth disease of cattle, to overcome unconsciousness, in the treatment of typhoid, spleen related problems, in the treatment of spermatorrhoea, sciatica, piles, obesity, nasal bleeding, liver disorders, kidney diseases, leprosy, hydrocoele, head ache, gout, gonorrhea, food poisoning in cattle, as an nervine and heart tonics. It was much interesting to note that some plants or their separate parts were being used to treat different ailments, so the numbers of the plants used to treat different diseases exceeded to the total numbers of the plants enumerated and documented in the ethno medico botanical investigation of the selected study area, Thus a total 69 disease and health problems are treated indigenously in the study area (Table 1.1). Some of the plants and their indigenous use in presented in Figure 1.1.

Table 1.1: Relevant Applications of the Various Plants Species in the Remote Localities of Ghat-Chamoli, Uttaranchal

Sl.No.	Biological and Curative Property	Plants Used
1.	Abortive	*Abrus precatorius*
2.	Anemia	*Chenopodium album*
3.	Antihelmentic	*Bauhinia variegata, Cissampelos pareira, Acorus calamus, Pleurospermum brunonis*
4.	Antiperiodic	*Olea glandulifera*
5.	Anti-poisoning	*Oxalis corniculata*
6.	Antiseptic	*Dioscorea bulbifera, Jurinea macrocephala*
7.	Arthritis	*Vitex negundo*
8.	Birth pain	*Ranunculus laetus, Gloriosa superba*
9.	Blood pressure/purifier/Blood sugar	*Withania somnifera, Hedychium spicatum, Tinospora cordifolia*
10.	Body pain/swelling	*Datura stramonium, Smilex glaucophylla*
11.	Bone fracture	*Abrus precatorius, Boehmeria rugulosa, Buxus wallichaina, Carpinus viminea, Coelogyne cristata, Vigna mungo*
12.	Burns	*Cuscuta reflexa, Urtica dioica*
13.	Cold and cough	*Sorbus aucuparia, Taxus wallichiana, Zingiber officinale, Betula utilis, Piper longum, Pistacia khinjuk, Punica granatum, Adhatoda vasica, Cinnamomum tamala, Ocimum sanctum, Origanum vulgare, Piper nigrum, Prunus persica, Urena lobata*
14.	Colic	*Rumex nepalensis*
15.	Constipation	*Cassia fistula, Plantago himalaica, Thymus linearis*
16.	Cooling	*Fragaria nubicola, Rubus foliolosus*
17.	Cut and wounds	*Anaphalis contorta, Artemisia nilagirica, Cannabis sativa, Dactylorhiza hatagirea, Rheum australe, Dioscorea bulbifera, Eupatorium adenophorum, Euphorbia royleana, Micromeria biflora, Reinwardtia indica, Symplocos paniculata*
18.	Diabetes	*Trigonella foenum-graecum*
19.	Diarrhea	*Bauhinia variegata, Geum elatum, Indigofera atropurpuria, Mangifera indica, Mentha arvensis, Mentha piperita, Paris polyphylla, Trachyspermum ammi*
20.	Digestive/purgative	*Amomum subulatum, Angelica glauca, Carica papaya, Ficus palmata, Hippophae rhamnoides, Aegle marmelos*
21.	Dislocation of bones	*Rheum australe*
22.	Diuretic	*Coriandrum sativum, Corydalis govaniana, Curculigo orchioides, Polygonum macrophyllum*
23.	Dog bite	*Araesma jacquemontii*

Contd...

Table 1.1–Contd...

Sl.No.	Biological and Curative Property	Plants Used
24.	Dysentery	*Cannabis sativa, Rheum emodi, Rubia cordifolia, Erythrina suberosa, Mesua ferrea*
25.	Eczema	*Anemone vitifolia, Calanthe tricarinata, Geranium wallichianum, Heracleum canescens, Indigofera atropurpuria*
26.	Emetic	*Cythula tomentosa*
27.	Eye diseases	*Berberis umbellata, Clematis barbellata, Solanum nigrum*
28.	Fever	*Ajuga bracteosa, Megacarpia polyandra, Mesua ferrea, Paeonia emodi, Picrorhiza kurrooa, Pistacia khinjuk, Sida cordata, Swertia chirayta, Tanacetum longifolium, Thalictrum foliolosum, Viola canescens, Jurinea macrocephala*
29.	Food poisoning in cattle	*Urginea indica*
30.	Gall stone	*Bergenia ciliata, Macrotyloma uniflorum, Taraxacum officinale*
31.	Gastric	*Pleurospermum angelicoides, Zanthoxylum armatum*
32.	Gonorrhea	*Quercus leucotrichophora*
33.	Gout	*Vitex negundo*
34.	Hair tonic	*Arnebia benthamii, Emblica officinalis, Prunus cerasoides, Sapindus mukorossi*
35.	Headache	*Gaultheria trichophylla*
36.	Heart tonic	*Rhododendron arboreum*
37.	Hydrocoele	*Vervascum thapsus*
38.	Hysteria	*Nardostachys jatamansi, Valeriana wallichii*
39.	Infested wound of cattle	*Caltha palustris*
40.	Insect repellent/Insecticide	*Nicotiana rustica, Chenopodium ambrosioides, Lyonia ovalifolia*
41.	Jaundice	*Boerhavia diffusa, Calanthe tricarinata, Curculigo orchioides, Solanum viarum*
42.	Kidney diseases	*Tribulus terrestris*
43.	Leprosy	*Onosma emodi*
44.	Lice repellent	*Boenninghausenia albiflora, Nicandra physalodes*
45.	Liver disorders	*Portulaca oleracea*
46.	Malarial fever	*Roylea cinerea*
47.	Milk enhancing	*Asparagus curillus, Pueraria tuberosa*
48.	Mouth diseases/refresher/ sore/blisters	*Pyracantha crenulata, Osmanthus fragrans, Callicarpa macrophylla, Begonia picta*
49.	Muscular pain	*Achyranthes aspera, Corylus jacquemontii, Hyoscymus niger, Ricinus communis*
50.	Narcotic	*Datura stramonium, Nicotiana rustica*
51.	Nervine tonic	*Centella asiatica*
52.	Nose bleeding	*Cynodon dactylon*
53.	Obesity	*Withania somnifera*

Contd...

Table 1.1–Contd...

Sl.No.	Biological and Curative Property	Plants Used
54.	Piles	*Polygonatum verticillatum*
55.	Psychomedicinal	*Vervascum thapsus, Betula utilis, Origanum vulgare, Prinsepia utilis, Pueraria tuberosa, Selinum vaginatum*
56.	Rheumatic pain/Rheumatism	*Urena lobata, Aconitum atrox, Aesculus indica, Allium sativum, Trigonella foenum–graecum*
57.	Sciatica	*Ranunculus pulchellus*
58.	Skin diseases	*Anemone vitifolia, Calotropis procera, Skimmia laureola, Ampelocissus rugosa, Arisaema jacquemontii, Azadirachta indica, Cassia tora, Cedrus deodara, Citrus medica, Clematis kanguli, Cynoglossum glochidiatum, Drymaria diandra, Elaeagnus parvifolia, Mallotus philippensis, Melia azadirachta, Myrica esculenta, Parthenoessus rubiosa, Pinus roxburghii, Podophyllum hexandrum, Saussurea lappa, Saussurea obvallata, Taxus wallichiana, Valliris solanacea*
59.	Snake bite	*Allium cepa, Bupleurum longicaule, Cythula tomentosa, Galinsoga parviflora, Leucas lanata*
60.	Spermatorhoea	*Bombax ceiba*
61.	Spleen infection	*Rhamnus virgatus*
62.	Stomach ache	*Terminalia bellerica, Aconitum heterophyllum, Ainsliaea aptera, Cassia fistula, Equisetum arvense, Megacarpia polyandra, Terminalia chebula*
63.	Strains	*Curcuma domestica*
64.	Tonic	*Aconitum heterophyllum, Dactylorhiza hatagirea, Habenaria aitchisonii, Malaxis muscifera, Mucuna nigricans, Roscoea purpurea, Saraca asoca, Typhonium diversifolium, Withania somnifera, Ziziphus nummularia*
65.	Tooth ache	*Anemone obtusiloba, Delphinium denudatum, Dephne papyracea, Ephedra gerardiana, Juglans regia, Potentilla fulgens, Zanthoxylum armatum, Myrica esculenta*
66.	Typhoid	*Calanthe tricarinata*
67.	Unconsciousness	*Morina longifolia*
68.	Urinary complaints	*Sida cordata, Valeriana wallichii, Salvia hians, Salvia lanata*
69.	W&M disease of cattle	*Trichosanthes tricuspidata*

Indigenous methods of health care, their effectiveness and established safety have been an integral part of the human survival in the inhospitable terrains of Indian Himalaya. Traditional treatment of several ailments in poorly developed societies runs parallel to modern health care system. Herbal heritage of Himalaya has been harnessed since time immemorial and with the wide acceptance of herbalism this wealth may be useful tool for improving the socio-economic conditions of marginal communities and low income group people. This prospect is much useful in the areas, having extremes of diverse geophysical landscapes coupled with multitude of climatic adversities and a natural struggling interrelationship of humankinds with their surrounding. Himalayan states in the Indian subcontinent are known for their specific, socio-cultural practices and folk life adapted to environmental conditions. As a result, with a series of trials and errors, the native folk learned adopted and passed through a useful and tested repository of traditional health care knowledge.

Folk life subsisted with traditional agro-pastoral activities in the remote villages merely receive modern health care facilities. However, recent developments in the modern health care industries have enhanced the extraction of raw materials from these areas. As a result several localities have been emerged as an important collection centre for wild medicinal and aromatic plants. As a result several plants having useful properties and being used in indigenous knowledge system are depleting. Subsequently, the traditional knowledge is also depleting due to scarcity of such plants and acculturations.

It was also noted that most of the plants used in the ethnomedicobotany of study area are commonly growing in the surrounding forest, agro forestry premises and some of them were even cultivated enough to fulfill the natives requirement. *Withania somnifera*, *Mesua ferrea*, *Piper longum* and *P. nigrum* were the plants not growing naturally in the study area but procured from nearby crude drug market. Plants growing in the high altitude areas are collected during favorable season or in the course of transhumance traveling. Some of the traditional knowledge bearers are enough experts to collect the plants in off season from the surrounding areas. While going in depth of this practice was noticed that the peoples using various plants for different ailments are well known about their habitat specificity.

The well established indigenous knowledge of folk communities and to compensate these communities legally for this knowledge has been a complex matter. However, protection of the intellectual property of the native peoples may be useful option to help them from being exploited. Such legal status securing approaches may be useful for absolute documentation of doses and prescriptions as practiced by these communities as well as may also serve as baseline information for future clinical trials. In addition, the contribution of intellects from all walks of life, particularly a sociologist, anthropologist, ecologist, traditional medicine man, an agriculturist and statistician along with ethno botanist may be more applicable for drawing accuracy and specificity. Vulnerability of resources might be strongly being influenced by the anthropogenic disturbances. It is therefore, the composition of such economically important wealth specially used by native communities for a remedial purpose in traditional manner is also needs to be monitored.

What to Do With?

Finding of the present study indicated that still a significant part of rural population residing in remote areas facing the lack modern health care facilities only rely on indigenous, readily available and low cost remedies. Simultaneously application of the plants may be attributed to poor living condition, poverty, easy availability in surrounding areas and elixirity to overcome ailments. In the selected study area, modern developmental infrastructure merely percolate in the remote areas, alternative in general and indigenously developed in particular (through a series of trials and errors) system of health care have well acceptance. However, the myth about this system, emotional attachment of such knowledge bearer to his knowledge and oral possession hinders this knowledge to be used widely or in commercial scale. All the facts about this knowledge remain to be passing orally from one to another generation. Also, the bearer of this knowledge remains quite secretive due to disbelief, that if it has been told others the effect of such remedies will degrade. In addition, the native knowledge bearer feels that no one else should get any kind of benefit from his/her intellectual property. In order to promote the ethno medico botany attempt are needed to document this practice including the series of investigation beginning from treatment to final cure. As well as the bearer of this knowledge are required to understand importance of their knowledge in the global drive of herbalism. It is essential

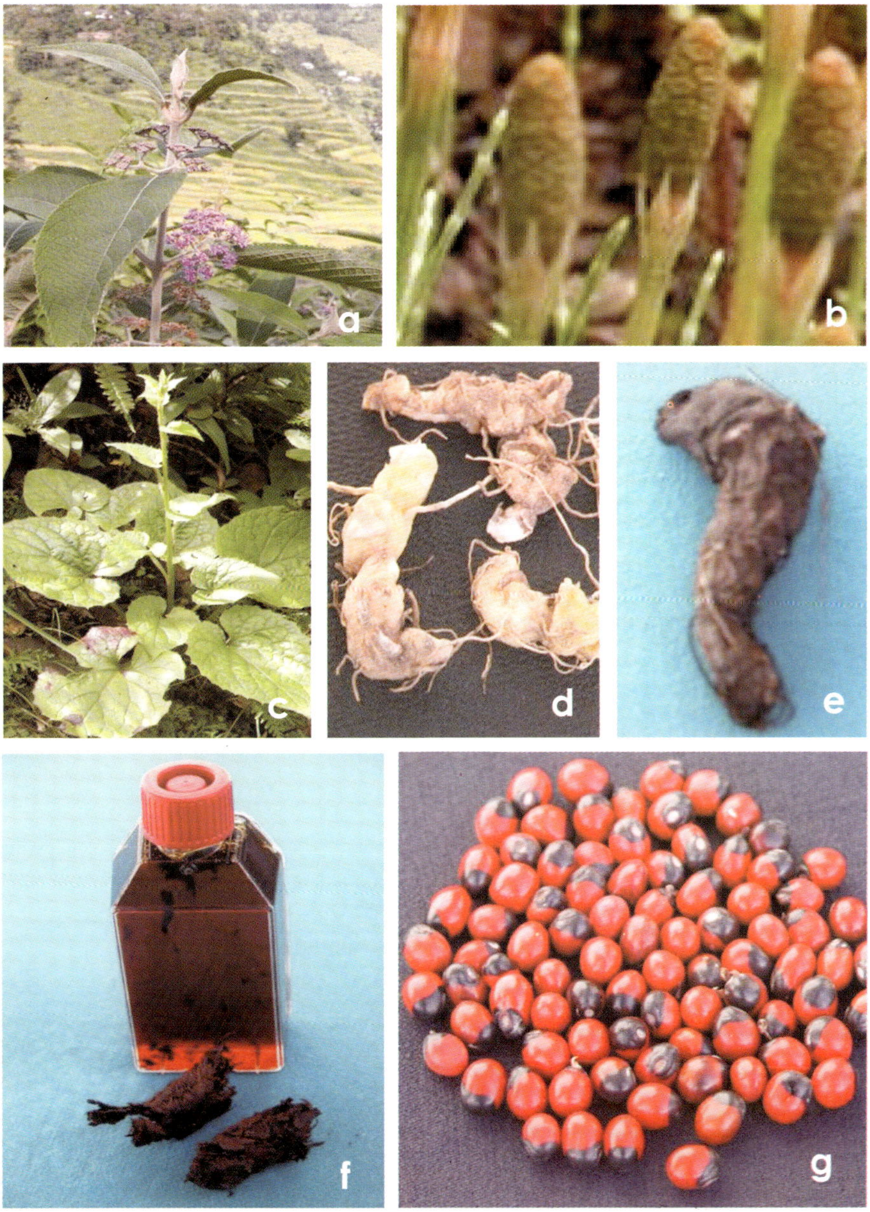

Figure 1.1: Different Plant Species Used by the Native Communities of Ghat Block for Curing Various Health Problems

a. *Callicarpa macrophylla* (bark is used to cure mouth sores), b. *Equisetum arvens* (whole plant is used in stomach ache and muscular pain), c. *Ainsliaea aptera* (roots are used for acute stomach ache of children), d. roots of *Polygonatum verticillatum* (used in piles), e. root of *Aconitum balfaurii* (an age old remedy for rheumatism), f. oil colored with roots of *Arnebia benthamii* and used as hair tonic and g. seeds of *Abrus precatorious* (seeds are used as abortive).

that the provision of incentives to the bearer of this knowledge is quite important. Initiatives towards the rejuvenation of the traditional health care systems should be supplemented with automation, provision for patenting and benefit sharing if the new noble products are developed.

It is widely known and accepted to the grass root level that ethno medico botany is equally relevant and effective. However, number of patient visiting to a traditional practitioner, how many of them has been treated and benefited successfully what was the entire treatment schedules, what to do's and what not to do's, a detail record of a series of results or clinical trial is merely recorded.

The native communities are accustomed to use the plants for variety of ailments and as a health care products etc. However, population pressure, out migration and poor living standard has enforced acculturation in traditional knowledge. This knowledge base has been much important for the humankind. In brief, above all considerations are quite essential for sustainable development of ethnomedicobotany. It is quite important to ensure public involvement for the conservation and sustainable utilization of the plants widely used in ethnomedicobotany.

Acknowledgements

We are thankful to the Director, Herbal Research and Development Institute, Gopeshwar-Chamoli for extending key facilities. Thanks are due to Dr. D. S. Rawat, Plant Taxonomist, for confirming the taxonomical identity of the collected specimens. Critical support from Dr. V. P. Bhatt, Dr. M. S. Rawat and Dr. M. Upadhyay is acknowledged. Hemlata thanks Mr. Vinod Bisht, Mr. Vineet Purohit and Miss Neelam Bisht for their help during the course of this study.

References

Farnsworth, N.R. and Soejarto, D.D., 1991. Global importance of medicinal plants. In: *The conservation of Medicinal Plants*, (Eds.) O. Akerele, V. Heywood and H. Synge. Cambridge University Press, Cambridge, U.K., pp. 25–51.

Gaur, R.D., 1999. *Flora of the District Garhwal North West Himalaya (with ethnobotanical notes)*. Trans Media Srinagar (Garhwal).

Hooker, J.D., 1872–1897. *The Flora of British India*, 1–7 Vols., Oxford.

Jain, S.K. and Rao, R.R., 1977. *A Handbook of Field and Herbarium Methods*. Today and Tomorrow, New Delhi.

Naithani, B.D., 1984–1985. *Flora of Chamoli*, 2 Vols. BSI, Howrah.

Osmaston, A.E., 1927. *A Forest Flora for Kumaon*. Govt. Press, Allahabad.

Raizada, M.B. and Saxena, H.O., 1978. *Flora of Mussoorie*. Bishen Singh Mahendra Pal Singh, Dehradun.

Shiva, V., 1996. *Protecting Our Biological and Intellectual Heritage in the Age of Biopiracy*. The Research Foundation for Science, Technology and Natural Resources Policy, New Delhi, India.

Subrat, N., 2002. Ayurvedic and herbal products industry: an overview. In: *Paper at a Workshop on Wise Practices and Experiential Learning in the Conservation and Management of Himalayan Medicinal Plants, Kathmandu, Nepal*, 15-20 December 2002, supported by the Ministry of Forest and Soil Conservation, Nepal, the WWF-Nepal Program, Medicinal and Aromatic Plants Program in Asia (MAPPA), IDRC, Canada and the WWF-UNESCO People and Plants Initiative.

Ten Kate, K. and Laird, S.A., 1999. *The Commercial Use of Biodiversity*. Earthscan, London, UK.

Medicinal Plants: Conservation, Cultivation and Utilization (2007) *Pages 11–15*
Editors: A.K. Chopra, D.R. Khanna, G. Prasad, D.S. Malik and R. Bhutiani
Published by: DAYA PUBLISHING HOUSE

Chapter 2

Medicinal Plants of India: Need for Their Preservation

Maya Ram Uniyal
Director, Farm, Maharishi Ayurvedic (NEPZ) Products, Noida – 201 305, U.P.

India has had a glorious past in respect of the science of life, like Ayurveda, which not only deals with medicine, but enables as to lead a healthy and happy life. It is an established fact, that man learnt the art of healing, with the help of natural resources from the animals in the primitive age. Thus, the history of medicine begins with the very appearance of the living being on earth.

Fortunately, our country represent practically the whole world in respect of climate and soil. Its widely varying topography provides a large variety of different climates and zones. The medicinal flora the country is rich enough to meet the demands of medicinal plants not only of our own country, but for large parts of the world too, if it is properly managed.

Most of the medicinal flora growing wild in the forests in cultivated lands (as weeds) in the alpine zones and desert areas is unwittingly destroyed every year due to lack of technical knowledge and crude extraction methods. The shepherds, buffalo-graziers, tribals and villagers, collect the medicinal plants in forests and waste lands and utilize them for their own domestic purposes, or sell them in the nearby markets for a mere song. The valuable medicinal wealth of the forests is further extracted by the contractors in the name of fodder, fuel and minor products on permits from the forest department on a nominal payment of loyalty. In this competitive race for extraction of the maximum produce among the contractors, no one bothers about the future. This naturally adversely affects the quality and quantity of the potential drugs and some of the very valuable species, are either being eliminated rapidly or pushed back into unfavourable environment, to be replaced by other more lucrative products.

It is a well recognized fact, that the medicinal value of large number of plants growing wild in the country, is not properly grown even to scientists. In view of this situation the Ministry of Health and

Family Welfare, Government of India, established the Central Council for Research in Indian Medicine and Homeopathy, in 1969 for the improvement of indigenous system of medicine.

The council has been launching projects to explore the medicinal flora of the country, through surveys of medicinal plants units, working in various states. The teams under this project, collect details relating to flora, fauna, mineral wealth, medicinal practices, life and food habits, of the local people.

After a study of available literature and practical experience, during some of these surveys, the author feels that this arduous task of forest products, with special reference to the medicinal plants, is not an easy job. It requires systematic planning, with collaboration of several Government departments, like Health, Forest, Agricultural industries, Foreign Trade and Planning. Joint groups should be set up by the Government of India with the help of experts of the concerned departments of the centre and the states. This would provide, not merely cheap and effective medicines, but also employment to large number. Genuine drug would be available for Pharmaceutical and other industries in the country and yet spare something to be exported abroad.

The following is an illustrative list of medicinal plants, found in India. The list contains only those plants which are neglected at present and, are not included in the particulars of the auction lists, of most of the forests but are being extracted regularly, ruthlessly by the clever contractors for nothing, though they are of great importance for medical science and industries. The attention of the scientists and forest authorities is invited, to consider the planned propagation, proper protection and skilfull extraction of the valuable minor products.

Table 2.1

Sl.No.	*Botanical Name*	*Sanskrit/Trade Name*	*Part Used*
1.	*Abrus precatorius* Linn	Gunga/Ratti	Seed, Root
2.	*Abutilon indicul* (L) Sw	Atibala	Whole plant
3.	*Achyranthus aspera* Lion	Apamarg	Seed, whole plant
4.	*Adhatoda vasica* Nees	Vasa	Root, bark, whole
5.	*Adiantum lunulatum* Burm	Hanspadi/Hansraj	Whole plant
6.	*Aegle marmelos* Correa	Bilva/Bel	Fruit, bark
7.	*Ailanthus excelasa* Roxb	Araluka/Arlu	Bark of stem and root
8.	*Alastonia scbolaris* R.Br.	Saptparna	Bark
9.	*Angelica glauca* Bdgew	Coraka/Chora	Root
10.	*Argemone mexicana* Linn	Satyanashi/Chok	Root, Seed
11.	*Andrographis paniculata* Nees	Kalmegh	Whole plant
12.	*Astercantha lonifolia* Nees	Talmakhana	Seeds
13.	*Bacopa monnier* (L) Pannel	Brahmi/Jalneem	Whole plant
14.	*Baliospermum montanum* Muell	Danti	Root and Seed
15.	*Barleria prionitis* Linn.	Sahchara	Whole plant
16.	*Berringtonia acutangula* (L) Gaertin	Samudraphal	Seed
17.	*Bauhinia variegate* Linn.	Kanchnar	Bark and Flower
18.	*Bergenia ligulata* (Wall) Brgl	Pasanbheda	Rhizome

Contd...

Table 2.1–Contd...

Sl.No.	Botanical Name	Sanskrit/Trade Name	Part Used
19.	*Blepharis edulis* Pers	Utingana	Seed
20.	*Boerhavia diffusa* Linn	Punarva	Whole plant
21.	*Buchanania lanzan* Spreng	Priyal/Ghirangi	Seed
22.	*Butea monosperma* (Lam) Kunts	Palas	Gum, Seed, Flower
23.	*Caesalpinia crista* Linn	Lataktanj	Seed
24.	*Callicarpa macrophylla* Vahl.	Priyangu	Seed
25.	*Calotropis gignata* (L) R.Br.	Arks	Flower, Root
26.	*Calotropis procera*	Arka/Madar	Flower, Root
27.	*Cassia occidentalis* Linn	Kasmard	Seed
28.	*Cassia tora* Linn	Chakramard	Seed
29.	*Celastrus paniculatus* Willd	Malkagni	Seed
30.	*Centella asiatica* (L) Urban	Mandukparni/Bhari	Leaves
31.	*Cissampelos pereira* Linn	Patha	Whole plant
32.	*Citrullus calocynathis* Schorad	Indreyan	Fruit
33.	*Clerodendrum phlomides* Linn.f	Arni	Whole plant
34.	*Clerodendrum serratum* (L) Moon	Bharangi	Root
35.	*Clitoria ternatea* Linn	Aparajita	Seed, Whole plant
36.	*Coccinea cordifolia* Cogn.	Bimbi	Whole plant
37.	Convolvulus pleuricaulis Chaisy	Shankhpushpi	Whole plant
38.	*Crataeva nurvala* Buch-Ham	Varun	Bark, Leaves
39.	*Cryptolepis bocbanani* Roem and Schult.	Krishna sariva	Root, stem
40.	*Curculigo orchioides* Gaerth	Kalimnsli	Root
41.	*Cyperus rotundus* Linn.	Mustak	Root
42.	*Cyperus pangorei* Rottb	Nagar motha	Rhizome
43.	*Desmodium gangeticum* De.	Salparni	Whole plant
44.	*Dermatachya bipinnata* Stapf.	Kusha	Whole plant
45.	*Eclipta alba* Hassak	Bharangrag	Whole plant
46.	*Euphorbia nerifolia* Linn	Sauhi	Latex
47.	*Euphorbia dacuncueloides* Linn	Satala	Whole plant
48.	*Euphorbia thymifolia* Linn	Dudhi	Whole plant
49.	*Evulvulus alsinoides* Linn	Sankhapuspi	Whole plant
50.	*Ficus beggalensis* Linn	Vat	Bark, Root
51.	*Ficus bispida* Linn	Plaksha	Fruit
52.	*Ficus racemosa* Linn	Udumber	Fruit and leaves
53.	*Ficus religiosa* Linn	Asvatha/Pipal	Bark/Fruit/Leave
54.	*Fumaria parviflora* Lam	Parpata/Satara	Whole Plant

Contd...

Table 2.1–Contd...

Sl.No.	Botanical Name	Sanskrit/Trade Name	Part Used
55.	*Gloriosa superba*	Kalihari	Root
56.	*Gymnema sylvestre* R.Br.	Gurmar	Leaves
57.	*Gyandropsis gynandra* (L) Brigves	Hul-Hul	Seed, Whole plant
58.	Habenaria intermedia D.Don	Ridhi	Root
59.	*Holarrhena antidysenterica* Well	Kutj	Bark, Seed
60.	*Jasminum arborescena* Roxb	Chemeli	Flower, Leaves
61.	*Jasminum officinale* Var *Grandiflorum*	Jati	Flower, Leaves
62.	*Lawsania inermis* Linn	Mehndi	Leaves, Seed
63.	*Leucas cephalotes* Sprung	Dronpuspi	Whole plant
64.	*Lillium poly phyllum* D.Don	Kshir Kakoli	Root
65.	*Luppia nodiflora* Mich.	Jalpippali	Whole plant
66.	*Luffa acutangula* Roxb	Deodali	Whole plant
67.	*Madhuca indica* J.F. Gmiel	Mahuva	Flower, Seed
68.	*Microstylis muscifera* Ridi	Jivak	Root
69.	*Microstylis wallichlii* Lindi	Jivak	Root
70.	*Mimosa pudica* Linn	Lajvanti	Seed, Whole plant
71.	*Mucuna prurita* book	Kapikachu	Seed, Root
72.	*Operculina turpethum* (L) Silva	Trivrit, Nishoth	Root
73.	*Paederia foetida* Linn	Gandhaprasarni	Whole plant
74.	*Peristrophe bicalyculata* Nees	Kakjangha	Whole plant
75.	*Phaseolus radiatus* Linn	Mudgaparni	Whole plant
76.	*Phaseolus trilobus* Ait	Masparni	Whole plant
77.	*Phyllanthus niruri* Linn	Bhumi akalki	Whole Plant
78.	*Pluchea lanceolata* Oilver and Hiern	Rasana	Leaves
79.	*Plumbago zeylanica* Linn	Chitrak	Root, bark
80.	*Polygonatum cirrhifolium* Royal	Mahameda	Rhizome
81.	*Premnalatifoliaver macronata*	Aganimanth	Bark
82.	*Prunus ceraloid* D. Don	Padam	Wood
83.	*Pueraria tuberosa* De	Widarikand	Tuber
84.	*Randia dumctorum* Lam	Madam	Fruit
85.	*Rhus parviflora* Roxb.	Samakdana	Seed
86.	*Salmalia malabarica* Schult and Endl.	Salmali	Gum, Flower, Bark
87.	*Sciendapsus officinalis* Schott	Gajpippali	Fruit
88.	*Scirpus kysoor* Roxb	Kaseruk	Tuber
89.	*Sida cardifolia* Linn	Bala	Whole plant
90.	*Sida rhombifolia* Linn	Khairati	Seed, Whole plant

Contd...

Table 2.1–Contd...

Sl.No.	Botanical Name	Sanskrit/Trade Name	Part Used
91.	*Solanum indicum* Linn	Vrihati	Whole plant
92.	*Solanum nigrum* Linn	Kakmanchi	Whole plant
93.	*Sphaerenthus indicus* Linn	Mundi	Fruit
94.	*Tinospora cordifolia* (Willd) Miers	Guduchi	Whole plant
95.	*Tribulus terrestris* Linn	Gokharu	Seed and fruit
96.	*Trichosanthes dioica* Roxb	Patrol	Whole plant
97.	*Uraria picta* Desv.	Prishnaparni	Whole plant
98.	*Vitex negundo* Linn	Nirgundi	Seed, Leaves, Bark
99.	*Zanthoylum alatum* Roxb	Tumbru	Seed
100.	*Alectra parasitica*	Kusthari	Whole plant

Acknowledgement

The author is thankful to the Director, Central Council for Research in Ayurveda and Sidha, New Delhi for providing necessary facilities and encouragement from time to time. Grateful thanks are due also to the forest authorities and worked for their kind cooperation.

Medicinal Plants: Conservation, Cultivation and Utilization (2007) *Pages 17–24*
Editors: A.K. Chopra, D.R. Khanna, G. Prasad, D.S. Malik and R. Bhutiani
Published by: DAYA PUBLISHING HOUSE

Chapter 3

Angiospermous Seeds of Medicinal Importance in Gujarat State

Premendra Singh, S. Sisodia and Jinesh Shah*
Department of Botany, Faculty of Science, The Maharaja Sayajirao University of Baroda, Vadodara – 390 002

ABSTRACT

India is one of the richest floristic regions of the world and is well known for its ancient heritage regarding medicinal plants and plant drugs since time of the Rigveda. India has immense medicinal plant diversity and is situated in the tropical zone and one of 12 mega biodiversity countries having a vast variety of flora and fauna. The plants as medicine are used in different systems of medicine, as in Ayurveda, Allopathy, Unani, Homeopathy and even in other systems. Despite all these advantages, we have lost our medicinal biodiversity and many herbs are on the verge of extinction due to over exploitation. It was also experienced that more destruction was caused by unscientific methods of harvesting, collection, transportation and storage. Hence, it was felt necessary to utilize the medicinal plants in a judicious manner. Different plant parts, including seeds, are being used, singly or in combination with other herbal parts, for treating various human diseases. The present paper produces a brief account of the main angiospermous seeds that find frequent use in the medicine.

Introduction

Seed is product of a fertilized ovule, consisting of an embryo, enclosed in the testa which is derived from the integuments. Food reserves may or may not be contained in the endosperm. Seeds are

* Corresponding Author.

ever a positive and creative force. They are the germ of life, a beginning as well as end they are the fruit of yesterday's harvest and the promise for tomorrow's sowing (Freeman, 1961). Seeds, the great staple food of the world, feel people more than any other type of food. The endosperm or cotyledons, with rich food reserve for the developing embryo and seedlings offers man and animals a highly nutritious food that can be easily stored (Kozlowski *et al.*, 1972). The mature seed normally consists of, (a). Seed coat or testa, which mainly provide protection against attack by microorganisms or insects, mechanical injury and desiccation and helps in seed dispersal (Bhatnagar *et al.*, 1972, Singh 1985). (b) Endosperm, a storage tissue which provides nutrition for embryo and the young seedling and (c) Embryo which comprises partially–developed young sporophyte (Esau, 1993). There are innumerable variations in the seed size, shape, Colour and surface. The seed range in size from tiny dust particles, as found in some orchids, to large double–coconut (*Ledoicea maldivica*). Fresh weight of an orchid seed may be about 25mg, and that of a double–coconut about 6kg. The seed Surface may be smooth, wrinkled, striate, ribbed, furrowed, reticulate, tuberculation, alveolate, hairy, pulpy or having patterns like Finger prints. In certain plants the seed are so characteristic that they help identifying or variety (Bhojwani *et al.*, 2001). Seeds are mostly brown or brownish. The brown and black colours cover half of the total seeds: the Conspicuous colour such as red, green, yellow and white are infrequent but usually with diagnostic value. (Kozlowski *et al.*, 1972). Appendages have drawn maximum attention. The appendages include wings, arils, caruncles, spines, tubercles, hairs and elaiosomes. Early investigation into seed anatomy lay around type, size and placement of embryo, quantity and quality of food reserves.

Classification of Seeds

Depending on the presence or absence of endosperm.

1. Albuminous or endosperous, where endosperm is absent, as in cereals and castor plant.
2. Ex-aluminous or non-endosperous where endosperm is absent, as in bean and cucurbits.

Economic Importance of Seeds

Seeds are probably more valuable than any other part of the plant for man as well as for the plant itself. Seeds are produced by plants to ensure the perpetration of their types and for the Spread of the Species to newer area. The nine–tenths of the cultivated seeds are cereal grains, the bread stuffs of the world. By for the greater part of human food in the world consist of seeds; cereal seeds such as rice sorghum and millet are the staple food in South Africa and latin America. Barley, rye and oats also contribute to the world's food supply (Senti *et al.*, 1961). Legume seeds are the Second largest group of seeds that we use for food. All beans, peas and lentils have sample proteins. Some legumes, such as soyabeans, peanuts are high in oil and proteins, contents, as are some other seeds including those of ripe sesame and sunflower. Peanuts are considered as the world's second most important legume and are used mainly for their oil. To a much greater extent we eat entire seed (Senti *et al.*, 1961).

Medicinal Importance of Seed

Seeds are also used in treating a variety of human ailments and occupy an important particularity in unani and Ayurveda. They are used both as a single drug and as an ingredient of compound formulations (Siddigi *et al.*, 2001).

Today, Herbal medicines get very popular. Day by day it gain an importance due to preserve of many chemical in it. It's very useful in many diseases as direct or in powder form roasted, extract and decoction.

About Gujarat

Gujarat state is the western most part of India. The forest cover in the state is poor but it has fairly rich biodiversity. The state comprises of less than 10 per cent forest land of its geographical area. According to different studies on floral diversity, 2,205 species of angiosperm plants belonging to 905 genera of 156 families have been recorded so far out of 2,205 plant species, 748 plants were identified as medicinally important (Uma Devi, 1988).

Table 3.1

Sl.No.	Botanical Name	Uses
1.	*Abelmoschus esculentus* (Linn.) Moench	Coffee substitute, antispasmodic and sudorific.
2.	*Abelmoschus moschatus* Medic.	Flavour, tonic, stimulate and carminative, perfumery, antispasmodic, stomachic, demulcent, aphrodisiac, nervous disorders and hysteria.
3.	*Abrus precatorius* Linn	Affection of nervous system, sciatica, stiffness of shoulder joint, paralysis, abrotifacient, antiseptic, antitubercular, antidysenteric, skin diseases, ulcers, inflammation and antitumor.
4.	*Abutilon hirtum* G. Don.	Laxative and demulcent.
5.	*Abutilon indicum* (Linn.) Sweet	Laxative, demulcent, anticancer, properties, piles, chronic, cystitis, gleet and gonorrhoea.
6.	*Abutilon theophrastii* Medic.	Dysentery, fistula, Sore eyes, laxative, demulcent and useful in coryza.
7.	*Acacia suma* Buch–Ham.	Hypoglycaemic
8.	*Achyranthes aspera* Linn.	Emetic and hydrophobia.
9.	*Adenanthera pavonina* Linn.	Treating boils and inflammation.
10.	*Alangium slavifolium* (Linn.f.) Wang.	Haemorrhages
11.	*Albizia amara* Boivin	Piles, diarrhea and gonorrhoea.
12.	*Albizia lebbeck* Benth.	Piles, diarrhea, tonic and restorative.
13.	*Annona squamosa* Linn.	Oxytocic and uterotonic.
14.	*Apium graveolens* Linn	Stimulant, cordial, tonic, carminative, diuretic, emmenagogue, antiseptic, in bronchitis, asthma and liver.
15.	*Argemone mexicana* Linn.	Nauseous, cutaneous troubles, cathartic, cough, catarrhal, affections, asthma, pulmonary diseases, purgative, Narcotic, demulcent, applied locally and over skin diseases.
16.	*Argyreia nervosa* (Burm.f.)Boj.	Significant hypotensive and spasmodytic activity.
17.	*Asphodelus tenuifolius* Cav.	Diuretic, applied, externally to ulcers and inflamed parts.
18.	*Asteracantha longifolia* Nees	Gonorrhoea
19.	*Astragalus multiceps* Wall	Demulcent, colic and leprosy.
20.	*Avicennia officinalis* Linn.	Poultice to hasten, boils and abscesses.
21.	*Azadirachta indica* A. Juss.	Mouth ulcers, swelling gums, skin affections, leprosy, scrofulas, ulcers and wounds.
22.	*Balanites aegyptiaca* (Linn.) Delile	Whooping cough, colic, hypotensive, trating burns and freckles.
23.	*Baliospermum montanum* Muell-Arg	Drastic purgative, stimulant, rubifacient, hydrogogue, cathartic, rheumatism, antiseptic and snake.
24.	*Beuhinia vahlii* W. and A.	Aphrodisiac and tonic.

Contd...

Table 3.1–Contd...

Sl.No.	*Botanical Name*	*Uses*
25.	*Beta vulgaris* Linn.	Cooling and diaphoretic.
26.	*Borreria articularis* (Linn.f.) F.N.Williams	Demulcent, diarchoea and dysentery.
27.	*Brassica Campestris* Linn.	Dengue fever and rubbed on chest in bronchitis.
28.	*Brassica nigra* (Linn.) Koch	Stimulant, rubefacieus, vesicant and snake-bite.
29.	*Brassica oleracea* Linn.	Diuretic, laxative, stomachic and anthelmintic.
30.	*Bridelia stipularis* Blume.	Hemagglutinating properties.
31.	*Broussonetia papyrifera* Vent	Tonic and diuretic.
32.	*Brownea coccinea* Jacq.	Hemagglutinating properties.
33.	*Brucea javanica* (Linn.) Merill	Anthelmintic, antipyretic and papilloma.
34.	*Butea superba* Roxb.	Sedative, emollient, anthelmintic and piles.
35.	*Caesalpinia crista* Linn.	Febrifuge, antiperiodic, dispersing swelling, restraining, hemorrhage, curing discharge from ear and managing colic.
36.	*Cassia absus* Linn	Opthalmia, skin, troubles, cathartic and lowers blood pressure.
37.	*Cassia alata* Linn.	Eye troubles, diabetes, chylous urine, cough and asthma.
38.	*Cassia auriculata* Linn.	Eye troubles, diabetes, chylous urine, cough and asthma.
39.	*Cassia occidentalis* Linn.	Purgative, cough, whooping cough and external applications for curing skin troubles.
40.	*Carica papaya* Linn.	Vermifuge, emmenagogue and quench thirst.
41.	*Celastrus paniculata* Willd.	Aphrodisiac.
42.	*Celosia argentea* Linn.	Diarrhoea, eye trouble, painful micturition, cough and dysentery.
43.	*Chrozophora rottleri* Klotzsch.	Cathartic and purgative.
44.	*Cicer arietinum* Linn.	Antibilious biochenins and aphrodisiac.
45.	*Citrullus vulgaris* Schrad.	Diuretic and tonic.
46.	*Clerodendrum serratum* Linn	Aperient and relief in dropsy.
47.	*Clitoria ternatea* Linn	Purgative and aperient.
48.	*Colchicum luteum* Baker	Carminative, laxative, aphrodisiac, liver and speen.
49.	*Crotalaria juncea* Linn.	Purify blood and impetigo and psoriasis.
50.	*Croton tiglium* Linn	Apoplexy, insanity, convulsicns, obstinate, constipanitis colic, calculous affections and gout.
51.	*Crinum asiaticum* Linn.	Purgative, diuretic and emmenagogue.
52.	*Cucumis melo* Linn.	Diuretic, refrigerant and nutritious and urinary infections.
53.	*Cucumis melo* var. *utilissimus* Duthie and Fuller	Painful micturition and suppression of urine.
54.	*Cucumis trigonus* Roxb.	Bilious disorders.
55.	*Cucumis satvus* Linn	Diuretic, refrigerant and nutritious.
56.	*Cucurbita maxima* Duch	Taenicide and diuretic.
57.	*Cuscuta chinensis* Linn.	Demulcent and diaphoretic.
58.	*Cuscuta reflexa* Roxb.	Carninative in pains and stomachache and liver complaints.

Contd...

Table 3.1–Contd...

Sl.No.	Botanical Name	Uses
59.	*Dalbergia lanceolaria* Linn.f.	Rheumatic affections.
60.	*Datura metal* Linn.	Insanity, fever with catarrhal and cerebral complications, diarrhea and skin disease.
61.	*Daucus carota* Linn.var. savita DC	Aromatic, stimulant, diuretic, carminative, dropsy, kidney, antiestrogenic, antiprogestation, antihistaminic and antiacetcholime.
62.	*Delphinium ajacis* Linn.	Insecticidal and destroying lice in hair.
63.	*Dolichos lablab* Linn.var. typicus prain	Febrifuge, stomachic, antispasmodic and aphrodisiac.
64.	*Emblica officinalis* Gaerth	Asthma, bronethis and biliousness.
65.	*Euphorbia helioscopia* Linn.	Cholera and purgative.
66.	*Euphorbia thymifolia* Linn.	Stimulant, astringent, anthelmintic and laxative.
67.	*Foeniculum vulgrae* Mill	Flavouring, soups, other dishes, confectionery, pickles, useful in dieases of cheast, spleen, kidney, laxative, stomatic, stimulant, appetizer, curing biliousness and stomach disorders.
68.	*Garcinia dulcis* (Roxb.) Kurz.	Diarrhoea, dysentery and also uses in malaria.
69.	*Garcinia indica* Choisy	Astringent, demulecent, emollient, soothing, for cutaneous affections, mucus diarrhea, phthisis, skin diseases and ulcertions fissures of lips.
70.	*Gossypium arboretum* Linn	Gonorrhoea, gleet, chornic cystitis, catarrh and constipation.
71.	*Gossypium barbadense* Linn.	Demulcent, antidysenteric, rheumatic disease, scabies disease and swelling and burns.
72.	*Gossypium herbaceum* Linn	Demulcent, laxative, expectrorant, galactagogue, aphrodisiac, nervine tonic and headache.
73.	*Helianthus annuus* Linn	Cooking, salad, oil, diuretic, expectrorant propecties, bronchiant, laryngeal, pulmonary, affections, cough and colds.
74.	*Hibiscus abelmoschus* Linn	Stimulant, antiseptic, stomachic, cooling, tonic, carminative and aphrodisiac.
75.	*Hibiscus cannabinus* Linn.	Applied externally to bruises and paining organs.
76.	*Hibiscus sabdariffa* Linn.	Diuretic and antiscobutic.
77.	*Holarrhena antidysenterica* (Linn) Wall	Astringent, anthelmintic, stomachic, febrifuge, antipyretic, tonic, antidysenteric, amoebic dysentery, diarrhoea, bilious affections, fevers, bowel complaints, piles and intestinal worms.
78.	*Hordeum vulgare* Linn	Sattu, cooling drink, manufacture of beer, diuretic and demulcent drink.
79.	*Hygroryza aristata* Ness.	Urinary tract and biliousness.
80.	*Iberis amara* Linn.	Asthama and bronchitis.
81.	*Indigofera articulate* Gouan.	Anthelmintic.
82.	*Indigofera glandulosa* Willd.	Nutritive and tonic.
83.	*Indigofera trifoliate* L.	Restorative, astringent and aphrodisiac, rheumatism and leucorrhoea.
84.	*Inula racemosa* Hook.f.	Aphrosiaiac.
85.	*Ipomoea muricata* (Linn.) Jacq.	Cathartic.
86.	*Jatropha curcas* Linn	Sciatica, dropsy, paralysis, skin troubles, rheumatism and aborifacient.
87.	*Jatropha gossypifolia* Linn.	Purgative, emetic and body pain.
88.	*Lagenaria siceraria* (Mol.) Standl.	Dropsy and intestinal disorders.

Contd...

Table 3.1–Contd...

Sl.No.	Botanical Name	Uses
89.	*Lapidium sativum* Linn	Galactagogue, emmenagogue, diuretic, tonic, aphrodisiac, laxative, rubefacient, poultices and sprains.
90.	*Luffa acutangula* (Linn.) Roxb.	Emetic and purgative and skin disease.
91.	*Luffa acutangula* Linn. Roxb. Var. *amra* Roxb.	Emetic, expectorant and demulcent, and skin disease.
92.	*Luffa cylindrical* (Linn.) M.J. Roem.	Skin affections and anti cancer activity.
93.	*Lupinum albus* Linn.	Deobstruent, carminative and anthelmintic.
94.	*Madhuca indica* J.F.Gmel	Rheumatiism, skin affections, laxative, habitual constipation and piles.
95.	*Malva parviflora* Linn.	Demulcent and used in cough and the ulcers in bladder.
96.	*Mangifera indica* Linn	Asthma
97.	*Melia azedarach* Linn	Rhematism.
98.	*Melilotus indica* All.	Bowel complaints and infantile diarrhea.
99.	*Mesua ferrea* Linn	Embrocation, skin troubles, embrocation and rheumatism
100.	*Mimusops elengi* Linn	Anus of children in cases, constipation.
101.	*Momordica cochinchinensis* Spreng	Aperient, treatment of ulcers
102.	*Mucuna prurita* Hook	Tonic, aphrodisiac, leucorrhoea, profuse menstruation, paralysis and spermatorrhoea.
103.	*Myristical fragrans* Houtt	Carminative, stomachic, flatulency, nausea and vomiting.
104.	*Nelumbo nucifera* Gaertn.	Check vomiting, diuretic and refrigerant, skin disease, leprosy and antidote to poisons.
105.	*Nigella sativa* Linn	Carminminatative, stomachic, diuretic, emmenagogue, galactagogue, mild cases of puerperal fever, skin affections, antibacterial, activity, indigestion, loss of appetite, fever, diarrhea and dropsy.
106.	*Nymphaea stellata* willd	Stomachic and restorative.
107.	*Ocimum basilicum* Linr	Deroulcent, stimulant, diaphoretic, diuretic, prolonged constipation, piles, poultice, sinuses, gonorrhoea, dysentery and diarrhea.
108.	*Ocimum sanctum* Linn	Demulcent, genitor-urinary, antimicrobial and antimycotic effects.
109.	*Papaver somniferum* Linn	Aphrodisiac, enhance muscular, capacity, allay nervous, culinary purposes, diarrhea, dysentery and skin care.
110.	*Phaseolus mungo* Linn.	Diet in fever and strengthen the eye.
111.	*Phaseolus radiatus* Linn.	Paralysis, rheumatism, affections of nervous system, piles, liver disorders, cough and fever.
112.	*Plantago ovata* Forsk	Demulcent, laxative, dysentery, diarrhea, inflammatory, febtile condition, affections of kidneys, bladder, urethera, rheumatic, glandular and swellings.
113.	*Polygonum barbatum* Linn	Tonic, purgative and emetic.
114.	*Pongamia pinnata* Pierre	Gernicidal, applied in scabies, herpes, leucoderma, other cutaneous disease, internally, dyspepsia with sluggish liver, whooping, irritating and coughs.
115.	*Portulacea oleracea* Linn	Used as a vermifuge.
116.	*Psoralea corylifolia* Linn	Laxative, diuretic, diaphoretic, aphrodisiac, leucoderma, leprosy, psoriasis and inflammatory diseases of skin.

Contd...

Table 3.1–Contd...

Sl.No.	*Botanical Name*	*Uses*
117.	*Punica granatum* Linn	Stomachic.
118.	*Quisqualis indica* Linn	Anthelmintic.
119.	*Raphanus satvus* Linn	Expectrorant, peptic, diuretic, laxative, carminative, lithontriptic, emmenagogue and stimulant.
120.	*Ricinus communis* Linn	Purgative, counter-irritant in scorpion sting and conjunctivitis.
121.	*Salvadora persica* Linn	Diuretic, purgative, tonic and rheumatism.
122.	*Salvia aegyptiaca* Linn	Diarrhea and hemorrhotids and diseases of eye.
123.	*Sesamum indicum* Linn	Emollient, tonic, diuretic, lactagogue, useful in piles, ulcers, burns, scalds and poultice.
124.	*Sesbania bispinosa* W.F. Wight.	Mixed with flour are applied to ringworms and other skin diseases.
125.	*Sida cordifolia* Linn	Gonorrhoea, colic, tensmus, leucorrhoea, spermatorrhoea, bleeding piles, hematuria, cystitis, chronic, dysentery, facial paralysis, asthma, jaundice, calculi of liver, gall bladder and hemorrhage.
126.	*Solanum indicum* Linn	Dysuria, odontalgia and arachidiolein.
127.	*Solanum surattense* Burm.f.	Asthma, cough and toothaches.
128.	*Sorghum vulgre* (Linn) pers	Siuretic, demulcent and aphrodisiac.
129.	*Sterculia foetida* Linn	Laxative and carminative.
130.	*Streblus asper* Lour.	Epistaxis, piles, diarrheoa and leucoderma.
131.	*Strychnos nux–vomica* Linn	Nervime, stomachic, tonic, aphrodisiac, spinal respiratory, cardiac stimulant, dyspepsia, nervous system, remedy in chronic dysentery, atonic diarrhea, paralytic, neuragice, affections, mental emotion, epilepsy, chronic constipation, bowels, prolapsus, rectum, gout, chronic, hydrophobia, impotency, somnia, antidote, alcoholism and spermatorrhoea.
132.	*Strychnos potatorum* Linn	Alternative, demulcent, emetic, diabetes, tonic, diabetes, diarrhea, gonorrhoea, local application and abscess.
133.	*Tamarindus indica* Linn	Vaginal discharges, ulcers, giddiness and vertigo.
134.	*Tephrosia purpurea* pers	Scabies, dematosis, eczema, tonic, laxative, blood purifier, diuretic, deobstruent, antipyretic and worm infestation in children dropsy.
135.	*Thevetia peruviana* Merr.	Rheumatism and dropsy.
136.	*Tribulus terrestris* Linn	Backache, impotency, kindney gravel, dyspepsia, hepatitis, sexual weakness and diuretic.
137.	*Trichosanthes cucumerina* Linn	Antifebrile, anthelmintic and stomach.
138.	*Trigonella foenum-graecum* Linn	Mucilaginous, demulcent, diuretic, tonic, carminatve, aphrodisiac, colic, flatulence, dysenter, diarrhea, arorexia, cough, dropsy, enlargement of liver, spleen, rheumatism, lymphatism rickets, anaenia, diabetes and cooling drink.
139.	*Vernonia cinerea* Less.	Anthelmintic, alexipharmic, leprosy and chronic skin diseases.
140.	*Vitex negundo* Linn	Cooling properties, cutaneous disease and leprosy.
141.	*Withania coagulans* Dunal	Alternative, diuretic and emetic.
142.	*Withania somnifera* Dunal	Hypnotic, diuretic and coagulating milk.
143.	*Wrightia tinctroria* R. Br.	Anthelmintic, antidiarrhoeal, antidysenteric, astringet, febrifuge, seminal and weakness.
144.	*Zygophyllum simplex* Linn	Anthelmintic, eyes in opthalmia and leucoma.

Result and Discussion

It was observed that total 748 plant species were identified as medicinal plant out of 748 plant species 144 plant species seed are used as medicinal importance.

References

Bhojwani, S.S. and S.P. Bhatnagar, 2001. *The Embryology of Angiosperms*. Delhi, pp. 266–291.

Bhatnagar, S.P. and B.M. Johri, 1972. *Development of Angiosperm Seeds, Vol. 1: Seed Biology*. Academic Press, New York, London.

Esau, K., 1993. *Plant Anatomy*. Wiley Eastern, New Delhi.

Freeman, O.L., 1961. *Seeds, Year Book*. Agric. USDA, Washington, D.C.

Kozlowski, T.T. and C.R. Gunn, 1972. Importance and characteristics of seeds. In: *Seed Biology*, Vol. 1. Academic Press, New York, London.

Nautiyal, S.R. Kumar and A.. Husen, 2002. Thoughts and reflections status of medicinal plant in India: Some latest issues. *Ann. For.*, 10(1): 181–190.

Senti, F.R. and W.D. Maclay, 1961. Age-old uses of seeds and some new ones. *Year Book Agric.*, USDA, pp. 27.

Siddigi, T.O., B. Dhir, S.H.K. Peerzada and M. Iqbal, 2001. Angiospemous seeds of medicinal importance. *J. Econ. Taxon. Bot.*, p. 251.

Singh, A.P. and M. Parabia, 2003. Status of medicinal plants consumption by the pharmaceutical industries in Gujarat state. *Indian Forester*, February.

Singh, A.P. and M. Parabia, 2003. The floral diversity of Gujarat State: A review. *Indian Forester*, February.

Singh, R.D., 1985. Anatomical patterns of seed coat in some dicotyledonous families. *Trends Plant Res.*, p. 233-243.

Singh, U., A.M. Wadhwani and B.M. Johri, 1990. *Dictionary of Economic Plants in India*. ICAR Publ., New Delhi.

Uma Devi, 1988. Identification and status survey of medicinal plant of Gujarat. *Ph.D. Thesis*, Department of Biosciences, South Gujarat University, Surat.

Medicinal Plants: Conservation, Cultivation and Utilization (2007) *Pages 25–28*
Editors: A.K. Chopra, D.R. Khanna, G. Prasad, D.S. Malik and R. Bhutiani
Published by: DAYA PUBLISHING HOUSE

Chapter 4

Management of Viral Diseases of Ashwagandha

L.P. Awasthi, R.V. Singh, Pardeep Kumar and Shyam Singh
Department of Plant Pathology, N.D. University of Agriculture and Technology, Kumarganj, Faizabad - 224 229 (U.P.)

Introduction

Ashwagandha (*Withania somenifera* L.) a medicinal plant, is used in the preparation of various Ayurvedic medicines. It normally grows as a wild plant. Since a huge amount of raw material is needed for the preparation of drugs therefore it is being cultivated in herbal gardens at many places Recently we have visited a few herbal gardens and noticed that a large number of plants were found infected with different viruses. These viruses caused very severe losses in plant growth and vigorousness. Therefore keeping in view, identification, characterization and management of viruses infecting Ashwagandha plants was undertaken.

Materials and Methods

Host Range

The test plants were grown in pots in an insect free glass house. Symptomatic young leaves were collected from the field and then washed and gently blotted dry with blotting paper. The leaves were macerated with an equal volume of 0.1 m phosphate buffer pH 7.0. After grinding, the leaf pulp was squeezed through double layers of muslin cloth to get filtered standard extract of the leaves. Carborundum powder 600 mesh was dusted on the leaves of test plants before inoculation. Cotton pad soaked in standard extract was rubbed on the leaves of test plants. After inoculation plants were washed with water to remove excessive inocula and kept at 20-28°C in an insect free glass house. The inoculated hosts were observed for symptoms over a period of three weeks.

Transmission

The causal viruses could be transmitted mechanically and through insects. The methods of mechanical transmission and host range was followed as described earlier (Verma and Awasthi, 1978). For insect transmission the pure culture of aphids was maintained in net house. The aphids from pure culture were collected and put in the glass vials for pre-acquisition fasting. After 2 hours of pre-acquisition fasting aphids were placed an virus in affected leaf for 5-10 minutes for acquisition feeding. Stylet feeding was observed under stereoscopic binocular microscope. Ten aphids per seedling were used for this study. Such seedlings were covered with cages after acquisition access and placed in dark chamber overnight. Next day these seedling are sprayed with the insecticide to kill the aphids. The seedlings were placed in a glass house for observations for the appearance of disease symptoms. The percentage transmission of the virus on test seedlings was recorded.

Serological Relationship

Serological relatedness of virus with other viruses infected solanaceous plants and a few others was ascertained by DAC, ELISA (Clark and Bar Joseph, 1984). The viruses tested were, Tobacco mosaic virus, Potato virus X, Cucumber mosaic virus, Chilli mosaic virus, Brinjal mosaic virus and chrysanthemum mosaic virus.

Management

Healthy seeds of Ashwagandha were directly sown in 3 × 2m plot during 2004-05 with five treatments under Randomized Block Design with four replications. The leaves of *Azadirachta Indica, Clerodendrum aculeatum, C. inermi* and filaments of *Cuscuta reflexa* were collected and ground with the help of a grinder. The extracts were prepared by making the suspension of leaves/filaments in water. The suspension was strained through two folds of cheese cloth and the homogenate was clarified by centrifugation at 3000 rpm for min. The supernatant was diluted to 1:10 with water and used for spray an experimental plots. The first spray was done after 15 days of sowing. The rest nine sprays were done at weekly time interval following the first spraying. In control plots water alone was sprayed instead of antiviral substance. Observations were recorded or disease incidence, severity and per cent control.

Results and Discussion

Symptomology

The diseased plants exhibited typical mosaic mottling symptoms with mild puckering and stunted growth of plants. In severe cases flowering and fruiting was reduced.

Host Range

The caused virus had a narrow host range which include plant species of family Solanaceae, chenopodiaceae and cucurbitaceae. The mosaic symptoms were observed on Ashwagandha, Rushbarry and *Cucurbita moshata*. Whereas, Necrotic lesions were observed on *Nicotiana glutinosa* and *Chenopodium amaranticular*. Other host plants tested *viz., Cuumis melo, Luffa acutargula, Lycopersicon esculentus, Carica papaya* and *Vigna radiata* did not show any type of symptoms.

Transmission

The causal virus(es) can be transmitted mechanically from Ashwagandha to Ashwagandha plants. It was transmitted in a non persistent manner by several species of aphids. *Myzus persicae* (85 per cent), *Aphis crassivora* (80 per cent) and *A. gossypii* (82 per cent).

Table 4.1: Host Range of the Causal Viruses

Sl.No.	*Test Host Plants*	*Reactions*
1.	Ashwagandha (*Withania somenifera* L.)	Mosaic symptoms
2.	*Nicotiana glutinosa*	Necrotic local lesions
3.	*Rushbarry*	Mosaic symptoms
4.	*Chenopodium amaranticolor*	Necrotic local lesion
5.	*Cucumis melo*	No symptoms
6.	*Luffa acutangula* L.	No symptoms
7.	*Lycopersicon esculetum*	No symptoms
8.	*Cucurbita moschata* Ruch.	Mosaic symptoms
9.	*Carica papaya*	No symptoms
10.	*Vigna radiata L.*	No symptoms

Table 4.2: Transmission of Viruses on Ashwagandha Plants

Sl.No.	*Methods of Transmission*	*Transmission per cent*
1.	Sap Inoculation	90
2.	Insect	
	(i) *Myzus persicae*	85
	(ii) *Aphis crascivora*	80
	(iii) *A. gossipii*	92

Table 4.3

Treatments	*Disease incidence*	*per cent disease control*
Azadirachta indica	28.62	60.25
Clerodendrum aculaetum	24.94	65.36
C. inermi	31.92	55.67
Cuscuta reflexa	55.29	25.98
Control	72.00	-
SEm+	2.58	
CD at 5 per cent	7.21	

Serological Relationship

The virus strongly cross reacted with their polyclonal antisera in DAC ELISA. The virus(es) appears to be serologically related to TMV on the other hand it did not reach with Potao virus X, CMV. Chilli mosaic virus, Brinjal mosaic virus and Chrysanthemum mosaic virus. Many plant viruses were identified by DAC-ELISA by several workers (Ray *et al.*, 1999 and Singh *et al.*, 2005).

Management

Results indicated that the spraying of plant extract significantly reduced disease incidence when the sprays were given from seedling to maturity time. Minimum disease incidence of 24.94 per cent was recorded in *Clerodeudrum aculatum* followed by *Azadirachta indica* (28.62 per cent), *C. inermi* (31.92 per cent) and *Cuscuta reflexa* (55.29 per cent). In control plots disease incidence recorded was 72.0 per cent. On the other hand, maximum reduction in disease incidence found was 65.36 per cent in *C. aculeatum* followed by *A. indica* (60.25 per cent), *C. inermi* (55.67 per cent) and *C. reflexa* (25.98 per cent). Our findings were supported by Verma *et al.* (1988), Singh *et al.* (2004). Verma and Verma (1993) and Verma *et al.* (1994). Singh and Awasthi (2006) reported that the most effective botanical was *Clerodendrum aculeatum* leaf extract against mungbean yellow mosaic virus on mungbean and Urdbean followed by *Boerhaavia diffusa* and *Azadirachta indica*. Verma and Singh (1994) reported *C. aculeatum* as a possible prophytactic agent against natural viral infection in mungbean plants. Surendran *et al.* (1999) found the antiviral activity of *Azadirachta indica, C. infortunatum* against brinjal mosaic virus on its local lesion host *Datura stramonium*. Because of its phyto-chemical nature, it has many other advantages over chemicals, as as it is easily biodegradable, does not leave any residue, ecofriendly, non-phytotoxic, easily observed by the plants and very cheap.

References

Clark, M.F. and M-Bar-Joseph, 1984. Enzyme Immunosorbent assays in plant virology. In: *Methods in Plant Virology*. Academic Press, New York, pp. 51–85.

Ray *et al.*, 1999. Determined the serological features of PRSV by Direct antigen coated-enzyme linked Immunosorbent assay (PAC-ELISA) with *Polyclonal antisera*.

Singh, S., Awasthi, L.P. and Verma, H.N., 2004. Prevention and control of yellow mosaic disease of mungbean by application of aqueous root extract of *Boerhaavia diffusa*. *Indian Phytopath.*, 57(3): 303–307.

Singh, V., Rao, G.P. and Shukla, K., 2005. Response of commercially important papaya cultivars to papaya ring spot virus in eastern U.P. conditions. *Indian Phytopath.*, 58(2): 212–216.

Surendran, M., Shanmugam, V., Rajagopalan, B. and Ramanian, N., 1999. Efficacy of botanical on brinjal mosaic virus. *Plant Disease Research*, 14(1): 63–66.

Verma, A. and Singh, R.B., 1994. *Clerodendrum aculeatum* a possible prophylactic agent against natural viral infection in mungbean. *Ann. Plant Prot. Sci.*, 2(2): 60–63.

Verma, A. and Verma, H.N., 1993. Management viral disease of mungbean by *Clerodendrum* leaf extract. *Indian J. Plant Path.*, 11(1 and 2): 63–65.

Verma, H.N. and Awasthi, L.P., 1978. Antiviral activity of *Boerhaavia diffusa* root extract and the physical properties of the virus inhibitor. *Can. J. Bot.*, 57: 926–932.

Verma, H.N., Chowdhury, B. and Rastogi, P., 1994. Antiviral activity in leaf extracts of different *Clerodendrum* species. *Z. Pflanzenk Pflanzenschuz*, 91(1): 34–41.

Verma, H.N., Rastogi, P., Prasad, V. and Srivastava, S., 1985. A possible control of natural virus infection of *Vigna radiata* and *Vigna mungo* by plant extracts. *Indian J. Plant Path.*, 3(1): 21–24.

Medicinal Plants: Conservation, Cultivation and Utilization (2007) *Pages 29–35*
Editors: A.K. Chopra, D.R. Khanna, G. Prasad, D.S. Malik and R. Bhutiani
Published by: DAYA PUBLISHING HOUSE

Chapter 5

Ayurvedic Garden: A Novel Concept in Society for Education and Popularization of Medicinally Important Plants

Niraj N. Upadhyay*, Mitesh B. Panchal and Vishal K. Muliya
Department of Botany, Faculty of Science,
The Maharaja Sayajirao University of Baroda, Vadodara – 390 002

ABSTRACT

Botanical gardens are playing a vital role in conservation and education of plants in society. They create awareness in society about nature, plants and their habitats. Now a day "Herbal" term has become very popular. A lot of people are using herbal medicines for maintaining their health but there is no specific institute for education about plants used in ayurveda. Concept of Ayurvedic Garden includes lot many objectives like *ex situ* conservation of plants, education of medicinal plants, creating awareness for ayurveda etc. It includes gardening in such a way that it can reflect the groups of plants which are used for making various ayurvedic compositions. India being a land of Ayurveda, there should be at least one ayurvedic Garden. A lot many factors like compositions described in ayurveda, groups described in ayurveda, habitats of the plants, aesthetic beauty and lay out of the garden and interactions between the plants in term of allelopathy etc. should be taken in to consideration while designing the Ayurvedic Garden. Paper deals with proposed design with consideration of all possible factors.

* E-mail: nir_niraj@yahoo.com.

Introduction

Ayurveda, said to be a world medicine, is the most holistic or comprehensive medical system available (Tirtha, 1998). Before civilization, Ayurveda was practice only in the applied form (Gaur, 2006). Patvardhan *et al.*, (2003) had reviewed some reports of negligence of term Ayurveda in many review articles published in prior reviewed journals. Though Ayurveda remains one of the most ancient and yet living traditions practiced widely in India, Sri Lanka and other countries and has a sound philosophical and experimental basis. India is sitting on a gold mine of well recorded and traditionally well practiced knowledge of herbal medicine and it is rightly called the botanical garden of the world (Dubey *et al.*, 2004).

Botanical garden is a natural meeting ground for science, history, art and culture. Botanical garden can give professional opinion, advice, information and service to all the issue related to plants (Seibert, 1958). They are primarily outdoor collections of labeled living plants, the whole being more or less effectively landscaped, playing specific role in community (Avery, 1958). European institutions in 16th and 17th centuries were medicinal gardens, also called physics gardens or gardens of simples, whose principle role was to provide material for medical facilities in Italy, France, and other western countries (Wilson, 1992).

Ayurvedic Garden: A Novel Approach

Ayurvedic garden is a garden with medicinally important plants in very simple term but it is not having restriction to only collection and landscaping of medicinal plants. There are many factors like education of ayurveda, ethanobotanical knowledge, layout of garden, allelopathy, phenology of plants, aesthetics, simplicity etc. should be considered while designing ayurvedic garden.

Objectives of Ayurvedic Garden

1. To encourage systematic maintenance of various plant groups with their most appropriate Ayurvedic and pharmacological uses.
2. To promote research into the propagation and maintenance in cultivation of medicinal plant genotypes considered rare, threatened or endangered.
3. To promote public awareness of conservation issues and philosophies through educational and interpretive programmes.
4. To provide an advisory service to individuals (professional or amateur academic or commercial), that would locate medicinal plants for research, propagation, distribution or reintroduction.
5. To strengthen the ties among botanical gardens, Ayurved Universities, medical institutes, pharmaceutical industries etc.
6. To create and maintain an information network of rare, endangered and threatened native plants of India.
7. To provide a national focus for, and cooperate with, other organizations in matters concerning medicinal gardens and herbaria.
8. To display the living collections in an educationally useful and attractive setting that enables people to enjoy and appreciate the recreational, horticultural and medicinal values of Ayurvedic gardens.
9. To share knowledge acquired relative to Ayurvedic medicines through publications and other media.

Importance of Ayurvedic Garden

1. The aim of this garden is to improve knowledge and understanding of medicinal plants in order to promote excellence in use of ayurvedic medicine system.
2. Education is a key element of the Garden with information available about the evolution of the traditional use of medicinal plants in Ayurveda.
3. Staff and visitors can access the Garden's herbarium and extensive library to further assist with enquiries.
4. In the near future such a garden can also be considered as a world heritage site for the study of medicinal plants used in ayurveda, at a single place with their compositions in detail.
5. This garden can serve the society in having a collection of in depth knowledge of cultivation, collection, storing and utilization of medicinally important plants at a place where any person can access it for its application in daily life.
6. Such a garden can stand as reservoir where a person can easily introduced to an endangered but medicinally very important plant.
7. Thus such a garden can prove to give service to mankind along with the conservation and wise use of medicinally important plants.

Salient features of Ayurvedic Garden

1. There should be grouping of plants in such a way that it can reflect some ayurvedic formulations or group of plants with same property. A list of such groups taken from an ayurvedic text "*Aryabhishak*" authored by Late Shastri Shri Shankar Daji Fade (2005). A hypothetical layout is given is Figure 5.1.
2. There should be one area were medicinal plants should be arranged according to their uses in modern medicine but more emphasizing should be there on ayurvedic groups.
3. Each and every plant should be labeled with Sanskrit name, local name, Latin name with family and property in brief.
4. There should be a group label describing uses of that group, names of the plants used in that group in Sanskrit, Hindi, and scientific name with family.
5. Allelopathic interactions of the plants should be considered while preparing the layout.
6. There should be a Guide/Public Relation officer with good knowledge of ayurveda, medicinal plant, traditional medicine systems of India for guiding to visitor so garden will become real education and information center.
7. There should be a good library, research laboratory and a conference room.

Some of the Important Compositions Listed in Ayurveda

Kantaktrutiya

All three plants is having thorns (*kantaka*) but to common medicinal use. It includes *Fagonia schweinfurthii*, *Solanum xanthocarpum*, *Ocimum gratissimum*. Here *O. gratissmimum* is having allopathic effect so it should be put in a pot separately.

Kantkaritray

Kantkaritray is three plants along with Kantkari (*Solanum xanthocarpum*), other plant is *S. indicum* and *Tribulus terrestris*. Allelopathic effect is seen in *T. terrestris* so it should be planted separately.

Trikatu

Zingiber officinale, Piper nigrum and *P. longum* are forming group trikatu and it is increasing acidity of stomach, used in asthclma, cough, obesity, elephantiasis and for skin diseases.

Triphala

Phyllanthus emblica, Terminalia chebula, T. belarica is forming group triphala, a well known composition for gastrointestinal disorders. All these plants are tree and they are in group of Trivarga also so can be integrated with Trivarga.

Trivarg (Trikatu, Triphala and Chitrakmul)

Zinger, black Pepper, long Pepper, *Terminalia chebula, T. belarica* aonla and *Plumbago zeylanica* are ingredient of Trivarg and it should be separately displayed because of its popularity and usefulness.

Madhur triphala

Vitis vinifera, Gmelina alborea and *Phoenix dactylifera* are ingredients of Madhur Triphala where all these three fruits are sweet in taste and effect equal to Triphala. Here *V. vinifera* is having allelopathic effect so it should be in pot and its fallen leaves should be collected immediately.

Sugandhi triphala

Myristica fragrans, Syzygium aromaticum and *Elettaria cardamomum* are the ingredients of Sugandhit Triphala where their name itself indicate three fruits with aromatic odour.

It is used as spices.

Trijat or Trisugandh

Cinnamomum zeylenicum, C. tamala and *Elettaria cardamomum* are three plants with aromatic odour and pungent taste and used as spices.

Trimad

Cyperus scariosus, Embelia ribes and *Plumbago zeylanica* are three narcotic plants (Monier, 2002). *C. scariosus* is having allelopathic effect so it should be planted separately.

Trisamm

Terminalia chebula, Zingiber officinale and *Tinospora cordifolia* are the ingredients of trisamm.

Trikarshika

Zingiber officinale, Aconitum heterophyllum and *Cyperus rotundus* are three ingredients of Trikarshika with astringent effect. *C. rotundus* is having allelopathic effect so must planted separately.

Trikantak

Zingiber officinale, Tinospora cordifolia and *Fagonia schweinfurthii* are the three plants having strong effect like thorne (*Kantak*).

Katugranthi

This group of plants has *Ushna* effect and it include dried and fresh *Zingiber officinale, Allium sativum* and roots of *Piper longum.*

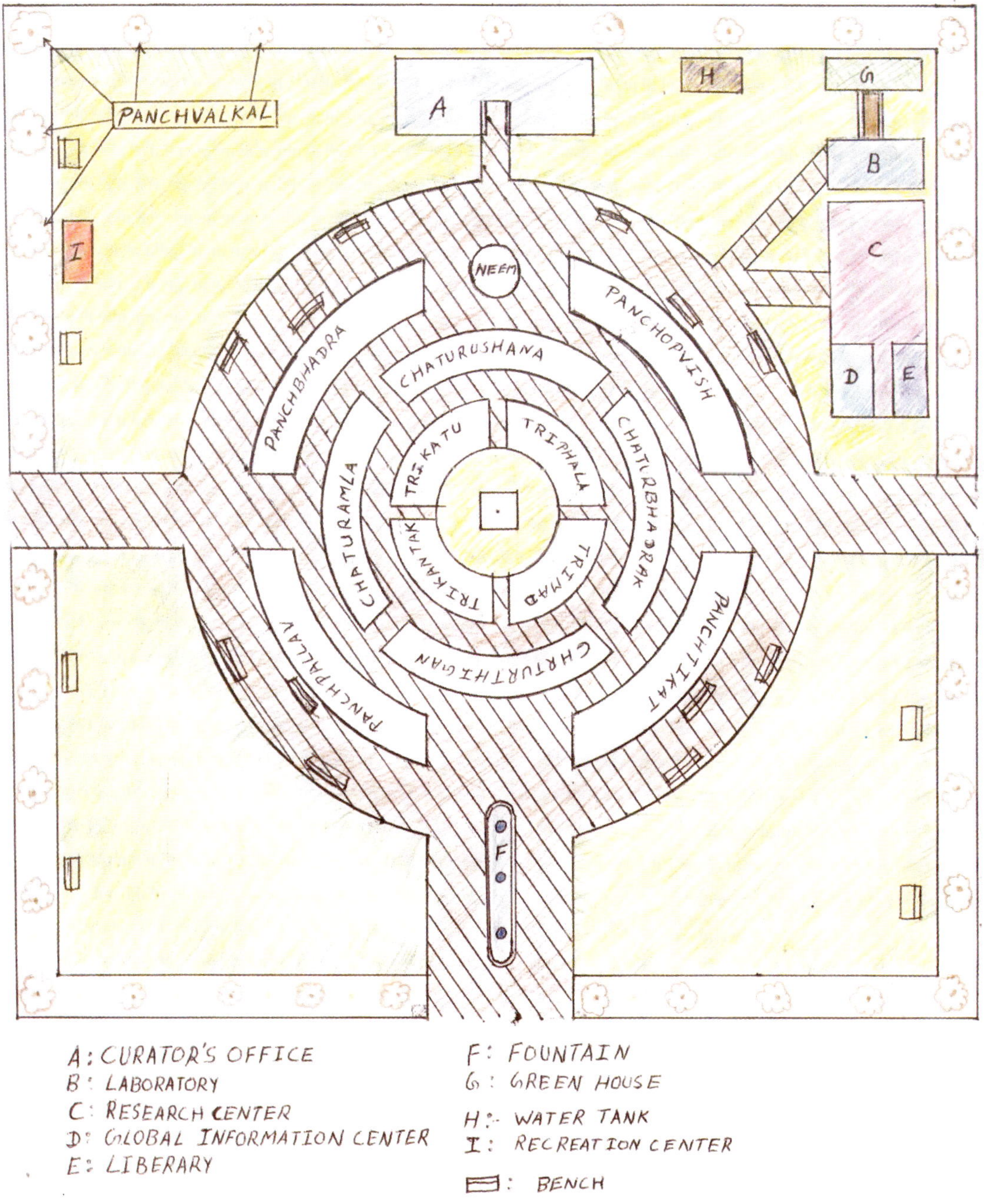
PANCHVALKAL
A
H
G
B
C
D
E
I
NEEM
PANCHBHADRA
PANCHOPVISH
CHATURUSHANA
TRIKATU
TRIPHALA
CHATURAMLA
CHATURBHADRAK
TRIKANTAK
TRIMAD
PANCHPALLAV
CHATURTHIGAN
PANCHTIKAT
F
A: CURATOR'S OFFICE
B: LABORATORY
C: RESEARCH CENTER
D: GLOBAL INFORMATION CENTER
E: LIBERARY
F: FOUNTAIN
G: GREEN HOUSE
H: WATER TANK
I: RECREATION CENTER
: BENCH

Figure 5.1

Chaturamla

Plants with sour effect are included in Chaturamla. *Citrus aurentifolia, C. medica, Garcinia indica* and *C. limon.* All this members are having allelopathic effect and they are shrubs and tree. So it should be separated from other groups.

Chaturushana

Chaturushna name indicates four *Ushna* plants *viz., Zingiber officinale* rhizome, fruit of *Piper nigrum,* fruit of *P. longum,* root of *Piper longum.*

Chaturbeej

It include four plant of which seeds (*Beej*) is useful and it includes, *Trigonella foenum-gracum, Lepidium sativum, Vernonia anthelmintica, Apium graveolens.*

Chaturjaat

All the plants in this group are having volatile oils. It is having *Ushna* effect. They are purgative used to prevent bad smell from mouth, *Kaffa* or *Vatta* condition. It includes *Cinnamomum zeylenicum, C. tamala, Elettaria cardamomum* and *Ochrocarpos longifolius.*

Chaturbhadrak

It includes *Zingiber officinale, Aconitum heterophyllum, Tinospora cordifolia, Cyperus rotundus* and used for curing fever. *C. rotundus* was listed by Holm (1969) as one of the ten worst weeds of the world so it should be planted in pot.

Chaturthikgan

This group is used for curing Gastero Intestinal disorders and to stimulate appetite. It includes *Phyllanthus emblica, Terminalia chebula, Piper longum* and *Plumbago zeylanica.*

Aushadhi Panhamrut

This group is having plants used for general tonic. It includes *Tinospora cordifolia, Curculigo orchioides, Zingiber officinale, Tribulus Terrestris* and *Asparagus racemosus.* In this group *T. Terrestris* is having allelopathic effect (El-Ghareeb, 1991) so it should be separated by bricks or it should be kept distinctly.

Panchtikat

Solanum xanthocarpum, Tinospora cordifolia, Zingiber officinale, Costus speciosus and *Andrographis panicuiata* are five bitter plants used for fever and other diseases.

Panchpallav

Mangifera indica, Syzygium jambolana, Feronia elephantum, Citrus medica and *Aegle marmelos.* Stem-bark of these plants are known as Panchpallav. They are having cooling and astringent effect so used as anti-diarrheal (Nanbahtt, 1955).

Panchbhadra

Fumaria officinalis, Tinospora cordifolia, Andrographis paniculata, Cyperus rotundus and *Zingiber officinale* are the ingredients of Panchbhadra which means five ospecious plants used for decoction. *C. rotundus* is having allelopathic effect so must planted separately.

Panchvalkal

Ficus benghalensis, F. siella, F. religiosa, F. glomerata and *Thespesia populnea* are latex containing plants were the stem-barks are having cooling effect.

Panchopvish

Calotropis procera, Euphorbia neriifolia, Gloriosa superba, Datura stramonium and *Nerium odorum* are five poisonous plants. These plants should be kept in such a way that common people can not reach it and there should be special precautionary notice for not touching these plants.

Shatoptvish

Calotropis procera, Euphorbia neriifolia, Gloriosa superba, Datura stramonium, Nerium odorum, Abrus precatorius and *Papaver somniferum* are the seven plants having poisonous effect. It includes group Panchopvish also.

Summary

India as the mother land of Ayurveda needs to have a living collection of plants mentioned in Ayurveda. It should be a premier institution for education, popularization, conservation, authentication and cultivation of Ayurvedic medicinal plants which reflect an ancient wisdom and glory of our marvelous heritage.

References

Al-Ghareeb, R.M., 1991. Suppression of annuals by *Tribulus Terrestris* in an abandoned field in the sandy desert of Kuwait. *Journal of Vegetative Science,* 2: 147–154.

Avery, G.S. (Jr.), 1958. Botanical gardens: What role today? An "Operation Bootstraps" opportunity for botanists. In: *Fifty Years of Botany,* (Ed.) W.C. Steere. McGraw-hill Company, Inc., New York.

Dubey, N.K., Rajesh Kumar and Tripathi, P., 2004. Global promotion of herbal medicine: India's opportunity. *Current Science,* 86(1): 37–41.

Gaur, B.L., 2006. Literary research in ayurveda: Need of hour. In: *Souvenir of 5th International Seminar on Ayurveda,* Gujarat Ayurved University, Jamnagar, pp. 41–43.

Holm, L.G., 1969. Weed problems in developing countries. *Weed Science,* 17: 113–118.

Monier, M.W., 2002. *A Sanskrit-English Dictionary.* Motilal Banarasidass Pub. Pvt. Ltd., New Delhi.

Nanbhatt, P., 1955. *Bhavprakash–Purvakhand.* Sastu Sahitya Vardhak Karyalay, Mumbai (in Gujarati).

Pade, S.D., 2005. *Aryabhishak.* Sastu Sahitya Vardhak Karyalay, Mumbai (In Gujarati), pp. 38–41.

Patvardhan, B., Chopra, A. and Vaidya A.D.B., 2003. Herbal remedies and the bias against Ayurveda. *Current Science,* 84(9): 1165–1166.

Tirth, S.S.S., 1998. *The Ayurveda Encyclopedia: Natural Secrets to Healing, Prevention and Longevity.* Sri Satguru Publications, New Delhi, pp. 3.

Wilson, E.O., 1992. *The Diversity of Life.* Harvard University Press, Cambridge, Massachusetts.

Medicinal Plants: Conservation, Cultivation and Utilization (2007) *Pages 37–42*
Editors: A.K. Chopra, D.R. Khanna, G. Prasad, D.S. Malik and R. Bhutiani
Published by: DAYA PUBLISHING HOUSE

Chapter 6

Isolation of Larvicidal Ingredient from the Leaves of *Catharanthus roseus* for Mosquito Control

M.F. Alam[1]*, A.K. Chopra[1] and V.K. Dua[2]
[1]Department of Zoology and Environmental Science, Gurukula Kangri University, Haridwar, India
[2]National Institute of Malaria Research (ICMR) F/S, BHEL, Haridwar, India

ABSTRACT

The larvicidal activity of *Catharanthus roseus* fractions were evaluated against early 4th instars larvae of different species of mosquitoes *viz., Anopheles stephensi, Culex quinquefasciatus* and *Aedes aegypti*. Results revealed that fraction code CAT-1 was more susceptible to dengue vector (*Aedes aegypti*) followed by malaria vector (*Anopheles stephensi*) and filarial vector (*Culex quinquefasciatus*). Fraction code CAT-1 showed 95 per cent, 91.2 per cent and 67.5 per cent mortality against *Aedes aegypti Anopheles stephensi* and *Culex quinquefasciatus* after 72 hours at 250ppm concentrations. Mean LC_{50} value of fraction CAT-1 was found 237.5ppm and 281.2ppm against the larvae of *Aedes aegpyti* and *Anopheles stephensi,* respectively.

Keywords: Larvicidal activity, Catharanthus roseus, Mosquitoes

Introduction

Mosquitoes not only cause nauisance by their bites but also transmit deadly diseases like malaria,

* E-mail: firoz.a@rediffmail.com.

filariasis, yellow fever, dengue and Japanese encephalitis, which contribute singnificantly to poverty and social debility in tropical countries (Jang *et al.*, 2002). Although eradication of these vectors was considered by the use of chemical insecticides, which are now being seriously questioned due to environmental pollution (Edward *et al.*, 1978); multiple resistance (Brown, 1986) and high operational costs. These factors have created the need for environmentally safe, degradable and target specific insecticides against mosquitoes. The search for such compounds has been directed extensively to the plant kingdom. The phytochemicals derived from plant resources can be used as an alternative to the synthetic insecticides (Mittal and Subarao, 2003). A large number of plant extracts have been reported to have mosquitocidal or repellent activity against mosquito vectors (Sukumar *et al.*, 1991). Recently Rajkumar, S and Jebanesan, A (2005) reported larvicidal and adult emergence inhibition effects of *Centella asiatica* Brahmi (Umbelliferae) against mosquito *Culex quinquefasciatus* and adulticidal activity against *Anopheles stephensi*.

Catharnthus roseus is an erect, much branched, annual or perennial herb, 60-90 cm height and it is distributed/cultivated as an ornamental plant in garden through out the India. Its medicinal value was known in 50 B.C. However, medicinal important of this plant in modern medicine has been realized only because of a chance discovery of anticancer activities in certain alkaloids of its leaves (Glossary of Indian medicinal plants with active principle 1915-81).

The present study was undertaken to investigate the larvicidal activity of different fractions of *Catharanthus roseus* leaves against *Anopheles stephensi, Culex quinquifaciatus* and *Aedes aegypti* due to good medicinal value and there has been no report on its activity against public health vectors.

Material and Methods

Catharanthus roseus Lin. (Apocynaceae) seeds were collected from locally B.H.E.L Campus Uttranchal, India. The leaves were washed properly, air dried in shade and powdered in Kitchen machine. 100 gram of leaves were sequentially extracted using Soxhlet apparatus (6hr) with petroleum ether, chloroform and methanol. Details of extraction procedure and their yields are depicted in Figure 6.1. The crude extracts thus obtained were evaporated to dryness under reduce pressure below 40°C and fraction was coded as CAT-1, CAT-2 and CAT-3.

Larvicidal activity was carried out of all the three fractions against early 4th instars larvae of *An. stephensi, Culex quinquifaciatus and Aedes aegypti as* described earlier (WHO, 1996). Twenty larvae of mosquitoes were placed in to 500 ml capacity glass beaker containing 250ml water. The mosquito larvae were initially exposed to 250ppm concentration of the isolated extracts and mixture of dog biscuit and yeast powder in the ratio of 3:2 were provided as nutrients. For each fraction test four replicated with parallel control were used at a time. Mortality of larvae was monitored after 24hrs, 48 hrs and 72 hrs. Preliminary larvicidal test revealed that petroleum ether fraction (CAT-1) showed good larvicidal activity. Therefore fraction (CAT-1) was further analyzed quantitatively at different dose *viz.*100, 150, 200, 250, 300, 350, 400, 450 and 500ppm concentrations for the estimation of LC_{50} and LC_{90} value using probit analysis methods (Finney 1971).

The mosquito larvae were obtained from well-established insectory at National Institue of Malaria Research, Haridwar (Uttranchal), All bioassay were performed according to standard methods (WHO procedure, 1996) in the laboratory at constant temp 26±2°C and relative humidity of (75±5) per cent.

Results

Larvicidal activity of isolated fraction code CAT-1, CAT-2 and CAT-3 from leaves of *Catharanthus roseus* were evaluated against mosquito larvae at 250ppm concentration.

Fractions code CAT-1, CAT-2 and CAT-3 showed 91.2,32.5 and 18.7 per cent larval mortality respectively against *Anopheles stephensi* after 72 hours at 250ppm concentrations details are given in Table 6.1. While Fraction code CAT-1, CAT-2 and CAT-3 showed 67.5,31.2 and 25.0 per cent larval mortality respectively against *Culex quinquefasciatus* at same concentration after 72 hours results are given in Table 6.2. The fraction code CAT-1, CAT-2 and CAT-3 produced 95.0,75.0 and 57.5 per cent larval mortality respectively against *Aedes aegypti* at 250ppm concentration after 72 hours. Results are tabulated in Table 6.3.

Table 6.1: Larvicidal Activity of *Catharanthus roseus* Fraction Against *Anopheles stephensi* 250ppm Concentration

Fraction Code	*No. of Mosquito Larvae*	*% Mortality (Mean ± S.D.)*		
		24 hours	*48 hours*	*72 hours*
CAT-1	20	42.5±6.4	73.5±8.5	91.2±4.7
CAT-2	20	20±4.0	31.2±4.8	32.5±6.4
CAT-3	20	0±0	10±4.0	18.7±4.7
CONTROL	20	0±0	0±0	0±0

Replicates (n)= 4

Table 6.2: Larvicidal Activity of *Catharanthus roseus* Fraction Against *Culex quinquefasciatus* 250ppm Concentration

Fraction Code	*No. of Mosquito Larvae*	*% Mortality (Mean ± S.D.)*		
		24hours	*48hours*	*72hours*
CAT-1	20	30.0±4.0	47.5±6.5	67.5±6.4
CAT-2	20	27.5±6.4	28.7±4.7	31.2±4.7
CAT-3	20	15.0±4.0	17.5±6.4	25.0±4.0
CONTROL	20	0±0	0±0	0±0

Replicates (n)= 4.

Table 6.3: Larvicidal Activity of *Catharanthus roseus* Fraction Against *Aedes aegypti* at 250ppm Concentration

Fraction Code	*No. of Mosquito Larvae*	*% Mortality (Mean ± S.D.)*		
		24hours	*48hours*	*72hours*
CAT-1	20	58.7±8.5	82.5±6.4	95.0±4.0
CAT-2	20	43.7±4.7	60.0±4.08	75.0±9.1
CAT-3	20	26.25±6.2	53.7±6.2	57.5±6.4
CONTROL	20	0±0	0±0	0±0

Replicates (n) = 4.

Results revealed that fraction code CAT-1 is more effective than other two fractions, which provided 95, 91.2 and 75 per cent larval mortality against *Anopheles stephensi, Culex quinquefasciatus* and *Aedes aegypti* after 72 hours at 250ppm concentrations.

The LC_{50} and LC_{90} values of active fraction code CAT-1 was evaluated against different mosquito larvae and results are given in Table 6.4. The results revealed that fraction code CAT-1 was found most effective against dengue vector (*Aedes aegypti*) than malaria vector (*Anopheles stephensi*) larvae with LC_{50} value 237.5 and 281.2ppm respectively.

Table 6.4: Larvicidal Activity of Fraction Code CAT-1 Against *Aedes aegypti* and *Anopheles stephensi*

Fraction Code	*Mosquito Species*	*Activity (ppm) (Mean ± S.D.)*	
		LC_{50}	*LC_{90}*
CAT-1	*Aedes aegypti*	237.5±6.4	365.5±10.8
	Anopheles stephensi	281.2±8.5	508.7±8.5

Replicates (n) = 4.

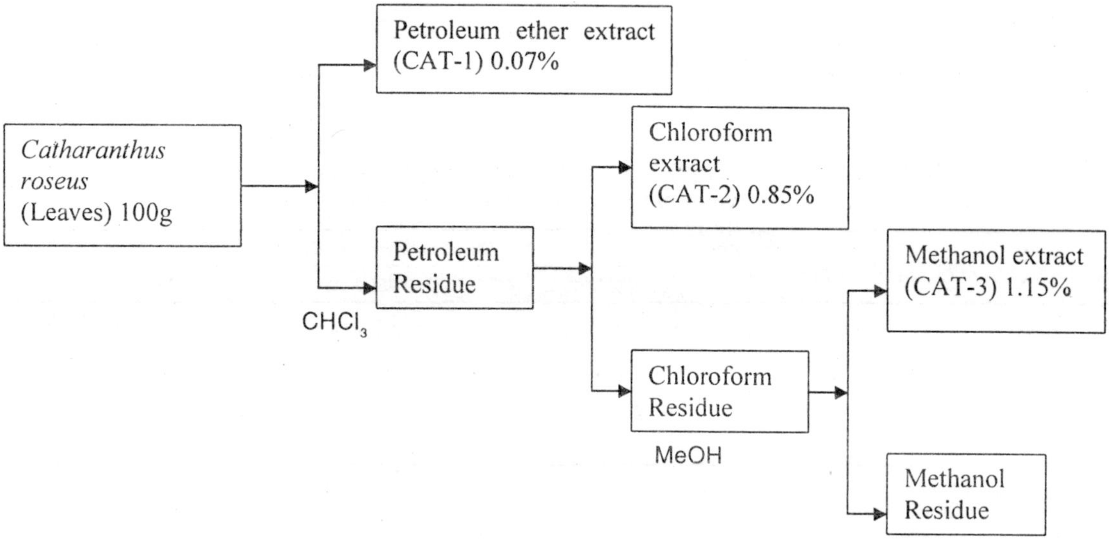

Figure 6.1: Extraction of *Catharanthus roseus* Leaves and their Yields

Discussion

Vector control is facing a threat due to the emergence of resistance in vector mosquitoes to conventional synthetic insecticide warning either counter measure to development of newer insecticide (Chandre, *et al.*, 1998). Botanical insecticides may serves as suitable alternative to synthetic insecticide in future as they are relatively safe, degradable and are redialy available in may areas of the world. Though several plants from different families have been reported for mosquitocidal activity, only few botanicals have moved from the laboratory to field use like neem base insecticide which might be due to the light and heat instability of photochemical compared to synthetic insecticide (Green *et al.*, 1991). According to Bowers *et al.*, 1995 the screening of locally available medicinal plants for mosquito control would generate local employment, reduce dependency on expansive imported insecticide and stimulate local effort to enhance the public health.

The petroleum extract of leaves of *Catharanthus roseus* has been found larvicidal activity against dengue vector (*Aedes aegypti*) and malaria vector (*Anopheles stephensi*) than filarial vector (*Culex quinquefasciatus*). The activity of the plant extract might be due to presence of various compounds like alkaloids, terpenoids and others like α-amyrine acetate and oleanolic acids.

Pizzarro, *et al.* (1999) studied the activity of the saponin fraction of *Agave sisalana* and estimated the LC_{50} and LC_{90} value against 3rd instar larvae of *Culex quinquefasciatus*, that were 183 and 408 ppm, respectively. Markouk, *et al.* (2000) evaluated the 16 extracts of four Moroccan medicinal plants for larvicidal properties against *Anopheles labranchiae* mosquito larvae and exhibited 9 extracts for high larvicidal activity with LC_{50} values (in the range 28 to 325ppm). Recently, Ansari, *et al.* (2005) reported the larvicidal activity of pine oil against *An. stephensi*, *Cx. quinquefasciatus* and *Ae. aegypti* with LC_{50} value 112.6, 85.7 and 82.1ppm, respectively.

The findings of the present study indicate that leaves of *Catharanthus roseus* possess larvicidal activity against mosquito vectors. Further investigations are needed to elucidate the pure compounds and test against wide range of mosquito species.

References

Ansari, M.A., Mittal, P.K., Razdan, R.K. and Sreehari, U., 2005. Larvicidal and repellent activities of Pine (*Pinus longifolia*, Family: Pinaceae) oil. *J. Vect Borne Dis.*, 42: 95–99.

Bowers, W.S., Sener, B., Evans, P.H. and Bingol F. Erdoganl, 1995. Activity of Turkish medicinal plants against mosquitoes *Aedes aegypti* and *Anopheles gambiae*. *Insect Sci. Applic.*, 16: 339–342.

Brown, A.W.A., 1986. Insecticide resistance in mosquitoes: A pragmatic review. *J. Am. Mosq. Cont. Assoc.*, 2: 123–140.

Chandre, F., Darriet, F., Darder, M., Cuany, A., Doannio, J.M.C., Pasteur, N. and Guillet, P., 1998. Pyrethroid resistance in *Culex quinquefasciatus* from West Africa. *Med. Vet. Entomol.*, 12: 359–366.

CSIR, 1915–81. *Glossary of Indian Medicinal Plants with Active Principle.* C.S.I.R, Part I (A–K).

Edwards, C.A., Veresh, G.K. and Ksueger, H.R., 1978. Pesticide residues in the environment in India. *USA Tech. Series* No. 32: 524.

Finney, D.J., 1971. *Probit Analysis*, 3rd ed. Cambridge University Press, Cambridge, pp. 9–158.

Green, M.M., Singer, J.M., Sutherland, D.J. and Hibbon, C.R., 1991. Larvicidal activity of Tagates minuta (Marigold) towards *Aedes aegypti*. *J. Am. Mosq. Control Assoc.*, 7: 282–286.

Jang, Y.S., Kim, M.K., Ahn, Y.J. and Lee, H.S., 2002. Larvicidal activity of Brazilian plants against *Aedesaegypti* and *Culex pipiens* (Diptera : Culicidae. *Agric. Chem. Biotechnol.*, 45: 131–134.

Markouk, M., Bekkouche K., Larhsini, M., Bousaid, Lazrek, H.B. and Jana, M., 2000. Evaluation of some Moroccan medicinal plant extracts for larvicidal activity. *J. Ethnopharmacol.*, Nov; 73: 293–297.

Mittal, P.K. and S.K. Subarao, 2003. Prospect of using herbal products in the control of mosquito vectors. *ICMR Bull.*, 33: 1–10.

Pizzarro, A.P.B., Oliveira-filho, A.M., Parente J.P., Melo, M.T.V., Santos C.E. and Lima, P.R., 1999. O aproveitamento do residuo da industria do sisal no controle de larvas de mosquitos. *Rev. Soc. Bras. Med. Trop.*, 32: 23–29.

Rajkumar, S. and Jebanesan, A., 2005. Larvicidal and adult emergence inhibition effects of *Centella asiatica* Brahmi (Umbelliferae) against mosquito *Culex quinquefasciatus* Say (Diptera : Culicidae). *African Journal of Biomedical Research*, 8: 31–33.

Sukumar, K., Parich, M.J. and Boobar, C.R., 1991. Botanical derivatives in mosquito control: A review. *J. Am. Mosq. Cont. Assoc.*, 7: 210–287.

WHO, 1996. Report of the WHO informal consultation on the evaluation and testing of insecticides. CTD/WHOPES/IC/96.1; 69.

Medicinal Plants: Conservation, Cultivation and Utilization (2007) *Pages 43–51*
Editors: **A.K. Chopra, D.R. Khanna, G. Prasad, D.S. Malik and R. Bhutiani**
Published by: **DAYA PUBLISHING HOUSE**

Chapter 7

Phenological Study of Naturalised Medicinal Herbs of Agra

Manjari Kumari and A.K. Singh
Department of Botany, R.B.S. College, Agra

ABSTRACT

In an assessment of five medicinal plants grown under field conditions on a sandy loam soil. Date of emergence flowering and fruiting varied widely with Genus of the medicinal plant. Maximum duration of leaf emergence were found in *Boerhaavia diffusa* and minimum in *Convolvulus arvensis*. And equal days for leaf emergence till flowering were found in same duration in case of *Ruellia tuberose* and *Pedalium murex*.

Pedalium murex (Vilaytigokhru) belongs the family (Pedaliaceae) its flowering and fruiting time: August to October and used in gonorrhea and spermatorrhoea. *Boerhaavia diffusa* (Santh) belongs the family (Nyctaginaceae) its flowering and fruiting time: Sept to November and used in blood impurities, asthma, vata and kapha. *Convolvulus arvensis* (Hirankhuri) belongs the family (Convolvulaceae) its flowering and fruiting time: February to April and used in possesses cathartic properties. *Ruellia tuberosa* belongs the family (Acanthaceae) its flowering and fruiting time July to October and used in emetic and sudorfic properties.

Introduction

Pedalium murex (Vilaytigokhru) (Plate 7.1A) belongs the family (Pedaliaceae) is a diffuse spreading or ascending much branched herb, 20-30 cm tall. Flowers yellow, fruits 4 spined (Sharma 1976). Rarely found in moist shady places. Flowering and fruiting time Aug-Oct. and used in gonorrhoea and spermatorrhoea. *Boerhaavia diffusa* (Santh) (Plate 7.1B) belongs the family (Nyctaginaceae) is a diffuse glabrous herb, 0.6-0.9 cm long. Flowers pink in colour and fruits clovate. Found in field, unused grounds gardens and along roadside. Flowering and fruiting time: Sept.-Nov. and used in blood impurities, asthma, vata, and kepha. (Kirtikar and Basu 1987) *Convolvulus arvensis* (Hiran Khuri) (Plate 7.2A) belongs the family (Convolvulaceae) is twining glabrous herb. Flowers pink or white and capsule globose. Found in cultivated field and in open grounds. Flowering and fruiting time February–April and possesses cathartic properties. *Ruellia tuberosa* (Plate 7.2B) belongs the family (Acanthaceae) is a erect branched, glabrous herb 55-64 cm tall. Flowers blue-violet, paired in the axile of leaves, capsule linear. Found in gardens and moist waste places. Flowering and fruiting time: July–Oct. and has a emetie, sudorfic properties. Phenology is an important function of forest ecosystem that relates the growth habit of a species with the physical environment. The phenological events and meaningful in describing and explaining seasonal aspect of ecological phenomenon (Leith 1973).

Phenology is generally described as the art of observing the phase of life cycle through the year (Leith 1973) these studies permit to construct a calendar for the growth activity of the plant especially the period of leaf emergence, appearance of mature leaves, flowering, fruiting, seed maturity and dispersal. There are many aspect of productivity which can be categorized, predicted and evaluated on the basis of phenological attributes (Leith 1973).

The present investigation was carried out in Agra in different season during the year 2004-2005.

Materials and Methods

Various important phases of life plants such as emergence of new leaves, leaf fall, flowering and fruiting etc. were recorded. The data are represented by phenograms of the type described by Singh (1967) and Agarwal (1973). The present investigation was carried out in Agra. Ten plant of each genus were selected and marked for phenological studies. Phenological data were recorded throughout the year. Following phenological events were noted in all plant species.

Table 7.1: Phenological Studies

Sl.No.	*Character*	*Observation*
1.	Emergence of new leaves	Appearance of new leaves and how long it continued.
2.	Vegetative Phase	Time period between emergence to flowering.
3.	Flowering	Time of flower initiation and its duration
4.	Fruiting	Time of fruit formation and how long they remain attached.
5.	Fruit fall	Time of fruit fall and its duration.
6.	Leaf fall	Time of leaf fall and its duration.

Various important phases of life plants such as emergence of new leaves, flowering, fruiting, fruit fall, leaf fall were recorded. The data are represented by phenograms of the type described by Singh (1967) and Agarwal (1973).

Phenological Events Represented by Phenograms

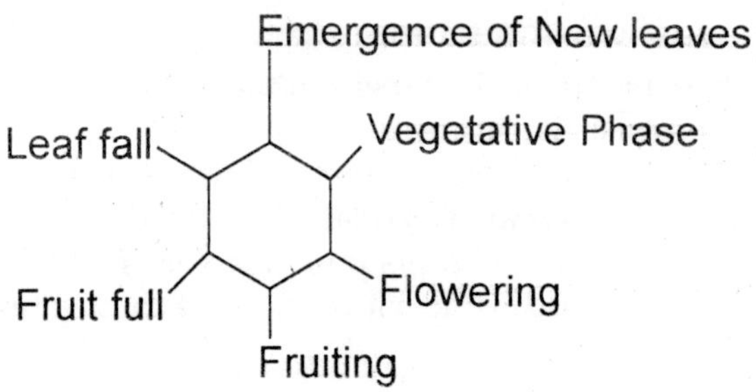

Result

Phenological observation of four genus have been described separately in this paper.

Leaf Emergence

New leaves occurs during the period of last week of July to August in case of *Pedalium murex* and

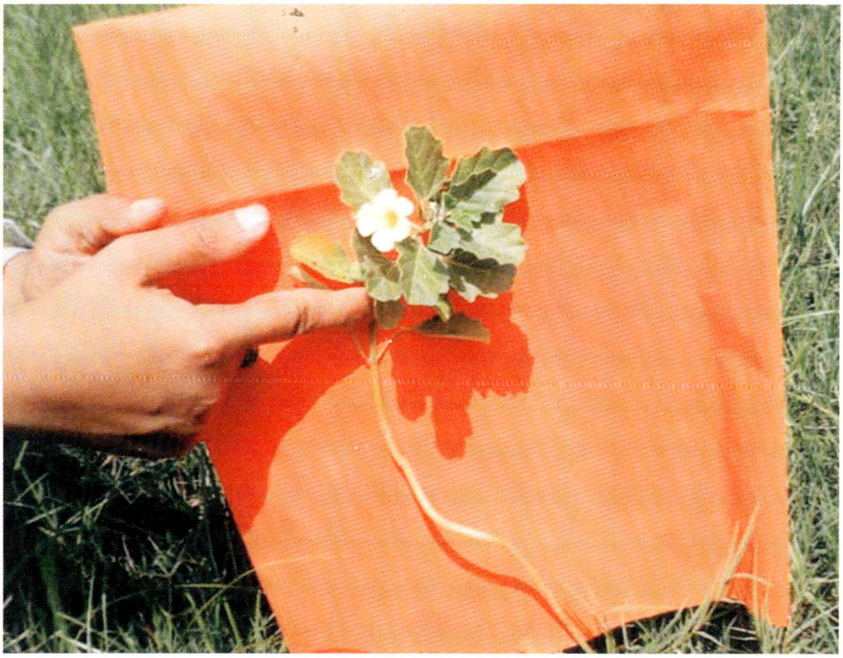

Plate 7.1A: ***Pedalium murex***

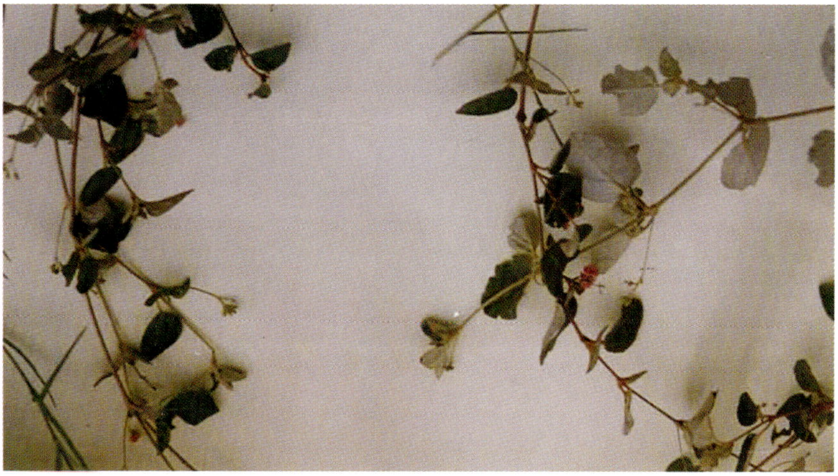

Plate 7.1B: ***Boerhaavia diffusa***

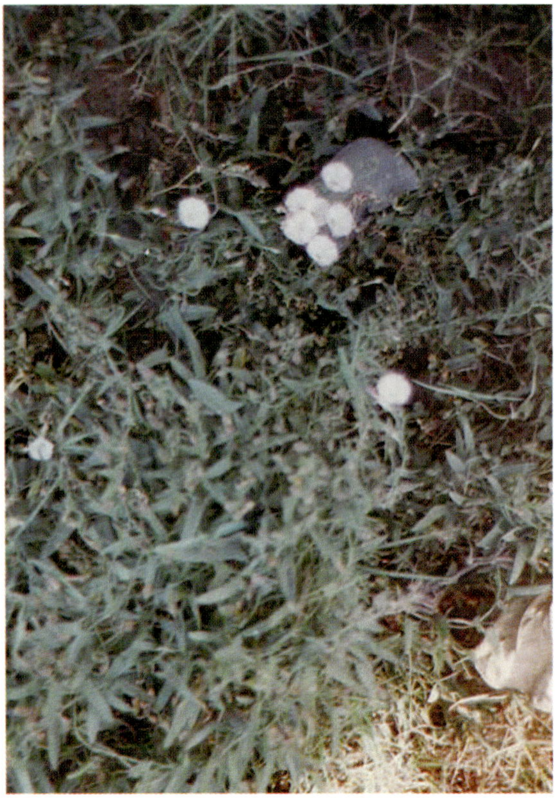

Plate 7.2A: *Convolvulus arvensis*

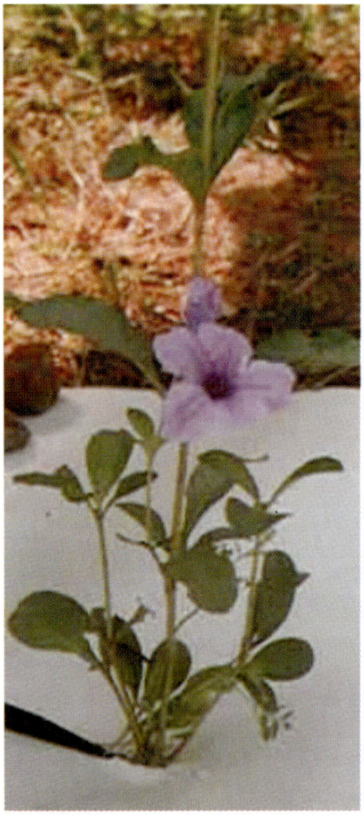

Plate 7.2B: *Ruellia tuberosa*

Ruellia tuberosa. While in case of *Boerhaavia diffusa* and *Convolvulus arvensis* start during the third week of Aug.-Sept. and first week of January respectively.

Maximum leaf emergence of *Pedalium murex. Ruellia tuberosa, Boerhaavia diffusa and Convolvulus arvensis* occurs during the period of August, September and January respectively (Tables 7.1 and 7.2) (Figure 7.2).

Flowering

In case of *Pedalium murex* flowering start in last week of August and same pattern followed by *Boerhaavia diffusa*. While in case of *Ruellia tuberose* flowering start in first week of November and continue till last week of October. While in case of *Convolvulus arvensis* flowering start last week of February and continue till last week of March (Tables 7.1 and 7.2) (Figure 7.2).

Fruiting

In case of *Pedalium murex* and *Boerhaavia diffusa* fruit formation occurs during the period of first week of September to second week of November and third week of September to third week of November.

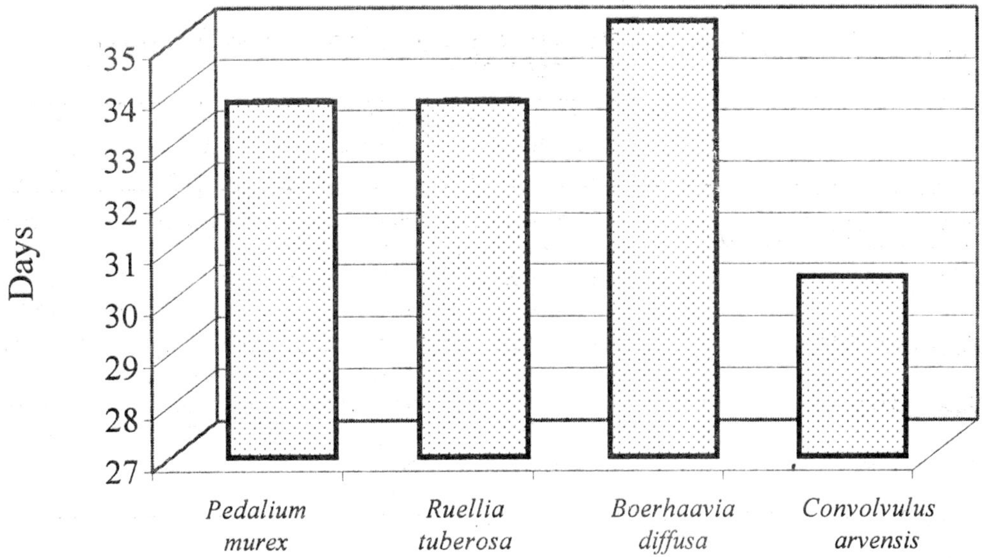

Figure 7.1: Leaf Emergence in Days (From Emergence to Flowering)

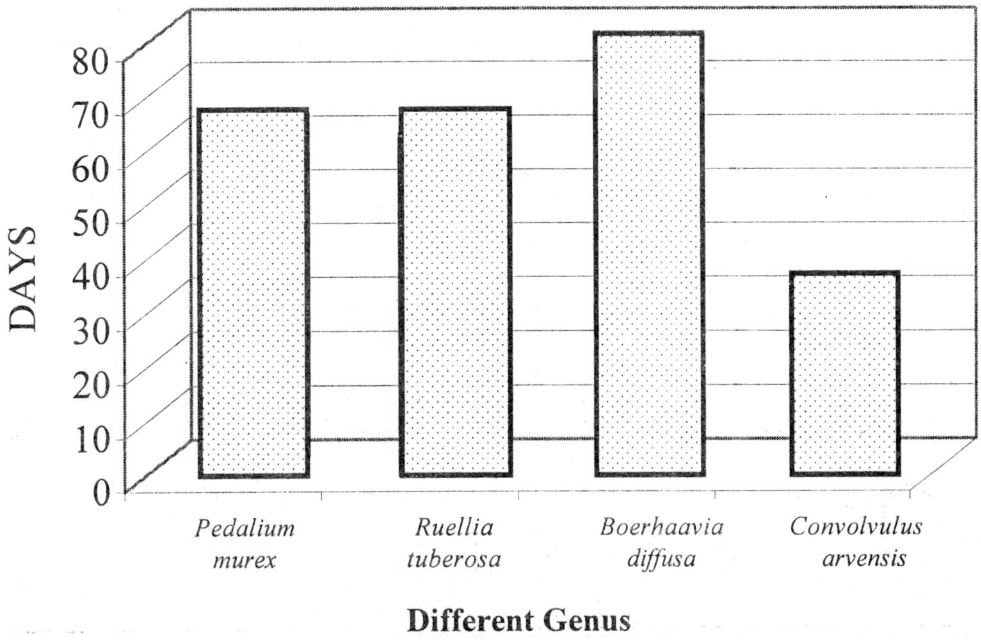

Figure 7.2: Variation in Duration of Flowering Period

While in case of *Ruellia tuberosa and Convolvulus arvensis* start during the first week of September to December and last week of April to May respectively (Tables 7.1 and 7.2) (Figure 7.3).

Table 7.1: Duration of Medicinal Plants for Appearance of Phenological Changes (Year 2004–2005)

Sl.No.	*Habit*	*Pedalium murex (in Days)*	*Ruellia tuberosa (in Days)*	*Boerhaavia diffusa (in Days)*	*Convolvulus arvensis (in Days)*
1	Leaf emergence (Duration) (From emergence to flow.) (Mean)	30-37 days 33.5	30-37 days 33.5	30-40 days 35	30 days 30
2	Flowering period	60-67 days 63.5	60-67 days 63.5	75-80 77.5	30-37 33.5
3	Time of fruit formation	70-75 days 72.5	110-115 days 112.5	55-60 days 57.5	30-37 days 33.5
4	Time of fruit fall	50-55 days 52.5	20-25 days 22.5	35-40 days 37.5	20-25 days 22.5
5	Time of leaf fall	25-30 days 27.5	40-45 days 42.5	35-40 days 37.5	35-40 days 22.5

Table 7.2: Respresentation of Changes in Medicinal Plants through Phenograms

Name of the Genus	*Jan*	*Feb*	*March*	*April*	*May*	*June*	*July*	*Aug*	*Sept*	*Oct*	*Nov.*	*Dec*
Pedalium murex												
Ruellia tuberosa												
Boerhaavia diffusa												
Convolvulus arvensis												

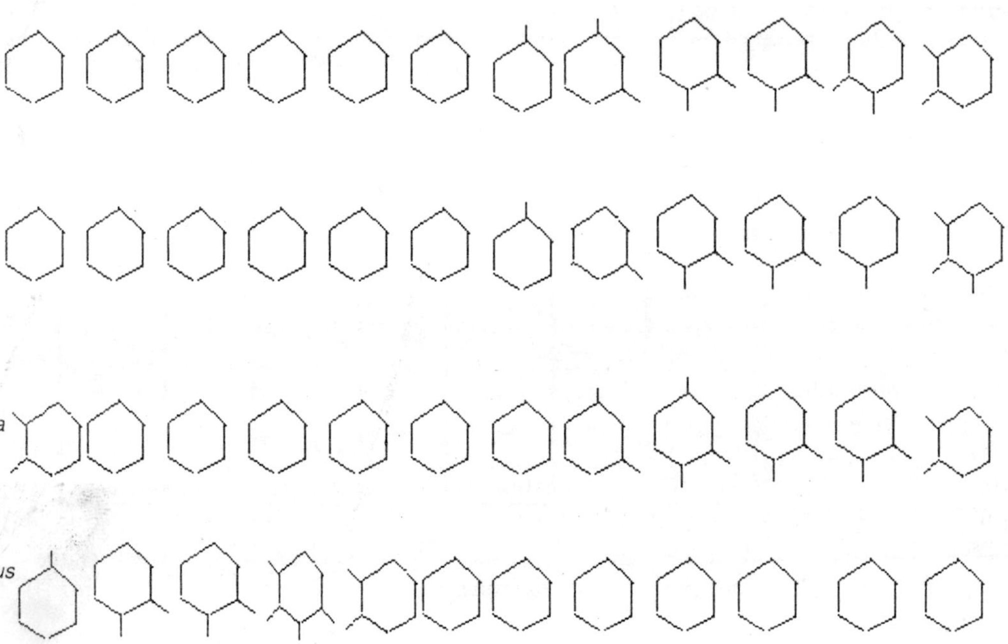

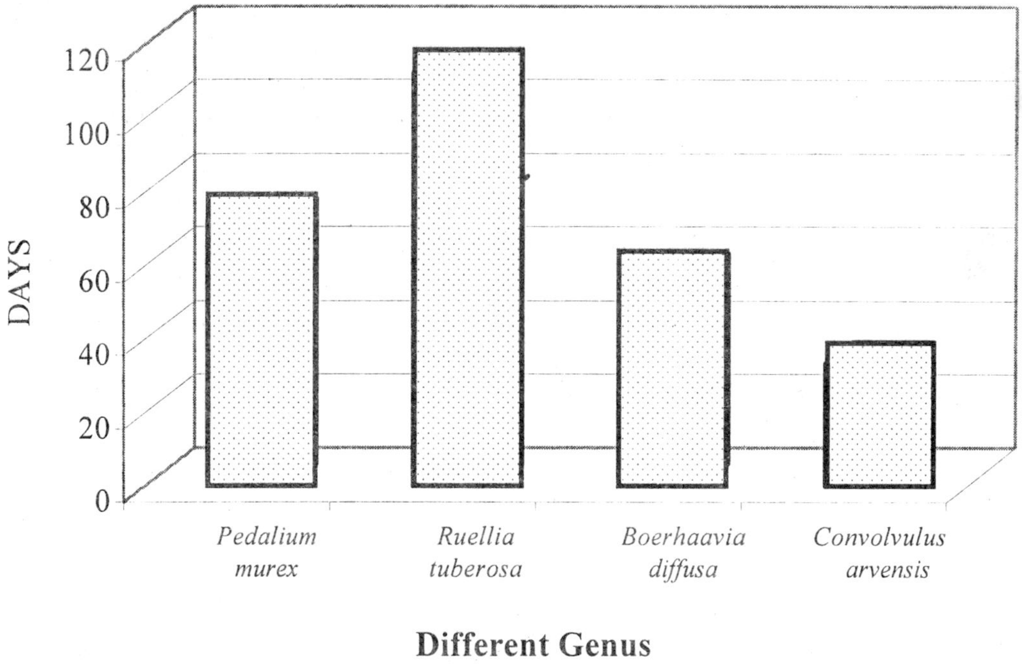

Figure 7.3: Difference in Days of Fruit Fall Formation

Fruit Fall

In case of *Pedalium murex* fruit fall start during last week of November–December. While in case of *Boerhaavia diffusa and Ruellia tuberosa* during the period of second week of December to second week of January and last week of December to second week of January. In case of *Convolvulus arvensis* start during the last week of April to May (Tables 7.1 and 7.2) (Figure 7.4).

Leaf Fall

In case of *Pedalium murex* leaf fall start in the month of December. While in case of *Boerhaavia diffusa and Ruellia tuberosa* start during the second week of December to third week of January and third week of December to last week of January. In case of *Convolvulus arvensis* it start the last week of April to last week of May (Tables 7.1 and 7.2) (Figure 7.5).

Discussion

Maximum days (35) of leaf emergence were taken by the plants of *Boerhaavia diffusa* and minimum (30 days) in the plants of *Convolvulus arvensis*. While plant of *Ruellia tuberosa* and *Pedalium murex* have taken equal days for their leaves emergence till flowering.

Longest period of flowering occur in *Boerhaavia diffusa* followed by *Ruellia tuberosa* and *Pedalium murex* both shortest duration was recorded in *Convolvulus arvensis*. On the other hand maximum days (70-75) for fruit setting was taken by *Pedalium murex* and minimum (30-37) in *Convolvulus arvensis*. Observations also revealed that fruit setting occurred later in plant of *Boerhaavia diffusa* in comparison to rest all three genus. While fastest/earliest fruit setting was recorded in plants of *Convolvulus arvensis*.

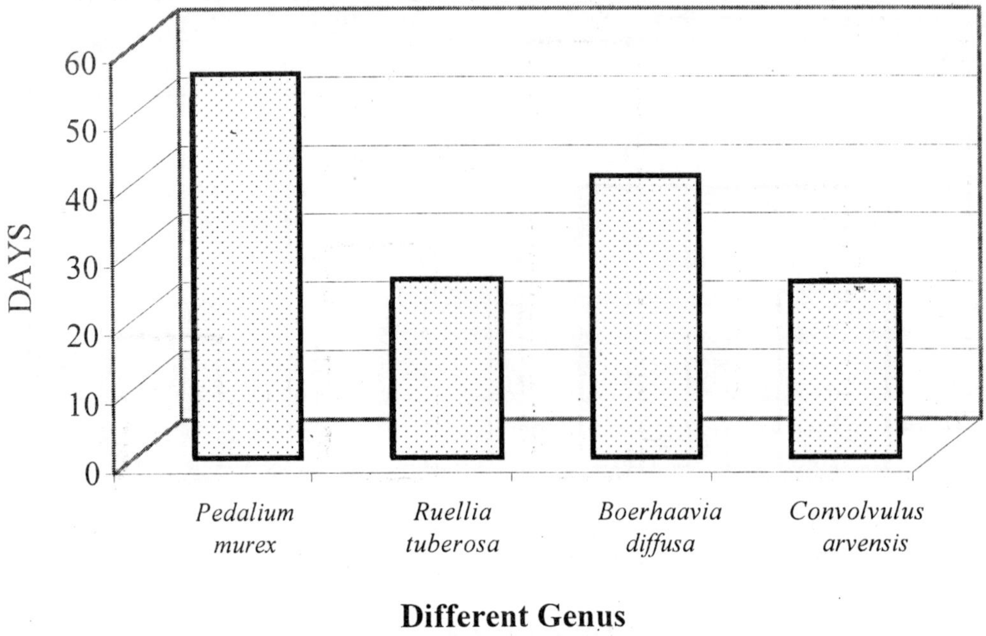

Figure 7.4: Difference in Days of Fruit Fall

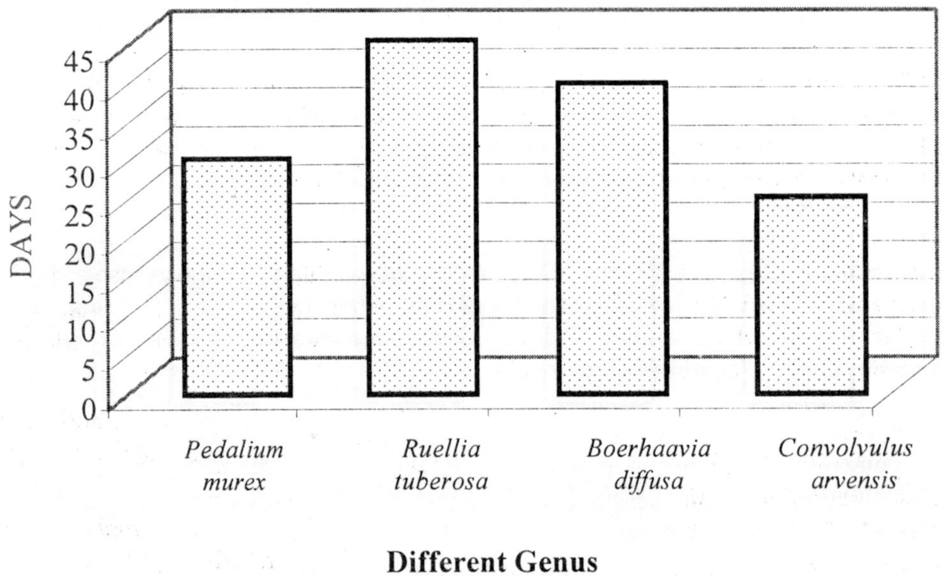

Figure 7.5: Variation in Leaf Fall Duration

Likewise max. days (50-55) for fruit falling were taken by genus *Pedalium murex* and duration of fruit fall of *Ruellia tuberosa* and *Convolvulus arvensis* remained equal.

Leaf falling occurred after starting of fruit falling in case of each experimental plants of present investigation. Hence fastest falling was recorded in *Pedalium murex* followed by *Boerhaavia diffusa* and *Convolvulus arvensis*. While slowest rate of leaf falling occurred in *Ruellia tuberosa.*

Acknowledgements

The author is grateful to Dr. A.K. Singh, Deptt. of Botany R.B.S College, Agra for suggesting the topic and guiding throughout the course of this study. I am also thankful to the principal, R.B.S College, Agra for providing field and laboratory facilities to carryout this work.

References

Agarwal, A.M., 1973. Ecological studies in the grassland of bhata solids of Bilaspur, (M.P.). *Ph.D. Thesis*, Ramshankar University, Raipur.

Kirtikar, K.R. and Basu, B.D., 1987. *Indian Medicinal Plants*, Vol. III. International Book Distributors, Dehradun, India.

Leith, H., 1973. Phenology in productivity studies. In: *Ecological Studies: Analysis of Temperate Forest Ecosystems*, (Ed.) David E. Riechle. Chapman and Hall Ltd., London, Springer-Verlag, Berlin-Heiadberng, New York, p. 29–46.

Sharma, A.K., 1976. Studies on the flora of Agra district. *Ph. D. Thesis*, Agra University, Agra.

Singh, J.S., 1967. Successional variation in composition plant biomass and net community production in grassland at Varanasi. *Ph.D. Thesis*, B.H.U.

Medicinal Plants: Conservation, Cultivation and Utilization (2007) *Pages 53–63*
Editors: **A.K. Chopra, D.R. Khanna, G. Prasad, D.S. Malik and R. Bhutiani**
Published by: **DAYA PUBLISHING HOUSE**

Chapter 8

An Ethnomedicinal Plants in Melghat of Amravati District: A Need for Conservation

U.S. Patil
Department of Botany, Bharatiya Mahvidyalaya, Amravati

ABSTRACT

The Amravati District is situated right in the centre of northern border of the Maharashtra state. The large Melghat tract is a hilly terrain of Satpura ranges, which is highly forested and occupies an area of about 4000 Sq.Kms. The Flora of Melghat contain valuable medicinal plants. Villages in Melghat have dominant population of Korku and Gond tribes.

The traditional healer are overexploiting their medicinal plants causing threat to the plant species. The preliminary survey made for such ethnomedicinal plants include: (1) *Andrographis paniculata* (Burm. F) Wall; (2) *Cissampelos pareira* L.; (3) *Clematis triloba* Heyne ex Roth.; (4) *Costus speciosus* (Koen.) Smith.; (5) *Curculigo orchiodes* Gaertn.; (6) *Dioscorea pentaphylla* L.; (7) *Gloriosa superba* L.; (8) *Leea macrophylla* Roxb.; (9) *Nervilia aragoana* Gaud; (10) *Oxystelma secamone* (L.) karst.

The medicinally important plants used by tribal medicinemen of the region are to conserved on priority basis. In the present paper the importance of these medicinal plants has been discussed with a view to create awareness of medicinal plants among the people.

Keywords: Ethnomedicine, Korku, Gond, Melghat, Amravati, Maharashtra.

Introduction

In recent years traditional drugs are receiving great attention all over the world, therefore, a great emphasis has been laid to revive the herital knowledge on the medicinal plants. The practices of traditional medicine are based on hundreds of years of belief and observations.

In some countries traditional medicine remains an integral part of the formal health system and exists on an equal footing with modern medicine (Akerele 1988).

The Amravati district lies between 20°30' and 21°46' south latitude and 70°37' and 78°27' east longitude. It occupies an area of 12,149.7 Sq. kilometer and has a population of 1,232,780 with 13 town and 1,968 villages (Amravati State Gazetteer, Amravati District). This district is right in the centre of the northern border of the Maharashtra state. The large Melghat tract is a hilly terrain of Satpura ranges, which is highly forested and occupies an area of about 4000 Sq.kms. Melghat have dominant population of Korku and Gond tribes. These tribals still depend on the knowledge of local 'Vaidu' or 'Bhagat' for primary health care. These local Doctors use seasonally available local flora for treating human diseases. They collect the herbal material available in the hilly areas and store it in the form of dried roots, rhizomes, corms, fruits, seeds etc.

Floristic Work

The floristic studies of Amravati district were pioneered by Late Prof. M.V. Mirashi (1975). Further Floristic investigation mostly concentrated on the forest of Chikhaldara by Dhore (1986, 2002). He reported the tree species of the area. The systematic exploration by Bhogaonkar (1999) also reported the new records of plant taxa from Amravati District. The ethnobotanical study of Korku tribes from Melghat has been undertaken by Padhye for the first time and he stressed the need of detailed investigation and phytochemical analysis of the indigenous wild medicinal plants (Padhye *et al.*, 1992).

Methodology

The field survey reported in this study was performed during the period of 2000 to 2002 and was conducted throughout Melghat. A good report was established with the local practitioners. The ethnomedicinal information about the plant species was confirmed through various sources.

The plant species are arranged in alphabetical order according to the botanical names followed by the local name, family, locality, habitat, flowers and fruits, description and Ethnomedicinal significance. Voucher specimens are deposited in the Department of Botany, Sant Gadge Baba Amravati University, Amravati.

Observations and Ethnomedicinal Significance

Andrographis paniculata (Burm.f.) Wall (Figure 8.1)

Local Name

Bhuinimba (G), Kirayat (H), Olenkirayat (M)

Family

Acanthaceae

Locality

Bhimkund (Chikhaldara)

Habitat

Spontaneously found in moist, shady places

Flowers

October–December

Fruits

October–December

Description

Wild, erect, glabrous, branched, annual herbs, Branches quadrangular, herbaceous. Leaves simple, lanceolate. Flowers in cymose panicle, small, white, pedicel short Fruit capsule, linear, oblong, Seeds, Yellowish brown.

Ethnomedicinal Significance

Stem and leaves constitute the drug. Dried powder of stem and leaves of this plant is used by the local tribes against worms specifically in kids. It is also given for the treatment of liver and digestive complaints, general debility, fever and excessive gas formation in stomach. The tribals of the region advise this plant for cure of Jaundice.

Cissampelos Pareira L. (Figure 8.2)

Local Name

Pahad mool (G), Akanadi (H), Paharvel (M).

Family

Menispermaceae

Locality

Ghatang

Habitat

Common in forest areas and at the low levels in the hills.

Flowers

July–October

Fruits

Cold Season

Description

Wild perennial twining, pubescent, herbaceous. Leaves simple, alternate, exstipulate, peltate, broad, ovate, base cordate. Flowers green, male flowers in cymose and female flowers in Pendulose raceme, yellowish pale green, bracteate, bract minute, pubescent.

Ethnomedicinal Significance

The entire plant has medicinal value. The root decoction is used to cure diarohoea and in case of urinary troubles. Leaves are externally applied in skin diseases. Korku tribes of the region also used roots to prevent abortion.

Clematis triloba Heyne (Figure 8.3)

Local Name

Bandersheti (G), Murhari (H), Rajani (M)

Family

Ranunculaceae

Locality

Khamla

Habitat

A fairly common climber on shrubs and also found trailing amongst grasses.

Flowers

October–February also in January

Fruits

October–February also in January.

Description

Wild perennial, climber, stem, weak sulcate with long internode. Leaves simple, slightly lobed shows three distinct lobes. Inflorescence axillary corymbose panicles. Flowers white. Fruit etario of acehene.

Ethnomedicinal Significance

Leaf paste is effective in skin diseases. The decoction of whole plant except root is given to curve asthma, whereas decoction of roots in alcohol distilled from *Madhuca longfolia* (Koen.) Macbr is used to stop menstruation by the local tribes.

Costus speciosus (Koen.) Smith (Figure 8.4)

Local Name

Nalguj (K), Keoo (H)

Family

Costaceae

Locality

Bela (Kalalkund)

Habitat

Not common, on slopes of hills.

Flower

July–September

Fruits

July–September

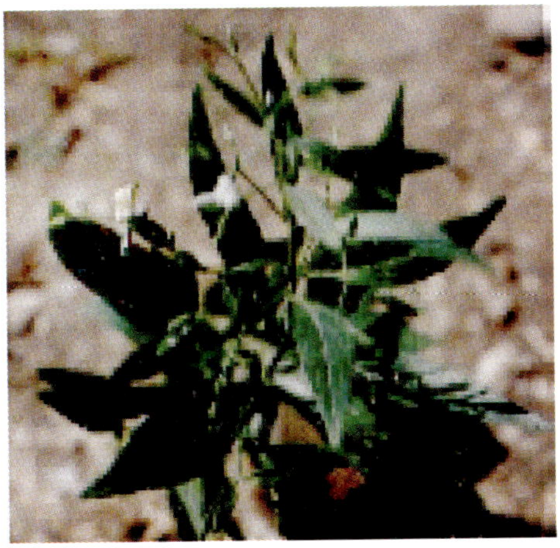

Figure 8.1: ***Andrographis paniculata*** **(Burm. F) Wall**

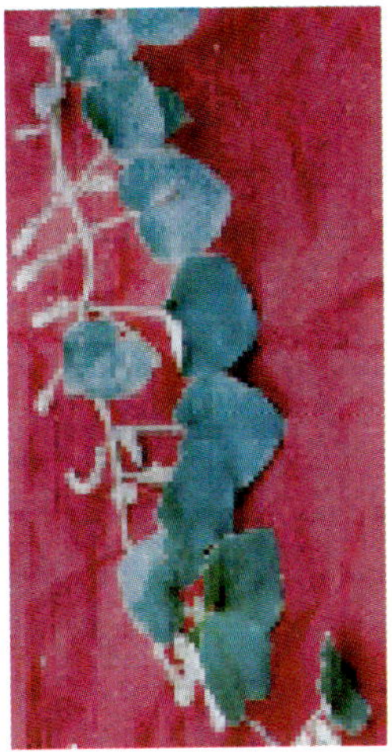

Figure 8.2: ***Cissampelos pareira*** **L.**

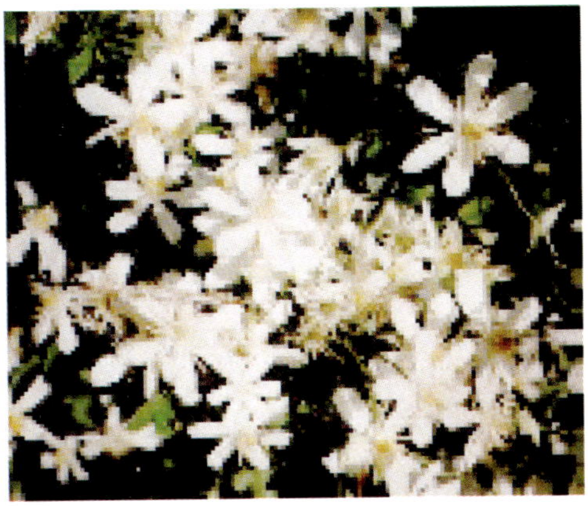

Figure 8.3: ***Clematis triloba*** **Heyne ex Roth.**

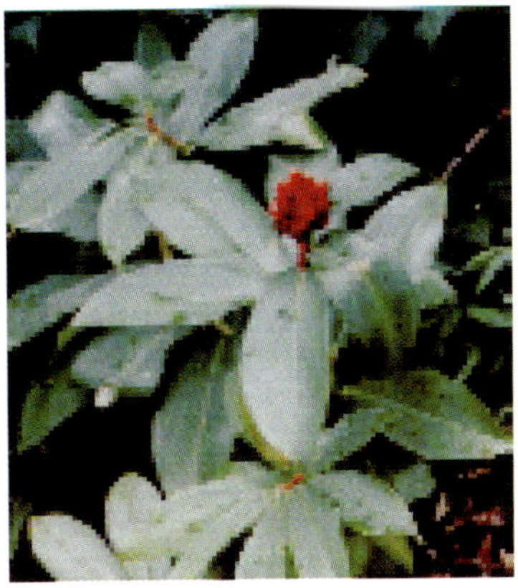

Figure 8.4: ***Costus speciosus*** **(Koen.) Smith**

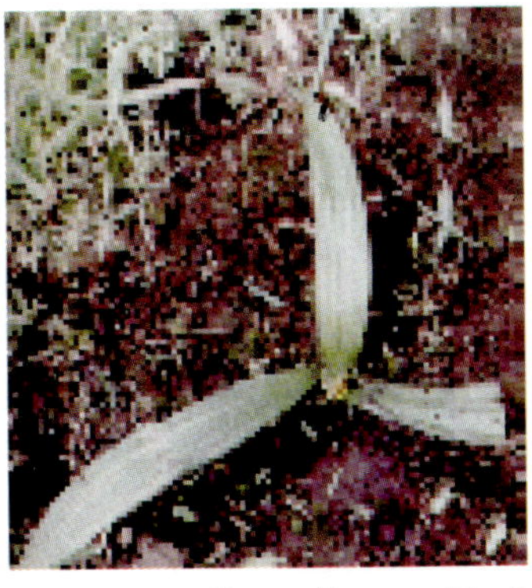

Figure 8.5: ***Curculigo orchiodes*** **Gaertn.**

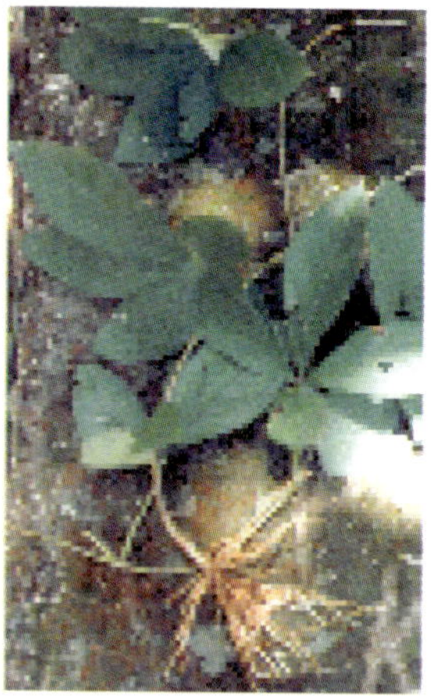

Figure 8.6: *Dioscorea pentaphylla* L.

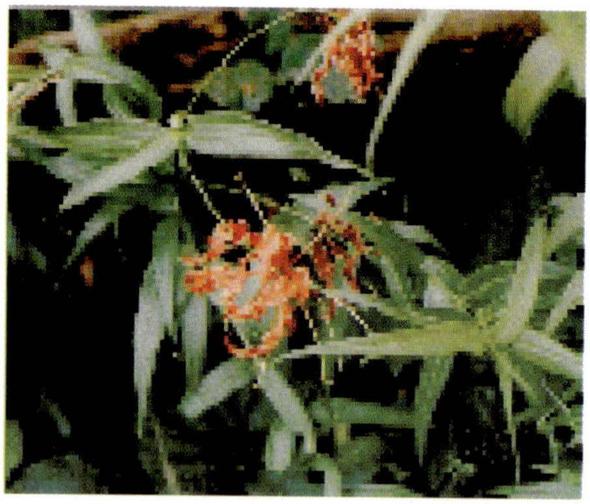

Figure 8.7: *Gloriosa superba* L.

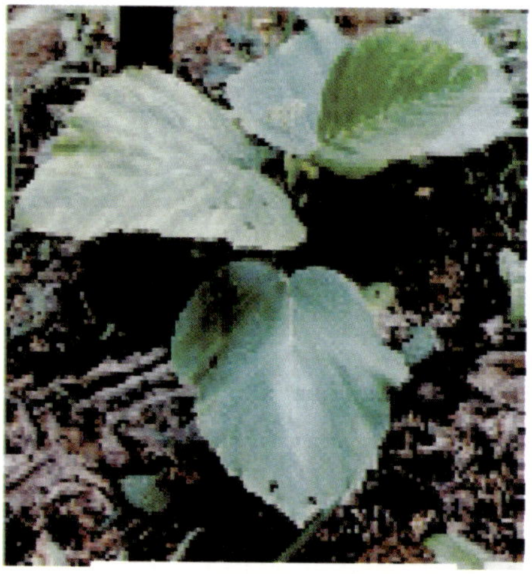

Figure 8.8: *Leea macrophylla* Roxb.

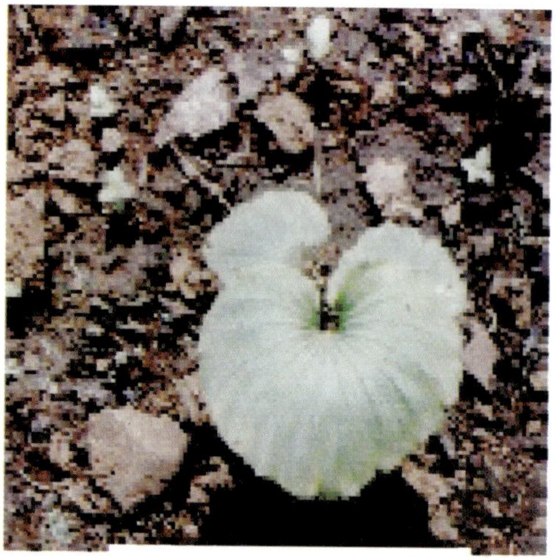

Figure 8.9: *Nervilia aragoana* Gaud

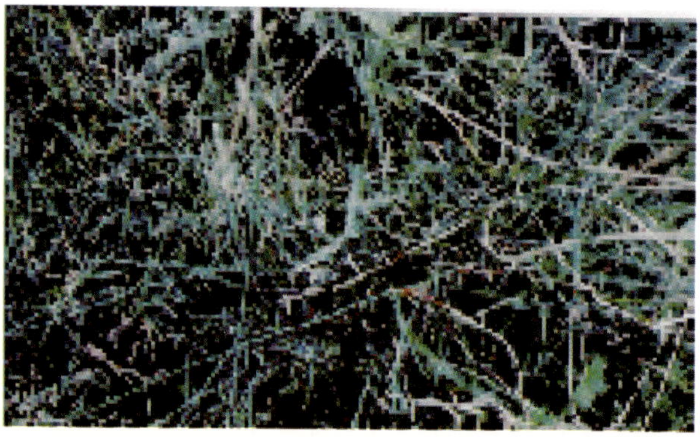

Figure 8.10: *Oxystelma secamone* (L.) karst

Description

Wild, erect, herbacious, rhizomatous. Leaves simple, sessile, broad, arranged spirally, oblanceolate, glabrous. Flowers white, red, large, many in terminal dense head. Fruit capsule subglobose, trignous, seeds black.

Ethnomedicinal Significance

In rheumatic pain Korku tribes boiled roots of this plants to evolve the medicated vapour and the affected parts are exposed to these vapours for relief. The root stock is also effective in fever, cough and other respiratory diseases. It is also claimed to acts as an antihelminthic.

Curculigo orchiodes Gaertn (Figure 8.5)

Local Name

Nelatatugadda (G), Kali Musli (M)

Family

Hypoxidaceae

Locality

Chunkhedi

Habitat

Common as forest undergrowth, among rocks and bushes.

Flowers

July–September

Fruits

July–September

Description

Annual tuberous herb with perennial root stock. Leaves simple, petiolate, linear, broad like palm. Flowers bright yellow, bisexual. Fruit capsular one to four seeded, capsule oblong. Seeds black, smooth.

Ethnomedicinal Significance

Tribal used tuberous roots of this plant in several combinations but mainly for the treatment of sexual impotency and veneral diseases and as a general health tonic. They also recommended about its role in asthma and jaundice.

Dioscorea pentaphylla L. (Figure 8.6)

Local Name

Utaran (K)

Family

Dioscoreaceae

Locality

Shirajbandh

Habitat

Common in forest areas

Flowers

August–October

Fruits

Cold season

Description

A wild twiner, with glabrous prickly base. Tubers long, Leaves alternate, pentafoliate. Flowers unisexual. Fruit capsular, 3–winged seeds small, winged.

Ethnomedicinal Significance

Tubers of this plants are effective against body swelling. Tubers are boiled in water and fumes given to the patient suffering from body swelling.

Gloriosa superba L. (Figure 8.7)

Local Name

Zagadya (k), Kalihari (H), Nagakaria, Kal-lavi (M).

Family

Liliaceae

Locality

Semadoh

Habitat

Occasionally found on slopes of hills

Flowers

June–October

Fruits

June–October

Description

A wild scrambling glabrous twiner, twins with the help of leaftip tendril. Root stock bifurcately branched. Stem herbacious. Leaves sessile, sublanceolate, spirally twisted at the tip to form tendril. Flowers are solitary, large, decorative. Fruit capsule, oblong, seeds small.

Ethnomedicinal Significance

Tuberous roots used against snake bite and scorpion sting. Very small quantity of root ingested to induce abortion. It is also effective in parasitical infection of skin. It is highly toxic in higher doses. It is also prescribed for ulcers, piles, leprosy and gonorrhoea.

Leea macrophylla Roxb. (Figure 8.8)

Local Name

Hattikand (K), Dholsamudra (H), Dinda (M)

Family

Leeaceae

Locality

Amadoha (Chikhaldara)

Habitat

Not very common, occurs as a forest undergrowth.

Flowers

July–September

Fruits

July–September

Description

Perennial, erect herb with thick fleshy tuberous roots. Stem racemosely branched. Leaves simple, Petiolate, broad, ovate, cordate at base. Flowers in corymbose cymes, greenish white. Fruit berries, globose, 3-6 chambered.

Ethonomedicinal Significance

Dried powder of the roots with coconut oil is used on wounds and sores. It is also prescribed against guinea worm and ringworm.

Nervilia aragoana Gaud (Figure 8.7)

Local Name

Dudhakand (M)

Family

Orchidaceae

Locality

Semadoha

Habitat

Cultivated

Flowers

May–June

Description

Wild, Leaf long, petiolate, cordate, hastate at the base, apex acute, margin undulating. Flowers greenish yellow.

Ethnomedicinal Significance

Tubers of this plant used to stimulate lactation. Korku tribes prefers to give decoction of tubers to the women after childbirth.

Oxystelma secamone (L) karst (Figure 8.10)

Local Name

Didam (k), Dudhialata (H), Dudhani (M)

Family

Asclepiadaceae

Locality

Biba

Habitat

Rare, occasionally found in sandy soil.

Flowers

July–January

Fruits

July–January

Description

Wild twining herb. Milky latex in stem and leaf. Leaves opposite, thin, simple, narrowly, lanceolate. Inflorescence cymose. Flowers white with purple ting, drooping in axillary umbellate cyme. Fruit etario of follicles, Seeds flat, ovate.

Ethnomedicinal Significance

It is a common practice in tribals of the region to use fresh plant to stimulate lactation in women after childbirth. They also claimed latex is effective in periodic fever.

Discussion and Conclusion

In the present investigation 10 medicinal plants have been reported which are used by Korku and Gond tribe of the region to cure their ailments. All the informants have agreed that more medicinal plants were in use in the past than those reported now. This has happened as a result of the continued deforestation, degradation and acculturization that took place in the area over several years. This situation gave way to the local loss of some medicinal plants and the associated knowledge. Most of the knowledge is owned by elders (picked up from the their fathers and grandfathers) who mainly use it to keep the well being of their respective families. Occasionally, they render help to other people within the community when a request comes. Most of these knowledgeable elders are men. Reported medicinal plants are restricted to certain pocket in Melghat forest. These medicinal plants definitely have a curative properties and can be used as a genuine source material in any formulations in pharmaceutical industry. It was observed that the plant species like *Andragraphis paniculata* (Burm.F) Wall, *Cissampelos pareira* L, *Cleamatis triloba* Heyne ex Roth, *Costus speciosus* (Koen) Smith, *Curculigo orchiodes* Gaertn., *Dioscorea pentaphylla* L. *Gloriosa superba* L, *Leea macrophylla* Roxb, *Nervilia aragoana*

Gaud, *Oxystelma secamone* (L) karst etc. are over exploited by herbal practitioners of the region and required to be brought under cultivation through medicinal farming. Thus, an alternative ex-situ conservation are required to be employed for such plants for their perpetual benefit to mankind.

References

Akerele, O., 1988. *Fitoterapia*, 59: 355–365.

Amravati State Gazetter, Amravati District, Directorate of Government printing and publications, Maharashtra State (1968): 1–834.

Bhogaonkar, P.Y. and V.D. Deverkar, 1999. Additions to the Flora of Melghat, Technical Bulletin, No., VIII, Directorate Project Tiger, Melghat Amravati, p. 1–67.

Dhore, M.A., 1986, 2002. *Flora of Amravati District with special Reference to the Distribution of Tree Species.* Amravati University Publication, Amravati, p. 1–404.

Mirashi, M.V. and J.B. Salpekar, 1975. Ornamental plants at Amravati. *The Botanique*, 6(4): 195–204.

Padhye, M.D., V.K. Deshmukh and V.J. Tiwari, 1992. Ethnobotanical Study of the Korku tribe of Amravati district, Maharashtra State, India. *Int. J. Pharmacognosy*, 30(1): 17–20.

Medicinal Plants: Conservation, Cultivation and Utilization (2007) *Pages 65–70*
Editors: A.K. Chopra, D.R. Khanna, G. Prasad, D.S. Malik and R. Bhutiani
Published by: DAYA PUBLISHING HOUSE

Chapter 9

Variability Measurements in Three Wild Collections of *Solanum nigrum* L. Complex

Manisha Dhasmana and R.K.S. Rathore
Department of Botany, Raja Balwant Singh College, Agra – 282 002, India

ABSTRACT

Solanum nigrum L. generally known as black-night shade is a newly emerging medicinal crop, which belongs to family Solanaceae. The plant is credited with emollient, diuretic and laxative properties and its decoction is regarded as an antisparmodic. The members of this group differ from each other on the basis of some important morphological characters and constitute a polyploid complex based x = 12.

The interrelationships of these species and races belonging to the same or different ploidy levels are still incompletely understood, so in the present investigation keeping in view the variable berry colour *i.e.* yellow, red and black, an effort has been made to identity the other three morphological characters fairly remain constant. The morphological differences indicated that three collections are different genotypes. Further studies an there breeding behavior are in progress.

Introduction

Solanum nigrum L. complex generally known as black nightshade is represented by a large number of genotypes, which are annual herbaceous weeds. According to Bey and Khan(1989) it constitute a polyploid series based on x = 12 chromosomes. They are herbaceous or suffrutescent weed found through out India in dry parts up to an elevation of 2,100m. The herb has a number of medicinal properties. It is antiseptic and antidysentric and is given internally for cardalgia and gripe. An infusion of the plants is used as an enema in infants having abdominal upsets, it is a household remedy for anthrax pustules and is applied locally. The plant is also credited with emollient, diuretic and laxative properties and its decoction is regarded as an antispasmodic and narcotic. Anonymous (1952), freshly prepared extract of the plant is effective in the treatment of cirrhosis of the liver, and also serves as an antidote to opium poisoning. An alcoholic extract of leaves is active against *Staphylococcus aures* and *E. coli*.

Infusion or decoctions of the plant after transient stimulation, depress the central nervous system and reflexes of the spinal cord. Small doses increases and large doses decreases, cardiac activity reduction in blood pressure. In China, leaves are applied to wounds and sores. The juice of fresh leaves is reported to produce dilation of the pupil. In the Philippines, the pounded leaves are rubbed on depigmented areas of the body for restoring the pigment.

Leaves and tender shoots of *S.nigrum* are boiled in the same way as spinach and eaten in many parts of India, especially by patients suffering from dropsy. Ripe fruits are used in pies and preserves. Berries are considered to posses tonic, diuretic and cathartic properties and are useful in anasarca and heart disease. They are domestic remedy for fevers, diarrhoea, ulcers and eye troubles. Keeping in view the above medicinal importance it needs to be ascertained their exact entity.

A lot of variability exists in the members of *S.nigrum* complex (Edmonds, 1977; Heiser *et al.*, 1979 Heiser *et al.*, 1979) such as plant habit, fruit colour and chromosome number. It is difficult to define the limit with in which they are genetically fixed and hence the genetically fixed and genetic relationship with in the group is considered important. Keeping in view the variable berry colour, under present investigation an effort has been made to differentiate type on the basis of their stomata, pollen grain and seed these morphological characters fairly remain constant.

Material and Methods

The plants of *Solanum nigrum* bearing black, yellow and orange berries were isolated from each other and grown separated in the Botanic Garden of our college. Next generation of these plants responded as true breeding type and strictly maintained their respective fruit colour on ripening. Five plants from each population were selected for measurements of their stomata from abaxial surface of leaves, pollen grains from first flush of flowers and seeds after extracting from berries and drying properly in the shade for two weeks. For microscopic measurements calibration of oculometer of.0 mm under the magnification of 10 x eye pieces and 10 and 40 x objective lenses respectively. For measurements of stomata size (length and width) of epidermal pealing from abaxial side of fully grown leaves were obtained and stained in Delafield's Hematoxylin and mounted in glycerine. Five slides from plants of each population were prepared four stomata from each slide were measured. Thus twenty observations for stomatal measurements were recorded. Like wise pollen grain from each plant selected from these variats were smeared on the slide, stained in acetocarmine mounted under the cover glass and measurements were recorded on four randomly selected pollen grains from each slide. For seed size, ten seeds were randomly selected from each population and measured on the scale. The average value for each parameter was calculated and statistical analysis was also done. These values are presented in the tabulated form and histograms for each parameter have been drawn as shown in Figures 9.4 to 9.6.

Result

A statistical comparison of the morphological characters of two species showed consistent difference between three wild collections (Table 9.1). The three wild collections of *S.nigrum* differ berries colour *i.e.* orange, yellow and black as shown in Figures 9.1–9.3.

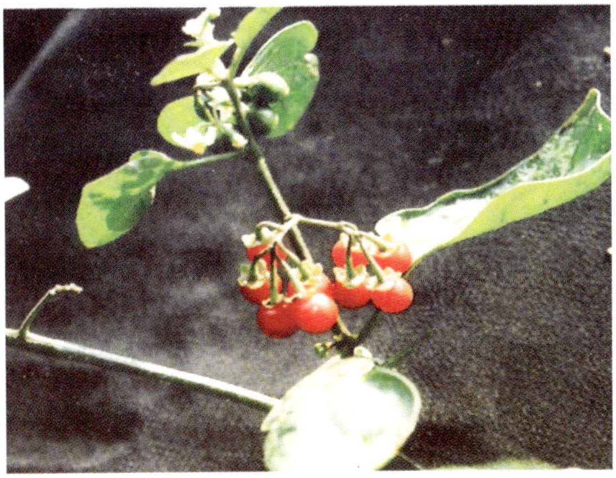

FIgure 9.1: *Solanum nigrum* (Orange)

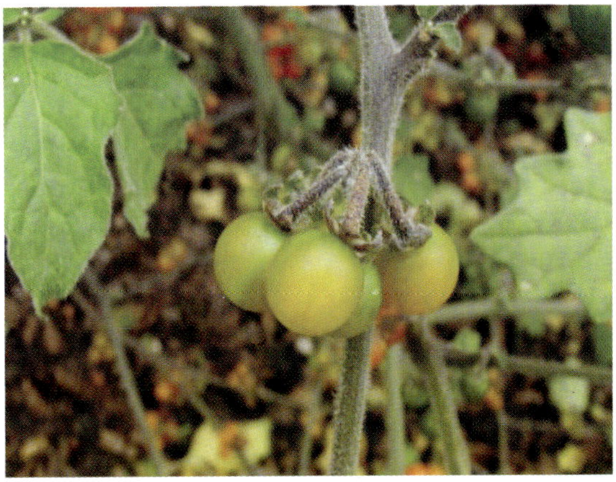

FIgure 9.2: *Solanum nigrum* (Yellow)

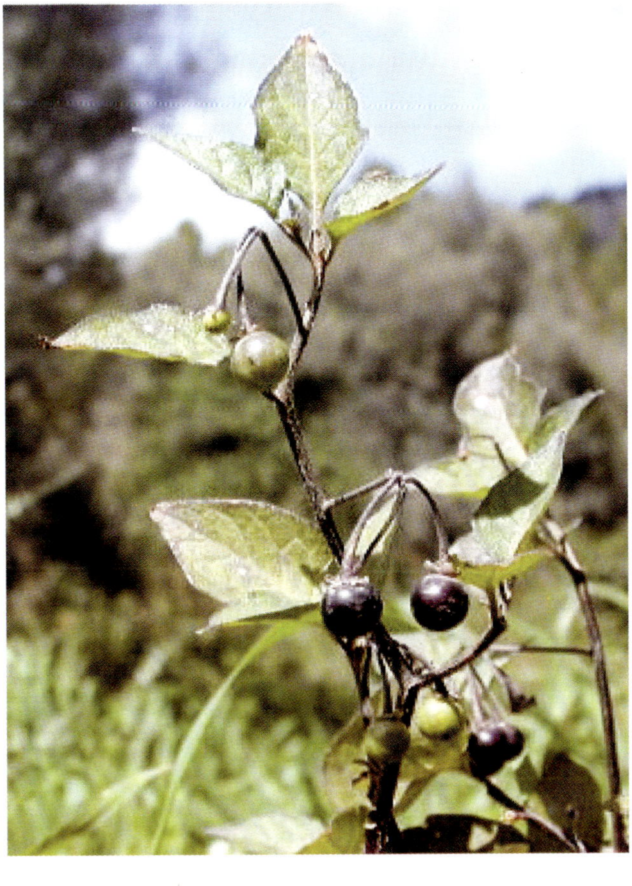

FIgure 9.3: *Solanum nigrum* (Black)

Figures 9.1–9.3: Plants of *Solanum nigrum* L. Complex Showing Variability in Berries Colour

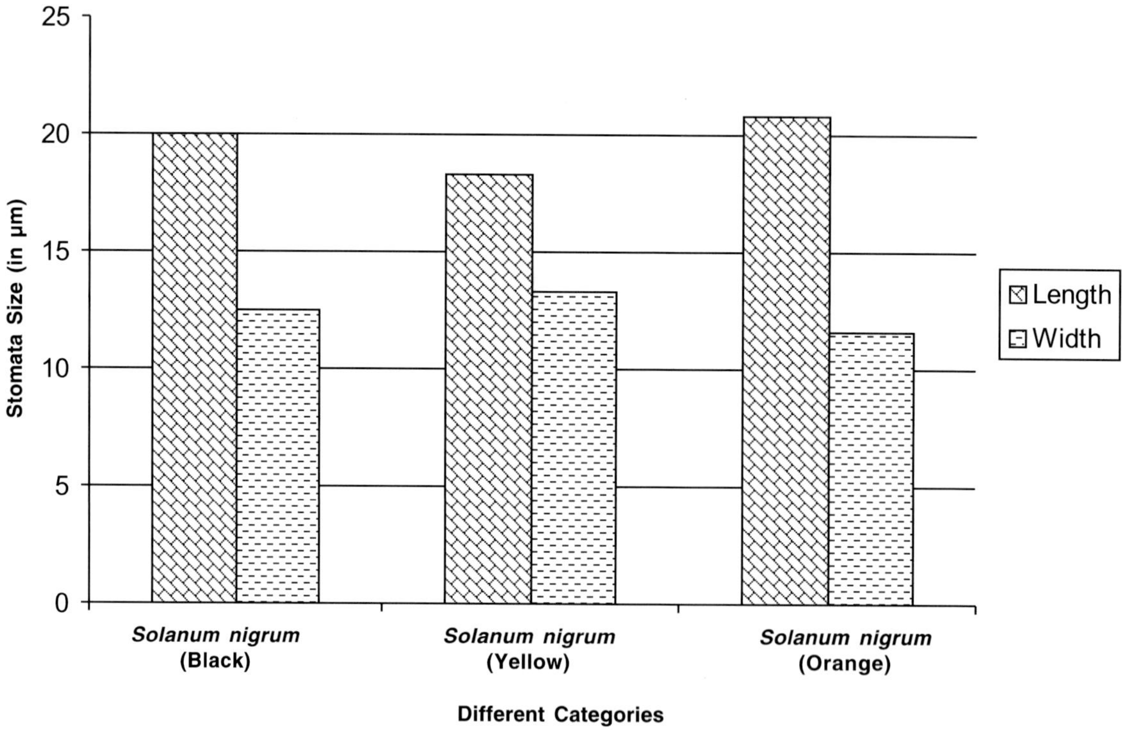

Figure 9.4: Comparative Size of Stomata in Three Genotypes of *Solanum*

Table 9.1: Comparative Size of Stomata, Pollen Grains and Seeds in Three Wild Collections of *Solanum nigrum* L. Complex

Genotypes		*Characters*					
		Stomata Size (µ)		*Pollen Grain Size (µ)*		*Seed Size (mm)*	
		Length	*Width*	*Length*	*Width*	*Length*	*Width*
Solanum nigrum (Black)	M S.E	20 (±0.95)	12.5 (±0.95)	16 (±0.53)	14.0 (±0.53)	1.58 (±0.02)	1.40 (±0.02)
Solanum nigrum (Yellow)		18.33 (±0.64)	13.33 (±1.28)	17 (±0.35)	15.5 (±0.35)	1.84 (±0.21)	1.51 (±0.19)
Solanum nigrum (Orange)		20.83 (±0.64)	11.66 (±0.64)	16 (±0.32)	13.5 (±0.21)	1.85 (±0.03)	1.40 (±0.02)

Stomata Size

In case of length longest stomata (20.83m) is recorded in *S.nigrum* (Orange) (11.6) hence later one recorded as shortest width of stomata size among all the genotypes.

Pollen Grains

In case of longest pollen (17) was recorded in *S.nigrum* (yellow), followed by *S.nigrum* (black) and

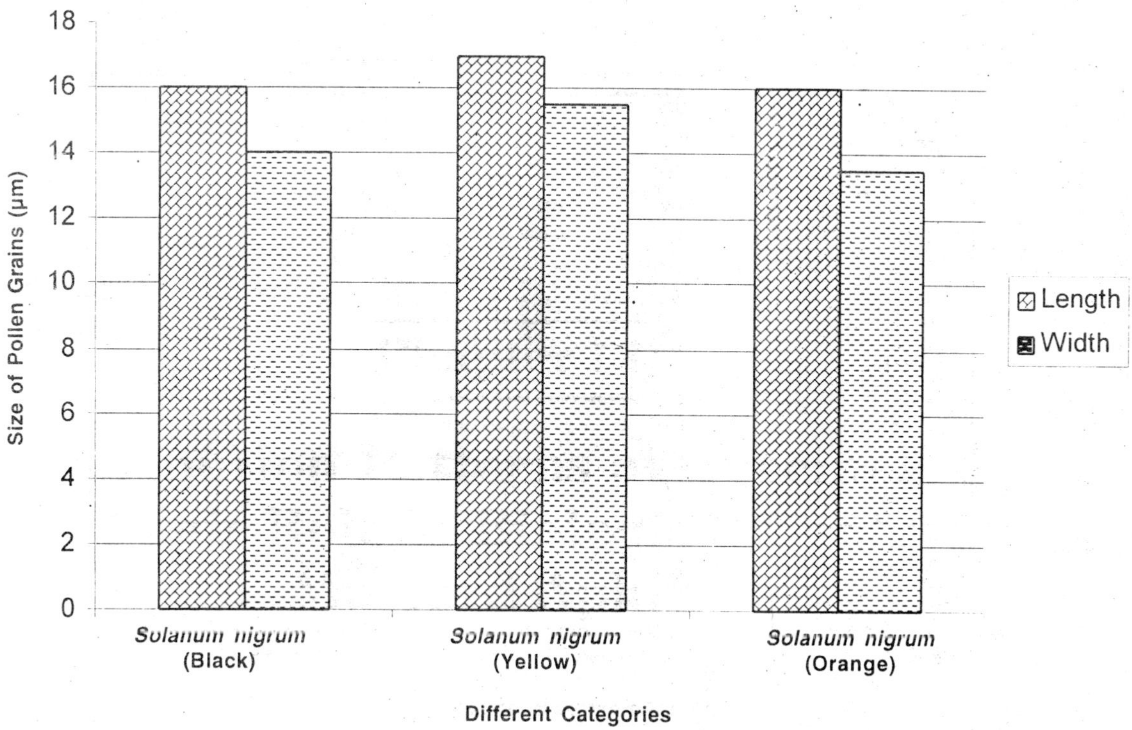

Figure 9.5: Comparative Size of Pollen Grain in Three Genotypes of *Solanum*

S.nigrum (orange) (16μ). Highest value (15.5) of width was recorded in *S.nigrum* (yellow) while followed by *S.nigrum* (black) (14μ) and lowest value was recorded in *S.nigrum* (orange) (13.5).

Seed Size

Longest seed (1.85mm) was recorded in *S.nigrum* (orange) followed by *S.nigrum* (yellow) (1.84mm) and shortest (1.58) in *S.nigrum* (black), Highest value of width was recorded in *S.nigrum* (yellow) (1.51mm) followed by *S.nigrum* (black) and *S.nigrum* (orange) (1.40mm).

Discussion

Solanum nigrum complex quite differs in all the six microscopic morphological characters to each other. The morphological differences have been confirmed by statistical comparison. The most important characters which *S.nigrum* can differentiate complex are colour of berry like orange, yellow and black. Greater size of stomata length (20.83μ) and seed size length (1.85mm) affects width of stomata (11.66μ) and seed size (1.40μ) in case of *S.nigrum* (orange), same pattern were followed by *S. nigrum* (black). Greater size of stomata length (20.00μ) and seed size length (1.58mm) affects width of stomata (12.50μ) in case of *S.nigrum* (black). This pattern shows that they posses some morphological homology. In case of *S.nigrum* (yellow) the size of stomata (18.33μ) were found to be reduced due to the increase in size of length (17μ) and width (15.5μ), among all three wild collections of *Solanum* this morphological pattern only occurs in *S.nigrum* (yellow). In case of increased length in stomata in *S. nigrum* (orange) and yellow seed length seems to be almost equal but in case of *S. nigrum* (black) there is a marked difference in length of seed size (1.58mm) as represented in Figures 9.4–9.6.

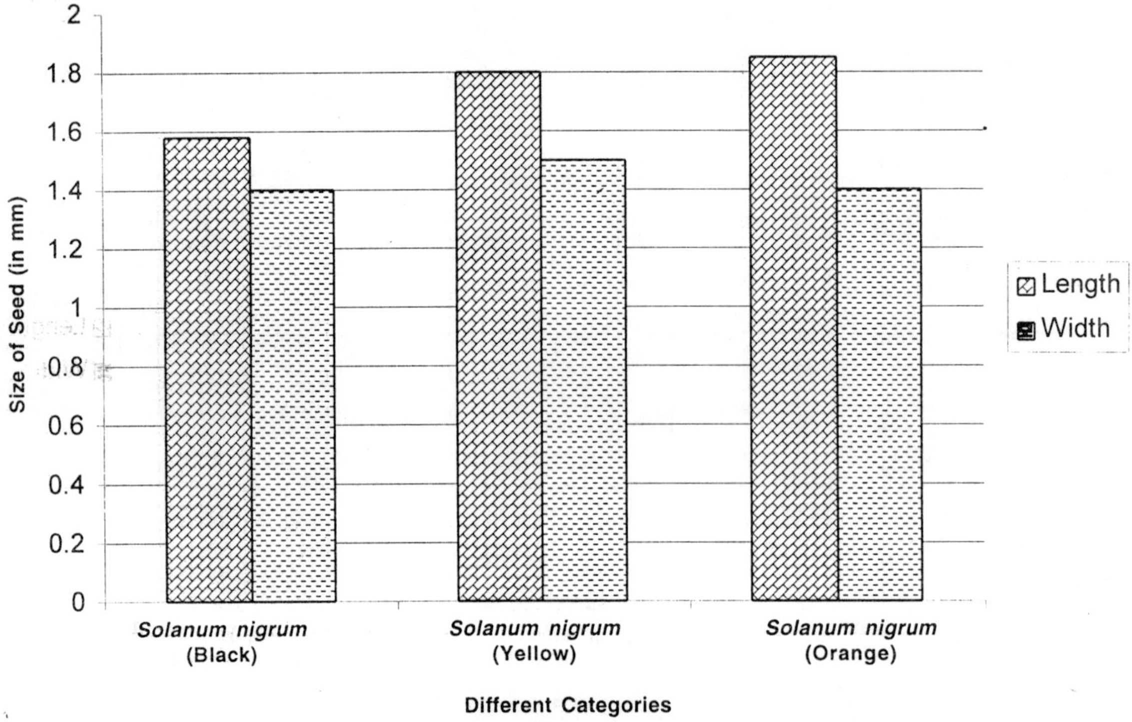

Figure 9.6: Comparative Size of Seed in Three Genotypes of *Solanum*

The present investigation shows that morphologically *Solanum nigrum* having yellow berries are vigorous in width of stomata, size of pollen grain and seed size in comparison to *Solanum nigrum* (black) and *Solanum nigrum* having orange berries. The morphological differences indicated that three collections are different genotypes. Further studies on their breeding behavior are in progress.

Acknowledgement

The author is grateful to Dr. R.K.S Rathore, Deptt.of Botany R.B.S College, Agra for suggesting the topic and guiding throughout the course of this study. The seeds of 11 cultures of *S.nigrum* obtained from University of Agriculture science GKVK, Banglore. Iam also thankful to the Principal, R.B.S College, Agra for providing field and laboratory facilities to carry out this work.

References

CSIR, 1952. *The Wealth of India: Raw Materials.* CSIR, New Delhi.

Edmonds, J.M., 1977. Taxonomic studies *Solanum*, sec. *Solanum* (Maurella). *Bot. J., Linn. Soc.*, 75: 141–178.

Heiser, C.B., Burton, D.L. and Schilling, E.E., 1979. Biosystematic and taxonomic studies of the *Solanum nigrum* complex in Eastern North America. In: *The Biology and Taxonomy of Solanaceae* Linn. Soc. Academic Press, London, 7: 513–528.

Beg, M.Z. and Khan, A.H., 1989. Morphological diversification and genetic isolating mechanism between some members of *Solanum nigrum* Complex.*Cytologia*, 54: 419–424.

Medicinal Plants: Conservation, Cultivation and Utilization (2007) *Pages 71–74*
Editors: A.K. Chopra, D.R. Khanna, G. Prasad, D.S. Malik and R. Bhutiani
Published by: DAYA PUBLISHING HOUSE

Chapter 10

Antibacterial Activity of Mixtures of Essential Oils

R.C. Dubey and Anika Rana
Department of Botany and Microbiology,
Gurukul Kangri University, Hardwar–249404

ABSTRACT

Mixtures of five essential oils namely, *Trachyspermum ammi, Cinnamomum zeylanicum, Syzygium aromaticum, Zingiber officinale* and *Curcuma longa* were assessed for their possible synergistic and antagonistic inhibitory effects against Gram–positive (*S. aureus* and *B. subtilis*) and Gram–negative (*S. typhi, K. pneumoniae* and *E. coli*) bacteria using filter paper disc diffusion method. Combinations of *C. zeylanicum, T. ammi* and *S. aromaticum* oils with the oil of *Z. officinale* separately produced remarkable antibacterial effect.

Keywords: Essential oils, Synergistic, Antagonistic, Antibacterial effect.

Introduction

It is estimated that there are 250,000 to 500,000 species of plants that thrives on earth and relatively small percentage of these are used as foods by both humans and animals. In India, botanical garden of the world a well established system of medicine *i.e.* Ayurveda is practiced since thousands of years. Increasing number of multi drug resistant microorganisms and side effects caused by synthetic chemicals greatly attracted people towards the use of eco-friendly and bio-friendly medicinal plants and their products for a healthy living and for the prevention and cure of human diseases. In present scenario medicinal plants are moving from fringe to the mainstream. Essential oils, secondary metabolites produced by plants are mixture of compounds, highly volatile and are characterized by the capacity to generate flavor or aroma and form the backbone of aromatherapy, described as Gandhachikitsa in Ayurveda (Ranade, 2002). Essential oils are extensively used in perfumes, flavours, cosmetics, pharmaceuticals etc. throughout the world. Inherent antibacterial (Hammer *et al.*, 2003; Dubey *et al.*, 2005), antifungal (Salguerio *et al.*, 2004; Pina *et al.*, 2004), antiviral properties of essential oils that make them highly valuable as skin stimulants, expectorants, diuretics antiseptics, and disinfectant agents have been well scientifically documented by many research scientists around the world.

Therefore, the present investigation was designed to evaluate the possible synergistic/or antagonistic inhibitory effects of equal combinations (1: 1) of different essential oils against certain pathogenic bacterial strains.

Material and Methods

Different parts of *T. ammi, C. zeylanicum, S. aromaticum, Z. officinale* and *C. longa* for the present study were obtained from Gurukul Kangri Pharmacy, Hardwar and the essential oils were extracted by the hydrodistillation of powdered plant material (washed and shade dried) using Clevenger's apparatus. The oils obtained were dried over anhydrous sodium sulphate and stored at 4°C.

Antibacterial Assay

Antibacterial effects of individual and equal combinations of essential oils were assessed against two Gram–positive (*B. subtilis* and *S. aureus*) and three Gram–negative (*S. typhi, K. pneumoniae* and *E. coli*) bacteria using filter paper disc diffusion method. All the six bacterial strains were maintained on nutrient agar slopes. Bacterial cells were subcultured in nutrient broth and incubated overnight at 37°C. Next, small amount (1 ml) of each culture were separately added into 100 ml sterile and cooled (40°C) molten agar medium and mixed gently. Seeded agar medium were poured into pre-sterilized Petri plates. On gelation, a 6 mm filter paper disc soaked with 10 μl of different essential oils (individual and mixtures) was placed separately on seeded agar medium. After diffusion the plates were incubated at 37°C. Inhibition zones caused by the mixtures of oils against pathogenic bacterial strains were measured after 24 h of incubation and compared with those produced by undiluted individual oils.

Results and Discussion

Antibacterial activity of essential oils of *T. ammi, C. zeylanicum, S. aromaticum, Z. officinale* and *C. longa* has been reported earlier by Dubey *et al.* (2005) and found the oils of *C. zeylanicum* and *T. ammi* as most effective and *S. aromaticum* as moderate inhibitor against certain pathogenic bacteria. In the present investigation we have tried to evaluate the antibacterial effects of pure individual oils and mixtures of oils (in equal ratio) and the results are shown in Tables 10.1 and 10.2, respectively.

Mixtures of oils resulted in remarkable variations as compared to individual oil against the bacterial strains. Activity of mixtures of *T. ammi* and *C. zeylanicum* with *S. aromaticum* was found to be antagonistic when compared with that of *T. ammi* and *C. zeylanicum* oils individually but the two combinations proved synergistic when compared with the antibacterial effects produced by the oil of *S. aromaticum*. Similar trend of activity was observed when *C. zeylanicum* and *T. ammi* oils were blended with the oil of *C. longa*.

These results were favored by Balchin and Deans (1998) who studied the different combination of essential oils and reported that the use of highly active essential oils with less effective ones reduced the activity of the strongest one.

Table 10.1: Antibacterial Effects of Undiluted Essential Oils

Essential Oils (Undiluted)	S. typhi	S. aureus	E. coli	K. pneumoniae	B. subtilis
		Inhibition percent (per cent)			
C. zeylanicum	94.0	92.0	100	100	97.5
T ammi	94.0	100	100	100	100
S. aromaticum	52.0	48.0	54.0	57.0	52.1
Z. officinale	35.3	39.0	45.0	39.0	51.0
C. longa	31.0	35.0	37.0	32.0	34.0

Table 10.2: Effect of Mixtures of Essential Oils on Bacterial Growth

Mixture of Oils (1 : 1)	S. typhi	S. aureus	E. coli	K. pneumoniae	B. subtilis
		Inhibition percent (per cent)			
C. zeylanicum + S. aromaticum	67.7	68.7	72.5	79.6	78.6
C. zeylanicum + C. longa	86.7	70.0	100	71.4	75.0
T ammi + C. zeylanicum	91.0	100	100	100	100
S. aromaticum + C. longa	100	80.0	100	100	90.3
S. aromaticum + Z. officinale	37.7	50.0	54.6	55.7	54.6
T. ammi + S. aromaticum	40.0	61.0	53.6	71.4	76.0
T. ammi + C. longa	47.7	67.7	77.1	80.7	100
T. ammi + Z. officinale	47.7	67.7	75.0	82.1	75.0
C. zeylanicum + Z. officinale	91.0	100	100	100	100
Z. officinale + C. longa	28.7	51.0	34.3	59.3	51.0

Combination of *T. ammi* and *C. zeylanicum* resulted in significant effects against all except *S. aureus* and *B. subtilis* where inhibitory activity was weak as compared to their individual effects.

Effective antibacterial results were obtained on mixing *T. ammi* oil with the oil of *Z. officinale,* however mixture was less effective against *S. typhi*. Similarly, on blending *Z. officinale* with *C. zeylanicum* the inhibitory effects were greatly enhanced. Mixture posed synergistic results against *S. aureus* and *B. subtilis*, while antagonistic effect was recorded against *S. typhi*. Antibacterial effect of *Z. officinale* was magnificently increased against all the bacteria.

Inhibitory effects of *Z. officinale* were enhanced against *S. aureus* and *K. pneumoniae* and reduced against *S. typhi* after mixing with the oil of *C. longa*. Against *B. subtilis* mixture was more effective when compared with those produced by the oil of *C. longa* alone. Mixing of *S. aromaticum* oil with *C. longa* and *Z. officinale* separately, tend to increase the efficacy of both the oils against all the bacterial strains.

Different bacterial strains acted differently against essential oils (individually and mixtures). Synergistic as well as antagonistic effects of mixtures of essential oils were noticed in this study that were supported by the work scientifically documented by many research scientists (Gulati *et al.*, 1990; Rath *et al.*, 2002; Ozcan and Erkmen, 2001). Effectiveness of mixtures of essential oils was also supported by Geda (1995) who reported that the oils in 1: 1 combination were more active than individually.

Therefore, it can be concluded from the present investigation that the essential oils can be useful in combating disease causing bacteria if used with suitable combination.

Acknowledgement

The authors are greatly thankful to General manager, Gurukul Kangri Pharmacy, Hardwar for providing necessary laboratory facilities required for the present study.

References

Balchin, M.L. and Deans, S.G., 1998. Studies on the potential usage of mixtures of plant essential oils as synergistic antibacterial agents in foods. *Phytother. Res.*, 12(7): 472–475.

Dubey, R.C., Rana, A. and Shukla, R.K., 2005. Antibacterial activity of essential oils of some medicinal plants against certain human pathogens. *Indian Drugs*, 42(7) 443–446.

Geda, A.K., 1995. Antibacterial activity of essential oils and their combinations. *Felt Wissenschaft Technol.*, 97(12): 458–461.

Gulati, B., Sinha, S.K., Bhattacharya, S.C. (ed.), Sen, N. (ed.) and Sethi, K.L. (ed.), 1990. Studies on some important species of *Ocimum*. In: *Proceedings of the 11th International Congress of Essential Oil, Fragrance and Flavours*, New Delhi, India, 12–16 Nov, 1989. *Chem. Analysis Str.*, 4: 197–206.

Hammer, K.A., Dry, L., Johnson, M., Michalak, E.M., Carson, C.F. and Riley, T.V., 2003. Susceptibility of oral bacteria to *Melaleuca alternifolia* (tea tree) oil *in vitro*. *Oral Microbiol. Immunol.*, 18(6): 389–392.

Ozcan, M. and Erkmen, O., 2001. Antimicrobial activity of essential oils of Turkish plant spices. *Eur. Food Res. Technol.*, 212(6): 658–660.

Pina, V.C., Rodrigues, A.G., Pinto, E., Costa, De. O.S., Tavares, C. and Salgueiro, L.R., 2004. Antifungal activity of Thymus oils and their major compounds. *J. Eur. Acad. Dermatol.*, 18: 73–78.

Ranade, G., 2002. Aromatherapy with special reference to Lavender. *Indian Per.*, 46(3): 273–275.

Rath, C.C., Dash, S.K. and Mishra, R.K., 2002. Antibacterial efficacy of six Indian essential oils individually and in combination. *J. Ess. Oil Bearing Plants*, 5(2): 99–107.

Salgueiro, L.R., Pinto, E., Gonclaves, M.J., Pina, V.C., Cavaleiro, C., Rodrigues, A. G., Palmeira, A., Tavares, C., Oliveira, S.C. and Oliveira, J.M., 2004. Chemical composition and antifungal activity of the essential oil of *Thymbra capitala*. *Planta Med.*, 70: 572–575.

Medicinal Plants: Conservation, Cultivation and Utilization (2007) *Pages* 75–79
Editors: A.K. Chopra, D.R. Khanna, G. Prasad, D.S. Malik and R. Bhutiani
Published by: DAYA PUBLISHING HOUSE

Chapter 11

Herbs, Health and Environment

Vinod Upadhyay
Hon. Advisor, Himalik Herbs India, Jwalapur, Haridwar – 249 407, India

ABSTRACT

The use of herbs for health care is as old as our culture. Plant worship is an old tradition in our society. The purpose of this worship probably was to preserve the plants and use them for health care and various other benefits, *viz.*, Environment protection. The object of this paper is to review the old system of utilizing herbal home remedies for prophylaxis and curative management of day to day ailments. If we are aware of the identity of plants, definitely we will protect them and beside being benefited we will plant them with more attention which will enrich our environment also.

Keywords: Herbs, Spices, Trees, Environment and Health.

Introduction

Since time immemorial herbs have been an integral part of Health care. After an era of chemical and synthetic drugs based health care programmes again there is great interest towards Ayurveda and it's method of Herbal health care. The insidious side effects of chemical based and synthetic medicines evoked a worldwide interest in the study of Traditional systems of medicine. Ayurveda which has a historical background of thousands of years mentions the utilization of Herbal, Animal and mineral products. In vedic era only herbal products were in prime use while in later period the mineral and animal products were also added but always processed or incorporated with herbs. Thus the prevalence of herbs from vedic era to present era of Herbal renaissance took various turns. 'Vedic Soma' the divine drink of immortality, the herbs used in the drink are yet unidentified.

The ancient thought of environmental and body purification has now come to a close scrutiny. Organization of great Yagyas (Herbal sacrificial fires) to purify environment and the purification of body and mind through Yoga (meditation and Ayurveda) are common practices since vedic period. Previous years have been very humiliating to mankind when we drifted away from nature. The synthetic and chemical products based life brought havoc to our health.

Materials and Methods

The very aim of Ayurvedic system is to protect the health of healthy person and to eradicate the disease of the ailing. Our cultural heritage was initiated through the learned saints who dwelled in forests. They had intricate relationship with plants and forests. This close association established by our learned forefathers was acquired in the form of Ayurveda. It is so deep rooted in our life that we used this knowledge in our kitchen as spices and condiments, in our kitchen gardens as essential medicinal plants and some trees for our environment which have medicinal value besides being ornamental.

A list of spices in kitchen, some very important plants to check day-to-day health problems in kitchen garden and for plantation around the community has been suggested. This programme is being propagated through various means just to review the old tradition existed in every home as Grandmother's recipes or folklore remedies. However, there are many more useful herbs but this selection of 45 species and plants fulfill the need to prevent major disorders which may be treated safely.

Table 11.1: Herbs, Health and Environment Series

Sl.No.	*English Name*	*हिन्दी नाम*	*Latin Name*	*Effective in*
(A) Spices in Kitchen				
1.	Ajowan*	अजवायन	*Trachyspermum ammi*	Indigestion, Pain
2.	Cardamom*	इलायची	*Elettaria cardamomum*	Anti-acid
3.	Black Pepper*	काली मिर्च	*Piper nigrum*	Cough-cold
4.	Cumin Seed*	जीरा	*Cuminum cyminum*	Promotes digestion
5.	Cinnamon Leaf*	तेजपत्र	*Cinnamomum tamala*	Diabetes, Face pack
6.	Cinnamon*	दालचीनी	*Cinnamomum zeylanicum*	Face pack, Pain
7.	Coriander*	धनिया	*Coriandrnm sativum*	Indigestion
8.	Long-pepper*	पिप्पली	*Piper longum*	Indigestion
9.	Fenugreek*	मेथी	*Trigonella foenum-graecum*	Diabetes, Hair tonic, Liver care
10.	Clove*	लवंग	*Syzygium aromaticum*	Anti-emetic
11.	Dry Ginger*	सोंठ	*Zingiber officinale*	Indigestion
12.	Fennel*	सौंफ	*Foeniculum vulgare*	Indigestion
13.	Nutmeg*	जायफल	*Myristica fragrance*	Diarrhoea, Acne, Anti-Gas
14.	Turmeric*	हल्दी	*Curcuma longa*	Anti-inflammatory, Cosmetic
15.	Asafoetida*	हींग	*Fernla narthex*	Gastric pain

Contd...

Table 11.1–Contd...

Sl.No.	English Name	हिन्दी नाम	Latin Name	Effective in
(B) Plants for Kitchen Garden				
1.	Sacred basil*	तुलसी	*Ocimum sanctum*	Anti-oxidant
2.	Aloe	ग्वार पाठा	*Aloe vera*	Cosmetic, anti-wrinkle
3.	Mentha*	पुदीना	*Mentha arvensis*	Indigestion, cough cold, Pain
4.	Rose*	गुलाब	*Rosa centifolia*	Constipation
5.	Bryophyllum	पत्थर चटा	*Bryophyllum pinnata*	Kidney, Bladder care
6.	Giloi	गिलोय	*Tinospora cordifolia*	Immunity
7.	Basella	उपोदिका-पोईशाक	*Basella rubra*	Salad
8.	Ashwagandha	अश्वगंधा	*Withania somnifera*	Indian Ginseng
9.	Asparagus	शतावरी	*Asparagus racemosus*	Galactogogue
10.	Sweet Flag*	वचा	*Acorns calamus*	Asthma, Speech disorder
11.	Akarkara*	अकरकरा	*Spilanthes acmella*	Dental care
12.	Brahmi, Gotu Kola*	मण्डूक पर्णी	*Centella asiatica*	Mental, Skincare
13.	Vasaca*	बांसा	*Adhatoda vasica*	Cough, T.B.
14.	Lemon grass*	आज्ञाघास	*Cymbopogon citrates*	Anti-pyretic
15.	Marigold*	गेंदा	*Tagetes erecta*	Haemostatic, wound healing
(C) Trees for Environment				
1.	Jamun*	जामुन	*Syzygium cumini*	Anti-diabetic
2.	Margosa tree	नीम	*Azadirachta indica*	Anti-septic
3.	Chebulic Myrobalan	हरड़	*Terminalia chebula*	Laxative, Rejuvinates
4.	Belliric Myrobalan	बहेड़ा	*Terminalia belerica*	Cough, Asthma
5.	Emblic Myrobalan*	आंवला	*Emblica officinalis*	Anti-oxidant, Vit. C
6.	Peepal	पीपल	*Ficus religiosa*	Environment care
7.	Banyan	बरगद	*Ficus bengalensis*	Astringent
8.	Bael*	बेल	*Aegle marmelos*	Colitis, Anti-diabetic
9.	Arjuna*	अर्जुन	*Terminalia arjuna*	Heart care
10.	Ashok	अशोक	*Saraca indica*	Female disorder
11.	Drum Stick Tree	सहजन	*Moringa oleifera*	Eye care
12.	Kachnar	कचनार	*Bauhinia variegata*	Gland care
13.	Purging Cassia*	अमलतास	*Cassia fistula*	Laxative
14.	Varun*	वरूण	*Crataeva nurvala*	Kidney care
15.	Shirish	शिरस	*Albizzia lebbeck*	Detoxify

*Contains Essential Oils

Infinite number of recipes are possible from among these three groups. To cover the major day to day disorders just see few examples:

Cold

Crush and keep 2 to 3 black pepper below tongue when acute symptom of cold, for relief.

Throat Infection

Add ½ tea spoon of Turmeric powder and 2 to 4 crushed black pepper in per cent cup of warm milk. Drink before sleeping and see the relief.

Indigestion/Pain

Take ½ teaspoon of ground Ajowan seed with warm water.

Anti-acid

Chew cardamom fruit.

Liver Disorder/Diabetes

Take 1 teaspoon of Fenugreek powder with water to prevent.

Burning and Indigestion

In summer take per cent teaspoon of coriander powder with cold water.

Indigestion-flatulence

Chewing fennel seed is a common practice.

Cosmetic

The paste of turmeric powder is applied on face and body to beautify complexion.

Gastric Pain

10 to 20 mg of asafetida with warm water and application of a thin solution on umbilicus and abdomen is suggested.

The hot infusion of Tulsi is a common cough and cold recipe. Aloe is every thing a cosmetic, anti-burn, a rejuvenator, anti-wrinkle, in liver disorder: Rose petals used to cure constipation. Bryophyllum leaf juice to prevent stone formation in kidney and bladder.

Giloy for immunity, Akarkara for dental Care, Brahmi for memory, Lemon grass tea for fever and Marigold petals to check bleeding.

Jamun vinegar is good for jaundice, Neem is a great phytobiotic, Amla the great immunity booster. Arjun is good for heart, Ashok for female disorder, Amaltas a good mild purgative.

Thus these grand mother's recipes may prevent many disorders.

Conclusion

When we take care of the plants our environment is protected and health is also preserved and promoted. Mother nature is always at our service to keep us fit.

References

Bedi, Ramesh, 1996. *Bedi Vanspati Kosh.* Kitabghar, New Delhi.

Bhandari, C.R., 1993. *Vanoshadhi Chandrodaya.* Chaukhambha Sanskrit Sansthan, Varanasi.

Lancaster, Percy, 1960. *Studies in the Sacred Plants of India.* National Botanical Gardens, (NBRI) Lucknow.

Muni, Brahma Swami, 1974. *Atharvavediya. Chikitsa Shastra.* Gyan Prakashan, New Delhi.

Sharma, Shiv Pt., 1929. *The System of Ayurveda.* Khemraj Shrikrishna Das, Bombay.

Singh, Daljit Hakin, 1974. *Unani Dravya Guna,* Part-III. Ayurved-Tibbi Academy, U.P., Lucknow.

Medicinal Plants: Conservation, Cultivation and Utilization (2007) *Pages 81–90*
Editors: A.K. Chopra, D.R. Khanna, G. Prasad, D.S. Malik and R. Bhutiani
Published by: DAYA PUBLISHING HOUSE

Chapter 12

Ecological Studies on Medicinal Plants of Neeru Watershed, (J&K)

Harish Chander Dutt
Department of Botany, University of Jammu, Jammu

ABSTRACT

Neeru watershed is situated in the Pir Panjal range of northwest Himalayas in J&K exactly from where the sub valleys of Dholadhar range bifurcates. Climatically the area represents almost whole of the state as the climatic conditions of the area range from sub-tropical to alpine. Neeru is a perennial stream of the area, which originates in alpine region and drain in Chenab in sub-tropical climatic conditions at 821 msl. The catchment area of Neeru watershed is 64,024 hectares and dominating forest sub-type is Moist deodar forest sub type 15/C1a. Among medicinal flora of the study area Asteraceae is the most dominant family. 194 medicinal plant species belonging to 161 genera have been collected from the area. In the present study phyto-sociological studies have been conducted for all the four seasons. Biological richness is studies by calculating diversity indices *viz.*, Margalefs, Menhinick's and Shannon Wieners indices. A biological spectrum for medicinal flora of the study area is also plotted and compared with Raunkiaer's normal biological spectrum. The soil of the area has also been analysed for physico-chemical parameters. The relations of soil; chemistry, meteorological data and altitudinal distribution of medicinal plants in the study have also been discussed.

Introduction

As new world is returning towards herbal medicines thus the distribution pattern, association relationships, soil chemistry and other ecological parameters related with the presences of medicinal flora becomes the thrust area to be considered by ecologists and conservationists. India has kept alive a number of traditional systems of medicinal whose origin can be traced to the ancient period. About 2000 plant species are described in various textbooks of Ayurveda, but in actual practice not more than 250–300 plant species are used. Kashmir has a long history of utilization of herbal drugs. These has been a continuously growing tradition of herbal treatment, and both Ayurvedic and Unani systems of medicines have played a major role in the health care systems of this region. Kaul (1997) discussed 23 medicinal herbs of western Himalayas as core group of medicinal herbs.

A good deal of work has been done on the ethnobotany and medicinal plants in India and abroad. Several reports on the Amchi system of medicine in Ladakh enumerating the herbs used by the local medicine practitioners (Amchis) have appeared in the recent past (Ragunathan, 1976; Satyavati *et al.*, 1976; Kurup, 1977; Dhar, 1980; Srivastava and Gupta, 1982; Visvanath and Mankad, 1984; Nawchoo and Buth, 1989; Chatterjee, and Pakrashi, 1991; Kaul *et al.*, 1995).

Study Area

Neeru watershed is situated between 32°08′24″–32°52′26″ North and longitude 75°48′38″ – 75°32′41″ East and extended in 64,024 hectares of the area in Pir Panjal range of northwest Himalayas. Neeru is a perennial main stream of the area. The stream is dual in origin (Originating from Kaplash Lake 4341 msl and Ashapatti Glacier 3300 msl) and drains in river Chenab at Pul Doda 821 msl. The area represents almost whole of the state of Jammu and Kashmir as the altitudinal range extend from sub-tropical to alpine temperate.

The rock formation exposed to the area is garnetiferous mica schists, geneisses, gametiferrous phyllites, slates limestone, granite, volcanic rocks, terrace, scree and glacial deposits.

The mean maximum annual temperature of the general area, as shown by the records at the weather station of India Meteorological Department is 24°C and the mean minimum annual temperature of the area is recorded as 8°C. Relative humidity at 0830 hrs never rises more than 85 per cent.

Materials and Methods

1. Plant species were collected in flowering stage for three consecutive years *i.e.*, April 2002–April 2005 by visiting the study area monthly.
2. Medicinal importance and ethnobotanical uses of the plant species was confirmed using different literature and books.
3. Phytosociological studies.

$$\text{Frequency} = \frac{\text{Total number of quadrates in which the species occurred}}{\text{Total number of quadrates studied}} \times 100$$

$$\text{Density} = \frac{\text{Total number of individuals of the species}}{\text{Total number of quadrates studied}}$$

$$\text{Basal Cover} = \frac{(\text{cgh})^2}{4\pi} \text{ (where cgh is circumference at ground height)}$$

$$\text{Relative Frequency} = \frac{\text{Frequency of a species}}{\text{Sum of frequency of all the species}} \times 100$$

$$\text{Relative Density} = \frac{\text{Density of a species}}{\text{Sum of densities of all the species}} \times 100$$

$$\text{Relative Dominance} = \frac{\text{Total basal cover of a species}}{\text{Total basal cover of all the species}} \times 100$$

4. Species Richness (Diversity indices)

   (*a*) Shannon-Wiener's Index (1949)

$$H = \sum\left[\frac{(ni)}{N} \log n \frac{(ni)}{N}\right]$$

where,

H: Index value

ni: Number of individuals of ith species

N: Total number of individuals of all species

(*b*) Menhinick's index (1964)

$$Db = \frac{S}{\sqrt{n}}$$

where,

S: Number of species

n: Number of individuals

(*c*) Margalef's index (1968)

$$Da = \frac{S - 1}{\text{Log } n\ (n)}$$

where,

S: Number of species

n: Number of individuals

Life forms and Biological Spectrum

The determination of life forms was preceded by detailed floristic studies. Raunkiaer's (1918) system as modified by Braun-Blanquet (1932) and Cain (1950) has been used in the present study for the classification of the vegetation on physiognomic basis.

Soil Chemistry

Soil analysis was done as suggested by Gupta 1999.

Observations

As most of the area in the Neeru watershed fall in forest land thus during the study period the forest types of the study area were explored and classified in accordance with the classification of Champion and Seth (1964). Sub type 12C1c of the area is the most dominant forest sub-type in the study area. This sub-type is represented by pure stands of *Cedrus deodara* with few countable trees of *Aesculus indica*. Although the area of this forest sub-type remain moist throughout year due to frequent rains but evidences of forest fires are common in this forest sub-type due to the availability of abundant resin. Acidic soils are characteristic features of this region.

The area of Neeru watershed from Pul Doda (821 msl) to Kaplash peak (4360 msl) represents sub-tropical to temperate climate. The area thus has all the floristic elements ranging from sub-tropical to temperate. 194 medicinal plants species belonging to 72 families have been collected from the area. Asteraceae is the most dominant family among medicinal flora with 18 genera and 20 species (Table 12.1).

Table 12.1: Names of Families, No. of Genera and No. of Species

Sl.No.	*Families*	*No. of Genera*	*No. of Species*
1.	Acanthaceae	1	1
2.	Acoraceae	1	1
3.	Aizoaceae	1	1
4.	Amaranthaceae	1	1
5.	Anacardiaceae	2	2
6.	Apiaceae	9	10
7.	Apocynaceae	1	1
8.	Araceae	2	2
9.	Araliaceae	1	1
10.	Asclepiadaceae	1	1
11.	Asteraceae	18	20
12.	Balsaminaceae	1	1
13.	Berberidaceae	1	1
14.	Betulaceae	1	1
15.	Boraginaceae	3	3
16.	Brassicaceae	7	8
17.	Campanulaceae	1	1
18.	Cannabaceae	1	1
19.	Caprifoliaceae	2	2
20.	Caryophyllaceae	2	2
21.	Commelinaceae	1	1
22.	Convolvulaceae	1	2
23.	Crassulaceae	1	1

Contd...

Table 12.1–Contd...

Sl.No.	Families	No. of Genera	No. of Species
24.	Cucurbitaceae	1	1
25.	Cyperaceae	1	1
26.	Dioscoreaceae	1	1
27.	Ericaceae	2	2
28.	Euphorbiaceae	2	3
29.	Fabaceae	3	5
30.	Fumariaceae	3	4
31.	Gentianaceae	1	2
32.	Geraniaceae	2	3
33.	Hypericaceae	1	1
34.	hidaceae	1	1
35.	Juglandaceae	1	1
36.	Juncaceae	1	1
37.	Lamiaceae	12	12
38.	Liliaceae	5	5
39	Loranthaceae	1	2
40.	Meliaceae	1	1
41.	Moraceae	1	1
42.	Morinaceae	1	1
43.	Oleaceae	1	1
44.	Oxalidaceae	1	1
45.	Papaveraceae	1	1
46.	Papilionaceae	1	1
47.	Phytolaccaceae	1	1
48.	Plantaginaceae	1	2
49.	Poaceae	3	3
50.	Podophyllaceae	1	1
51.	Polemoniaceae	1	1
52.	Polygalaceae	1	1
53.	Polygonaceae	5	8
54.	Primulaceae	2	2
55.	Punicaceae	1	1
56.	Ranunculaceae	8	12
57.	Rosaceae	7	11
58.	Rubiaceae	3	5
59.	Rutaceae	1	1

Contd...

Table 12.1–Contd...

Sl.No.	Families	No. of Genera	No. of Species
60.	Salicaceae	1	1
61.	Sapindaceae	1	1
62.	Saxifragaceae	1	1
63.	Scrophulariaceae	4	5
64.	Solanaceae	5	7
65.	Symplocaceae	1	1
66.	Taxaceae	1	1
67.	Thymealaeaceae	1	1
68.	Ulmaceae	1	1
69.	Urticaceae	2	2
70.	Valerianaceae	1	2
71.	Verbenaceae	1	1
72.	Violaceae	1	4
	Total	**161**	**194**

A total of 194 medicinal plant species have been grouped into various life forms (Table 12.2). Out of 194 medicinal plants collected from the study area, 52 species belong to Therophytes, 18 to Macro-phanerophytes, 51 to Hemicryptophytes, 15 to Nano-phanerophytes, 4 to Epiphytes, 15 to Geophytes, 6 to Hydrophytes/Helophytes, 1 to Lianas, and 32 to Chamaephytes.

Table 12.2: Total Percentage of Medicinal Plants of Different Life Form Classes

Life Forms	TH	HH	G	H	H	N	M	L	E
Raunkiaer's spectrum (%age life form in normal spectrum)	13.0	2.0	4.0	26.0	9.0	15.0	28.0	–	3.0
Study area (%age life form in study area)	26.80	3.09	1.13	26.28	16.49	1.13	9.27	0.51	2.06
Deviation from Raunkiaer's spectrum	+13.8	+1.09	+3.73	+0.28	+1.49	–7.21	–18.73	+0.51	–0.94

During the phytosociological analysis in the study area it has been observed that the medicinal plants like *Phytolaca acinosa, Verbascum thapsus, Taraxacum officinale, Aresemia jacqmontii* show the maximum during winter and *Justicea adhatoda, Salvia lanata, Hypericum perjoratum, Gnaphalium leuto-album, Rabdosia rugosa, Saussurea heteromalla* show the maximum during spring. *Arisaema jacquemontii, Indigofera heterantha, Xanthium strumarium, Phytolaca acinosa, Verbascum thapsus* show the maximum during summer. In autumn season *Commelina bengalensis, Verbascum thapsus, Phytolaca acinosa, Xanthium strumarium* and *Digitalis purpurea* show the maximum.

Biological richness was calculated using different diversity indices. During summer maximum values are found among all the three calculated indices (Table 12.3).

Table 12.3: Showing the Diversity Indices for Different Sites of the Study Area for all the Four Seasons of the Year 2003

Sites/Season	*Margalef's Index*	*Menhinick's Index*	*Shannon-Wiener's Index*
A/Winter	6.306	2.241	3.302
B/Winter	5.023	2.030	3.416
C/Winter	5.290	2.055	3.256
D/Winter	5.288	2.179	3.215
E/Winter	4.850	2.106	3.083
F/Winter	5.902	2.315	3.213
N/Spring	6.934	2.292	3.749
B/Spring	5.535	1.726	3.457
C/Spring	7.471	2.263	3.689
D/Spring	5.891	1.953	3.714
E/Spring	6.884	2.137	3.608
F/Spring	6.991	2.031	3.660
A/Summer	7.210	2.128	3.455
B/Summer	7.119	2.198	3.529
C/Summer	6.281	2.219	3.394
D/Summer	5.975	1.924	3.418
E/Summer	7.527	2.315	3.806
F/Summer	7.523	2.261	4.400
A/Autumn	6.093	2.266	3.481
B/Autumn	5.183	1.879	3.112
C/Autumn	5.001	1.792	3.127
D/Autumn	5.847	2.139	3.204
E/Autumn	5.443	2.090	3.183
F/Autumn	4.695	1.940	3.078

At maximum sites Sandy loam soils have been observed and moisture not more than 30 per cent in the study area. The soil temperature recorded in the study area not exceeds more than 22°C. pH ranges from 4.2 to 6.7 means that acidic' soils is the characteristic features of the soils of the study sites. Maximum value of Electric conductivity is recorded as 178µ mhos/cm. During chemical analysis organic carbon register the maximum value of 0.6 per cent, carbonate absent, bicarbonate 0.0244 per cent, magnesium 0.41 per cent, chloride 0.0177 per cent, sodium 2.28 per cent, potassium 4.02 per cent, phosphorus 0.04 per cent, sulphate 0.084 per cent, nitrate 5.01 per cent, Iron 6.2 ppm, copper 12.722 ppm, cadmium 0.089 ppm, zinc 1.1 ppm, nickel 9.27 ppm, cobalt 2.28 ppm, and lead 9.03 ppm (Tables 12.4 and 12.5).

Conclusions

In the present study 161 genera with 194 species of medicinal plants have been recorded. Dominant family among medicinal plants in the study area is Asteraceae with 18 genera and 20 species followed

Table 12.4: Physico-chemical Parameters of Soil (Macro-elements)

Sites	*Tarown*	*Paranoo*	*Baleru*	*Brampur*	*Sanii*	*Panjgram*	*Dhara*	*Kansru*	*Manthlu*	*Bheja*	*Duggi*	*Mothlu*
Altitude	1740-1850m	1180-1300m	1200-1300m	1600-1720m	1280-1380m	1500-1600m	1700-1860m	2400-2480m	2260-2360m	2020-2240m	1680-1780m	2060-2200m
Texture	Silt Loam	Sandy Loam	Sandy Loam	Sandy Loam	Silt Loam	Silt Loam	Loam Loam	Sandy Loam	Sandy Clay Loam	Sandy Loam	Sandy Clay Loam	Sandy Loam
Moisture (%)	25	20	15	30	25	20	20	25	30	20	20	25
Temperature (°C)	10	15	13	22	13	15	20	18	17	10	8	9
pH	6.5	4.2	6.1	4.5	5.5	4.5	6.7	6.2	6.5	5.5	5.3	6.5
Conductance (μMho/c)	18.9	123	117	112	19.5	18	19.4	168	178	18.7	136	102
Organic Carbon (%)	0.1	0.3	0.3	0.2	0.5	0.4	0.3	0.6	0.5	0.3	0.4	0.4
Carbonate (%)	Absent	Absent	Absent	Absent	Absent	Absent	Absent	Absent	Absent	Absent	Absent	Absent
Bicarbonate (%)	0.02135	0.01355	0.0244	0.0183	0.0122	0.0164	0.0244	0.01526	0.0183	0.0188	0.0171	0.0143
Calcium (%)	0.22	0.36	0.2	0.36	0.18	0.32	0.24	0.16	0.3	0.12	0.24	0.32
Magnesium (%)	0.32	0.35	0.19	0.41	0.25	0.29	0.25	0.38	0.25	0.38	0.19	0.25
Chlorides (%)	0.0053	0,0071	0.0177	0.0142	0.0124	0.0122	0.0088	0.0106	0.0126	0.0124	0.0117	0.0123
Sodium (%)	2.22	2.1	2.24	2.2	2.28	2.12	2.14	2.16	2.2	2.14	2.1	2.19
Potassium (%)	3.98	3.24	4.02	3.94	3.52	3.71	3.68	3.84	3.88	2.81	3.52	3.89
Phosphorus (%)	0.04	0.02	0.03	0.01	0.02	0.03	0.04	0.01	0.03	0.02	0.02	0.03
Sulphate (%)	0.076	0.084	0.068	0.044	0.0482	0.044	0.032	0.076	0.072	0.052	0.056	0.06
Nitrate (%)	1.1	1.5	3.03	2.03	2.52	2.01	3.03	4.02	2.02	1.5	5.01	3.01
Iron (ppm)	5.44	2.52	3.96	1.08	6.04	4.36	0.72	4.72	3.6	2.52	6.52	1.44

Table 12.5: Physico-chemical Parameters of Soil (Microelements)

Sites	*Tarown*	*Paranoo*	*Baleru*	*Brampur*	*Sanii*	*Panjgram*	*Dhara*	*Kansru*	*Manthlu*	*Bheja*	*Duggi*	*Mothlu*
Altitude	1740-1850m	1180-13700m	1200-1300m	1600-1720m	1280-1380m	1500-1600m	1700-1860m	2400-2480m	2260-2360m	2020-2240m	1680-1780m	2060-2200m
Copper (ppm)	12.722	6.988	5.016	3.297	12.224	4.032	3.777	1.989	2.614	0.85	0.934	5.771
Cadmium (ppm)	0.089	0.044	0.03	0.032	0.021	0.028	0.03	0.045	0.037	0.009	0.021	0.072
Zinc (ppm)	0.725	0.833	0.448	0.626	1.1	0.812	0.457	0.52	0.722	0.607	0.616	0.812
Nickel (ppm)	9.27	3.83	4.47	5.11	4.71	4.71	5.11	3.83	4.15	4.47	3.83	5.11
Cobalt (ppm)	1.2	0.97	1.19	1.95	2.28	2.17	1.41	0.86	1.73	1.19	1.52	2.28
Lead (ppm)	7.45	7.22	6.77	7.82	6.32	7.9	7.15	8.73	7.3	6.32	7.67	9.03

by Lamiaceae with 10 genera and 11 species, In the study area therophytic and chamaephytic medicinal plants show a great positive divergence from the Raunkiaer's normal spectrum, reflecting a thero-chamaephytic climate of the region. During the phyto-sociological analysis of the flora of Neeru watershed in winters, the medicinal species like *Taraxacuni officinale, Verbascum thapsus, Oxalis comiculata, Duchesnea indica, Phytolacca acinosa, Tegetus minuta, Hedera nepalensis, Colchicum luteum, Girardinia heterophylla, Arisaema jacquemontii* and *Bergenia cilliata* register a high V. Summer season shows maximum diversity of medicinal plants according to the calculated diversity indices, Edaphic factors more or less control the occurrence, composition and succession of forests within a climatic zone. Soil moisture had a direct relationship with soil temperature. Wetter soils were colder than the dry ones. The soils of the study area have been observed as acidic. According to the findings of Lucas and Davis (1961), nutrients *viz.*, Mo, Zn, Cu, Mn, Fe, Mg, Ca, S, K, P and N are available in the pH range of 5.5 to 6.5. Moreover, the dominating tree species of the area *Cedrus deodara* and many other floral elements bear a mycorrhizal association and all the soils of the study area are acidic in nature. Acidity promotes the weathering of rocks that release K, Mg, Ca and Mn and increase the solubility which facilitates absorption by the roots. The amount of rainfall and decomposition of organic matter in soils are major factors in lowering the soil pH.

Acknowledgements

Author is thankful to G.B.P.I.H.E.D., Almora for providing the funds for the project "Cultivation and Propagation of Traditional Herbs of Jammu". The present work is the part of the project.

References

Braun-Blanquet, I., 1932. *Plant Sociology* (Translated by G.D. Fuller and H.S. Conard). Mc-graw Hill, New York.

Cain, S.A., 1950. Life forms and phytoclimate. *Bot. Rev.*, 16: 1–32.

Champion, H.G. and Seth, S.K., 1964. *Forest Types of India*. Government of India Press.

Chatterjee, A. and Pakrashi, S.C., 1991. *The Treatise of Indian Medicinal Plants*, Vol. 1. Publication and Information Directorate, New Delhi.

Dhar, U., 1980. Plants of Kargil-Zanskar. In: *Ladakh: An Integrated Survey*, (Ed.) P. Kachroo. Kashmir University, Srinagar, India, pp. 48–51.

Gupta, P.K., 1999. *Soil, Plant, Water and Fertilizer Analysis*. Agro Botanica, Bikaner, India.

Kaul, M.K., Sharma, P.K. and Singh, V., 1995. Crude drugs of Zanskar (Ladakh) used in Amchi system of medicines. In: *Glimpses of Indian Ethnopharmacology*, (Eds.) P. Pushpangadan, Ulf Nyamn and V. George. TBGRI, Trivandrum, pp. 163–172.

Kurup, P.N.V., 1977. *Handbook of Medicinal Plants*. Central Council for Research in Indian Medicinal and Homeopathy, New Delhi.

Lucas, R.E. and Davis, I.F., 1961. Relationships between pH value of organic soils and availability of 12 plant nutrients. *Soil Sci.*, 92: 177–182.

Margalef, R., 1968. *Perspectives in Ecological Theory*. University of Chicago Press, 112 pp.

Menhinick, E.F., 1964. A composition of some species diversity indices applied to samples of field insects. *Ecology*, 45: 858–862.

Nawchoo, I.A. and Buth, G.M., 1989. Medicinal system of Ladakh, India. *J. Ethnopharmacology*, 20: 137–146.

Raghunathan, K., 1976. *Preliminary Techno-economic Survey of Natural Resources and Herbal Wealth of Ladakh.* CCRIMH Publication, New Delhi.

Raunkiaer, C., 1918. *Uber das biologishe.* Normal Spectrum. Kgl: Danksak. Vidensk. Selsk. Biol. Mddle, 1: 4.

Satyavati, G.V., Raina, M.K. and Sharma, M., 1976. *Medicinal Plants of India.* Indian Council of Medical Research, New Delhi.

Shannon, C.E. and Weiner, W., 1949. *The Mathematical Theory of Communication.* Urbana, Illinois, 117 pp.

Srivastava, T.N. and Gupta, O.P. 1982. Medicinal plants used by Amchis in Ladakh. In: *Cultivation and Utilization of Medicinal and Aromatic Plants,* (Eds.) C.K. Atal and B.M. Kapoor, New Delhi, pp. 103–106.

Visvanath, M.V. and Mankad, N.R., 1984. Medicinal plants of Ladakh (J&K). *J. Econ. Tax. Bot.*, 5: 401–407.

Medicinal Plants: Conservation, Cultivation and Utilization (2007) *Pages 91–100*
Editors: A.K. Chopra, D.R. Khanna, G. Prasad, D.S. Malik and R. Bhutiani
Published by: DAYA PUBLISHING HOUSE

Chapter 13

Assessment of Influence of SO_2 Pollution on Biochemical and Antioxidant Defense System of Medicinal Plant (*Azadiracta indica*): A Case Study

D.R. Khanna and Neetu Saxena
Department of Zoology and Environmental Sciences, Gurukul Kangri University, Hardwar, India

ABSTRACT

In the present study, the impact of increasing air pollution in the cities and its influence on the medicinal plant *Azadiracta indica* (Neem) is being assessed. The ambient SO_2 concentration was found to be in good correlation with the sulphur accumulation in the plant. The gaseous pollutant has adversely affected the nitrogen metabolism of the plant by decreasing the nitrate reductase enzyme activity. A positive correlation between SO_2 pollution and antioxidant enzymes, peroxidase and catalase was observed.

Keywords: Azadiracta indica, Nitrate reductase enzyme, Peroxidase, Catalase

Introduction

Azadiracta indica is a native tree of India, a tropical tree especially suited to semi-arid conditions. It belongs to the family Meliaceae. For centuries, *Azadiracta indica* has been held in high esteem in India because of its medicinal and insecticidal properties. Since ancient time Neem's various plant parts have been successfully used to control domestic insects, stored grain pests, crop pests and for human and livestock medicines. Neem is described as having amoebicidal, anti-allergic, anti-dermatitic, anti-inflammatory, anti-periodontitic, anti-tuberculus, anti-viral, anti-fungal, anti-feedant, larvicidal, bactericidal, insecticidal, spermicidal and wormicidal properties. The Neem and it's cornucopia of products–eco-friendly pesticides, medicines, cosmetics, birth control pills and ecological wealth–promise to rescue the world mired in poverty, overpopulation and environmental degradation and also offer the prospect of better food quality for developed countries beset with problems of toxic food residues and growing pesticide resistance.

In recent time, the surrounding environment of the plant has become polluted due to the anthropogenic activities such as automobile exhaust, refuse burning, pesticide pollution, industrial wastes etc. Transport has become the lifeline of our social and industrial progress. In the pursuit of accelerated industrialization and urbanization, the mushrooming of vehicles started on the city roads and highways in the last two decade, choking the major cities of our country. It has been estimated that in all the big cities of our country, about 800 to 1000 tons of pollutants are being ejected into the atmosphere every day (Rangarajan *et al.*, 1995).

Azadiracta indica is most affected by the automobile pollution as it is generally planted in residential areas and roadside areas. Photochemical oxidants such as SO_2, NO_x, and ozone are recognized as having phytotoxic effect on plants via generation of free radicals. The univalent pathway for reduction of molecular oxygen results in the generation of the superoxide anion radical (O_2^-), H_2O_2 and $OH^\bullet$ intermediates. In addition to direct oxidative degradation of lipids, destruction of intercellular and extracellular proteins, including enzyme inactivation or DNA damage, indirect toxic effects like mutagenicity and carcinogenicity have been related to oxygen radical formation (Richardson *et al.*, 1989).

Realizing the importance of Neem in national, regional and international perspective, there is an urgent need to locate, collect and study the diversity, pollution impact and quality status of the plant. In view of this, present study was conducted to study the effect of SO_2 pollution on the biochemical defense system of the plant.

Study Area

The study area of Bareilly is located in the northern part of India and falls in the state of Uttar Pradesh. The city lies between the latitudes of 28°10′ and 28°54′ and longitudes of 78°58′ and 79°47′ running over a distance of 97 km from North to South and about 76 km from East to West and covering an area of approximately 2540 square kms. The city is an important trade center in western U.P. as it lies in between Delhi and Lucknow and national highway no.24. passes through the city. The population of the city is about 30 lakhs. It has distinct tropical climate with a marked monsoonal effect.

There are many large and small industries working in Bareilly. Some of them are Camphor and Allied Products, C.B.Ganj; Synthetics and Chemicals Limited, Fatehganj (W); N.E.Railway Workshop, Izzatnagar; Hindustan Lever Limited, Bhojipura; IFFCO Limited, Aonla; J.K.Sugar Industries, Meerganj; Oswal Overseas Limited, Nawabganj; Bareilly Chemicals, Private Limited, Rampur Road, Bareilly and Brindavan Beverages Limited, Parsakhera. During last decade, the number of vehicles has increased tremendously to keep pace with public demand and hence contributed significantly to the air pollution problem of the city.

Material and Methods

To study the impact of SO_2 pollution, ten road intersections were selected, Railway station, Chowki chouraha, Kutubkhana, Dharamkanta, Sheel chouraha, Choupla, Kila, Pilibhit bypass and S.S. Nagar identified as SI, SII, SIII, SIV, SV, SVI, SVII, SVIII and SIX respectively (Figure 13.1). These sites are characterised by high motor vehicle density and frequent jams. Sampling site of Cantt has been taken as control site and identified as SX.

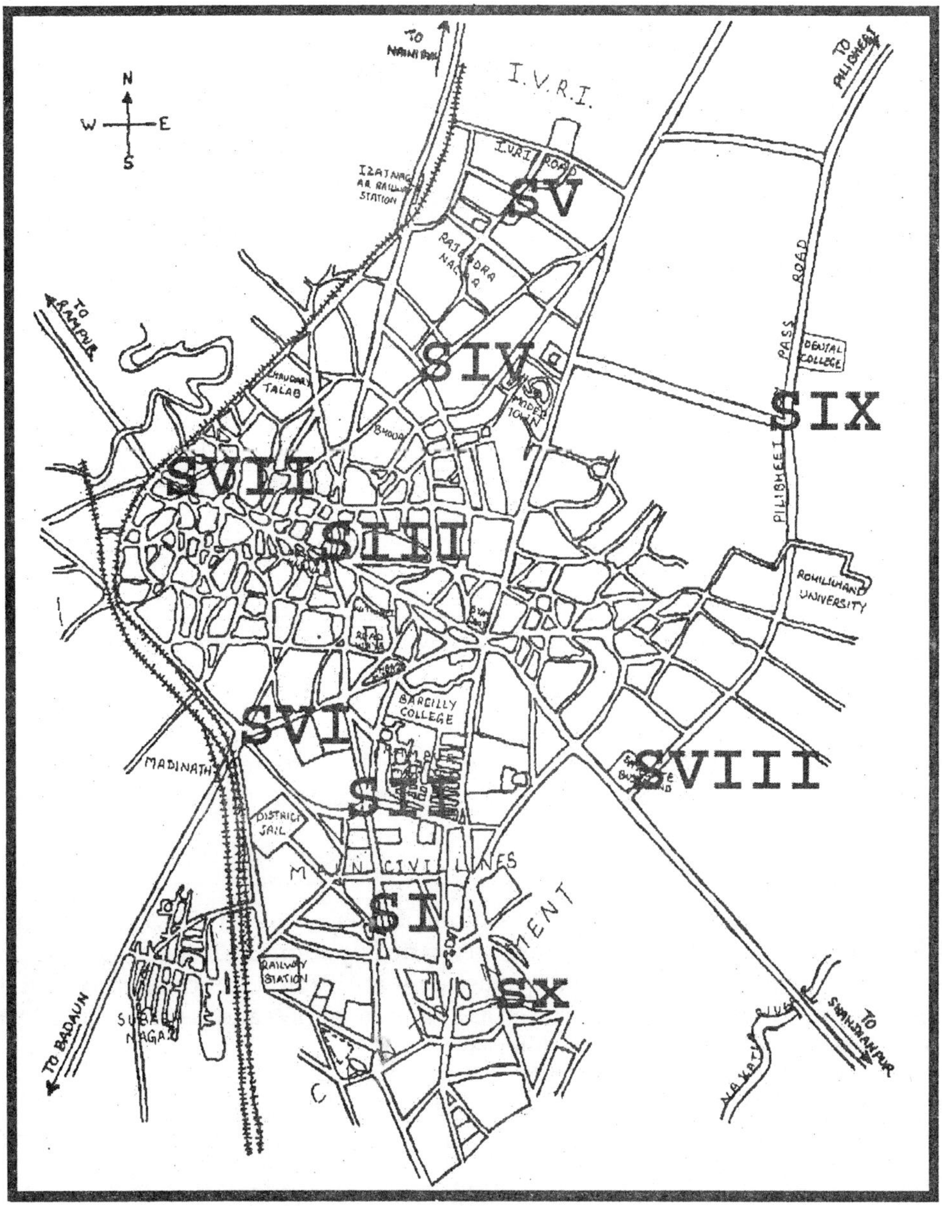

Figure 13.1: Location Map of Bareilly City

Ambient SO_2 Monitoring

HVS, having impingers in series with TCM as absorbing solution, was operated at an average air flow rate of 0.8 l m^3/min for collection of SO_2 for 8 hrs. The impinger samples were put in iceboxes and transferred to a refrigerator prior to analyze. The samples were analysed spectrophotometrically using West and Gaeke method (West and Gaeke, 1956; Saxena, 1990).

Samples of the plant leaves were collected in triplicates in the early hours of the day and following parameters were analysed.

Sulphur Content (as Sulphate)

Sulphur content in the leaves was estimated by the turbidity method of Garrido (1964) modified by Gavali *et al.* (2002). 0.1gm of dried leaves was digested in acidic potassium dichromate solution. The digestion medium was consisting of perchloric acid, nitric acid, ammonium monovendate and potassium dichromate solution. After digestion, volume of the sample was made upto 50 ml with distilled water. Aliquot of sample was taken and 0.5 ml of Tween 80–barium chloride solution was added, due to which turbidity develops in the sample. The absorbance was recorded at 420nm taking distilled water as blank. Standard graph was prepared by potassium sulphate. The amount of sulphate was deduced from the standard curve.

Nitrate Reductase Enzyme(NRA)

NRA enzyme was estimated according to the method of Srivastava (1975) and Shankar *et al.* (2000). Fresh leaf samples were grinded and added to the amber coloured bottles containing phosphate buffer (pH 7.4), propanol and KNO_3. Samples were incubated at 30°C for 30 minutes after which NED and sulphanilamide were added to the sample extract. NRA activity was estimated spectrophotometrically at 540 nm as milimoles $NO_2^{-}hr^{-1}gm^{-1}$ taking $NaNO_2$ as standard solution.

Peroxidase Enzyme (POD)

Peroxidase enzyme activity was determined by method of Putter (1974) and Van Assche and Clijsters (1990).

Extraction

The enzyme was extracted from the fresh samples in cold environment. The extraction medium was 0.1 M sodium phosphate buffer (pH 7.4). The extract was centrifuged at 5000rpm for 10 minutes and the supernatant was used as enzyme source.

Assay

Assay medium consisted of 1ml of 0.1 M sodium phosphate buffer (pH 7.4), 1 ml of guaiacol, 2 ml of distilled water and 1 ml enzyme. Reaction was started by addition of one drop of 3 per cent H_2O_2 and the absorbance was recorded spectrophotometrically at 470 nm at 15 second interval till absorbance increases. The enzyme activity was expressed as ΔOD $min^{-}gm^{-}$FW and was calculated by taking the difference of absorbance at 1 minute time interval.

Catalase Enzyme(CAT)

Catalase enzyme activity was measured according to the method of Barber (1980) and Thimmaiah (1999).

Extraction

The fresh plant material was grinded with 0.1 M phosphate buffer (pH 7.0) in a prechilled mortar and pestle. The extract was centrifuged at 10,000 rpm for 30 minutes at 4°C. The supernatant was used as the enzyme source.

Assay

Assay medium was prepared by mixing 3 ml of phosphate buffer (pH 7.0), 2 ml of 0.005M H_2O_2 and 1 ml of enzyme extract. The mixture was incubated at 20°C for 1 minute. After 1 minute, the reaction was stopped by adding 10 ml of sulphuric acid (0.7N) and the reaction mixture was titrated against 0.01 N $KMnO_4$ to find out the residual H_2O_2 until a faint purple color persists for at least 15 seconds. A blank was prepared by adding the enzyme extract to an acidified solution of reaction mixture at zero time. The enzyme activity was expressed as n moles of H_2O_2 used $min^{-1}gm^{-1}$ FW.

The data is represented as mean ± standard error. ANOVA test was applied to determine the significant differences at 5 per cent significant level.

Results and Discussion

In order to assess the effect of SO_2 pollution on the plant *Azadiracta indica*, monitoring of ambient SO_2 concentration at different intersections was carried out and the data have been presented in Figure 13.2. It was noted that the level of pollutant was maximum at site VII (89.45 μgm/m³). Site VII is characterised by intersection of railway line, narrow and congested roads, heavy traffic of trucks, buses and autos using diesel as fuel. The minimum level of SO_2 was observed at site X which is treated as control site. Site V shows the lowest SO_2 concentration (28.69 μgm/m³) as compared to other polluted sites. The concentration of SO_2 was above the CPCB recommended National Ambient Air Standard for residential area (80 μgm/m³) at site VII and VI. The observed high level of SO_2 may be explained by high traffic density in the city which is accompanied by slow-speed movement, frequent

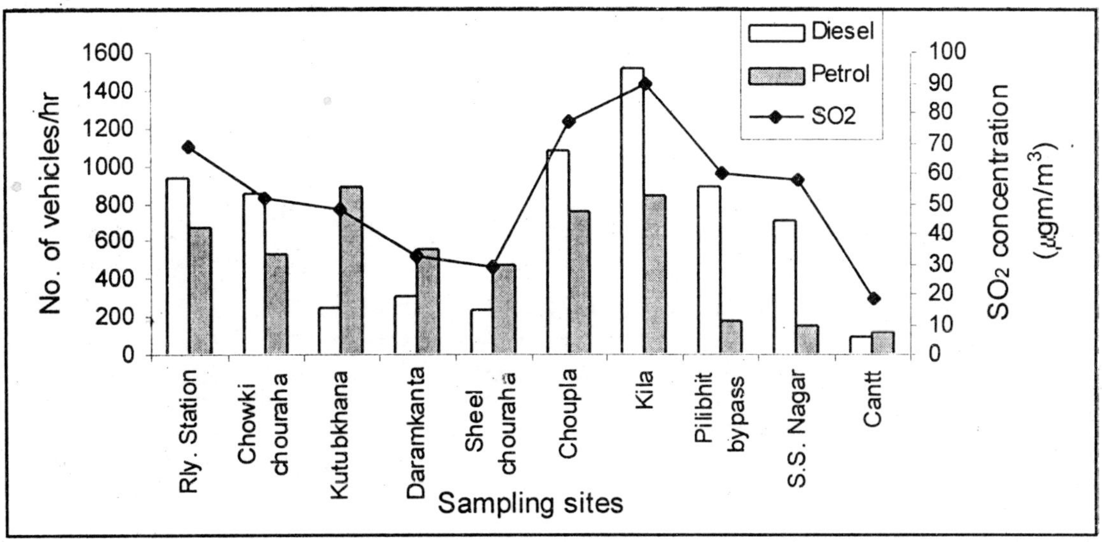

Figure 13.2: Ambient SO_2 Concentration (μgm/m³) and Vehicle Density (no. of vehicles/hr) at Different Sampling Sites

deceleration and acceleration of vehicles as well as undesirable and unnecessary idling time on the road (Jackson, 2005). The vehicular density, type of vehicles plying on the road, the road conditions, diffusion of the pollutant affected by the topography of high rise buildings on the either side etc. are some of the major factors, affecting pollutant ambient concentration on the roadside (Joshi, 1998). The concentration of primary pollutant showed a positive correlation with the traffic density at most sites indicating that the traffic pollution is the main culprit for urban pollution. The correlation coefficient for SO_2 and vehicles plying per hour at road intersections is found to be 0.92. In earlier studies also, automobiles were correlated to air pollution along the roadsides (Rangarajan *et al.*, 1995; Verma and Singh, 2004; Jackson, 2005).

A high sulphur content in leaves has been found at polluted sites having maximum at site VII (4.406 mg SO_4^- gm^{-1} dry wt.) and minimum at site V (1.890 mg SO_4^- gm^{-1} dry wt.) against 1.415 mg SO_4^- gm^{-1} dry wt. sulphur content at control (Table 13.1). There are significant differences ($p<0.05$) in sulphur content in leaves of different sites. The higher sulphur content at polluted sites is attributed to the high SO_2 concentration in the areas having a positive correlation of 0.945 between SO_2 concentration and foliar sulphur content (Figure 13.3). Raitio *et al.* (1995) also reported correlation in foliar sulphur concentration (total, organic and inorganic) with the estimated SO_2 concentration and distribution in air. Gavali *et al.* (2002) had studied the effect of SO_2 pollution on different plant species and had reported that tree species like Anogeissus, Azadiracta, Mangifera, Tamarindus acclimatised to pollution stress and can be treated as sulphur accumualtors.

Table 13.1: Sulphur Content as Sulphate (mg gm^{-1} dry wt.), Nitrate Reductase enzyme (n milimolesNO_2^- hr^- gm^- FW), Peroxidase enzyme (ΔOD min^-gm^-FW) and Catalase enzyme (n µmoles of H_2O_2 used $min^{-1}gm^{-1}$ FW) activity in *Azadiracta indica* at different sampling sites of Bareilly city

Site Code	*Sampling Site*	*Sulphur Content as Sulphate (mg gm^{-1} dry wt.)*	*Nitrate Reductase Enzyme (n milimolesNO_2^- hr^- gm^- FW)*	*Peroxidase Enzyme (ΔOD min^-gm^-FW)*	*Catalase Enzyme (n µmoles of H_2O_2 used $min^{-1}gm^{-1}$ FW)*
I	Rly. Station	2.952 ± 0.02^{a}	1.646 ± 0.008	0.615 ± 0.043	40.392 ± 0.519^{ab}
II	Chowki chouraha	2.542 ± 0.05	2.049 ± 0.016^{abc}	0.315 ± 0.124^{ab}	30.196 ± 1.193^{c}
III	Kutubkhana	2.256 ± 0.03	2.102 ± 0.039^{ade}	0.371 ± 0.006^{cd}	22.745 ± 1.092
IV	Daramkanta	2.113 ± 0.02	2.049 ± 0.039^{bdf}	0.358 ± 0.021^{c}	28.039 ± 0.707^{c}
V	Sheel chouraha	1.890 ± 0.03	2.025 ± 0.036^{cef}	0.206 ± 0.033	19.020 ± 0.707
VI	Choupla	3.617 ± 0.03	1.699 ± 0.045	0.864 ± 0.028	43.137 ± 0.519
VII	Kila	4.406 ± 0.02	2.157 ± 0.016^{g}	0.380 ± 0.140	38.039 ± 0.519^{a}
VIII	Pilibhit bypass	3.608 ± 0.04^{a}	2.337 ± 0.069^{g}	0.416 ± 0.023^{ae}	34.314 ± 0.519
IX	S.S. Nagar	3.279 ± 0.03	2.358 ± 0.015	0.475 ± 0.061^{bde}	38.431 ± 1.193^{b}
X	Cantt	1.415 ± 0.03	2.489 ± 0.055	0.137 ± 0.020	8.823 ± 2.503

* Values are represented as mean ± standard error.

** Values superscripted same alphabets within vertical columns are not significantly different at 5 per cent significance level.

The activity of Nitrate reductase enzyme was found to be lowest at site I (1.646 mmoleNO_2^- $hr^{-1}gm^{-1}$FW) and highest at site X (2.489 mmole$NO_2^-$$hr^{-1}gm^{-1}$FW). ANOVA ($p<0.05$) showed there is significant differences between the enzyme activity at different sites except some sites (Table 13.1). A

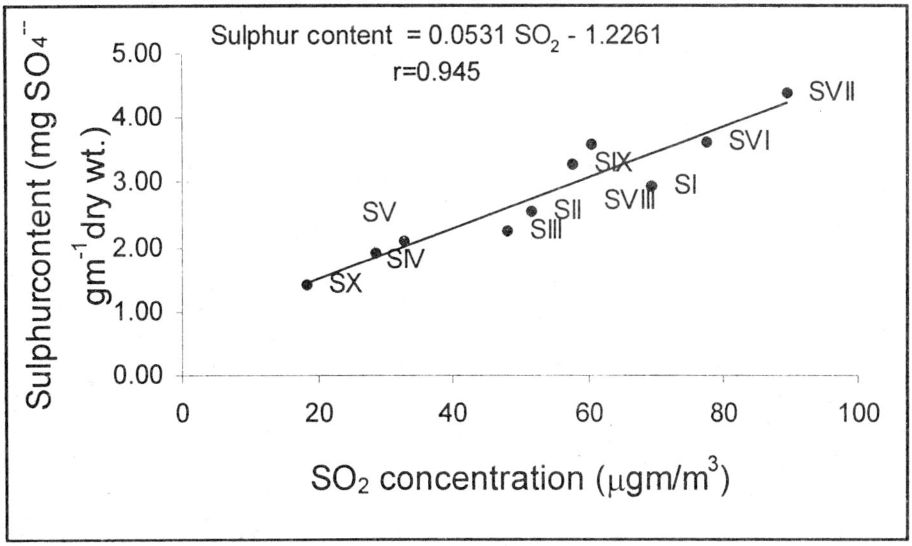

Figure 13.3: Correlation Between Ambient SO_2 Concentration (µgm/m³) and Sulphur Content (mg SO_4⁻gm⁻¹ dry wt.) in *Azadiracta indica* at Different Sampling Sites

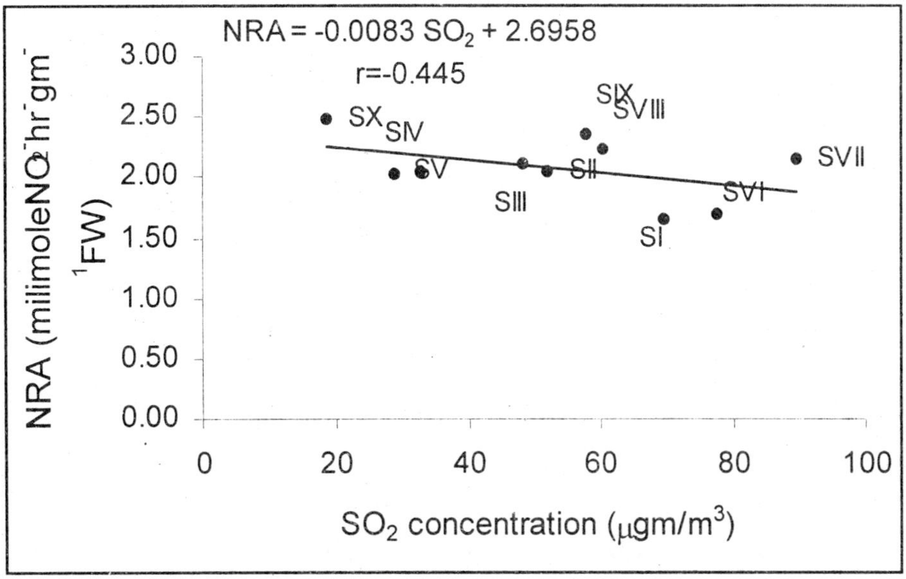

Figure 13.4: Correlation Between Ambient SO_2 Concentration (µgm/m³) and NRA Activity (milimoles NO_2^- hr⁻¹ gm⁻¹ FW) in *Azadiracta indica* at Different Sampling Sites

negative correlation of –0.445 has been found between ambient SO_2 concentration and NRA (Figure 13.4.). This shows that the SO_2 pollution reduces the NRA enzyme activity thereby affecting the nitrogen metabolism in the plant.

The SO_2 pollution has a stimulating effect on the stress enzymes, *viz.* Guaiacol peroxidase and catalase, which are found to be in a positive correlation (0.708 and 0.883 respectively) with the pollutant concentration (Figures 13.5 and 13.6). The activity of the Guaiacol peroxidase and catalase was maximum at site VI (0.864 ΔODmin^{-1}gm^{-1}FW and 43.137 µmole H_2O_2 used min.$^{-1}$gm^{-1}FW respectively) which has high SO_2 concentration. Among the other polluted sites, the peroxidase activity is minimum at site II (0.315 ΔODmin^{-1}gm^{-1}FW) and catalase activity is minimum at site V (19.020 µmole H_2O_2 used min.$^{-1}$gm^{-1}FW). The enzyme activity varies significantly ($p<0.05$) at different sampling sites, however some sites has shown non significant differences in the peroxidase and catalase enzyme activity according to ANOVA test (Table 13.1). SO_2 enters the leaf through the open stomata as readily as CO_2. In the cell wall, the SO_2 is first dissolved in water and its reaction products, hydrogen sulphite HSO_3^- and sulphite SO_3^- are then distributed inside the cell between chloroplast, cytosol and vacuole, in proportions which have been reported to be 96:3:1 (Larcher, 1995). The phytotoxic effect of SO_2 is greatly influenced by the ability of plant tissues to convert dissolved SO_2 into relatively non-toxic forms. The oxidation of SO_3^- to SO_4^{--} in plant cells can occur by enzymic mechanisms which involves the cellular enzymes such as peroxidase, cytochrome oxidase, catalase and ferredoxin NADP reductase (Malhotra and Khan, 1984). Bisulphite is photooxidized to less toxic SO_4^- and superoxide radical O_2^-. The superoxide radical can be dismutated by SOD to H_2O_2 and O_2. H_2O_2 is converted to H_2O and O_2 by peroxidase and catalase (Richardson *et al.*, 1989). Thus in the presence of HSO_3^- and SO_3^{--}, more O_2^- is formed by free radical chain oxidation reaction which also generates OH·. In order to arrest uncontrolled production of such free radicals, plants have developed natural scavengers. It is believed that the generation of oxy-free radicals is the principal biochemical event in responses of plants to any kind of environmental stress. Plants respond through increased activities and levels of antioxidant enzymes and metabolites, so that the oxy-free radicals are removed and minimum damage is done (Srivastava, 1998). Increased peroxidase enzyme activity that often results from fumigation of plants

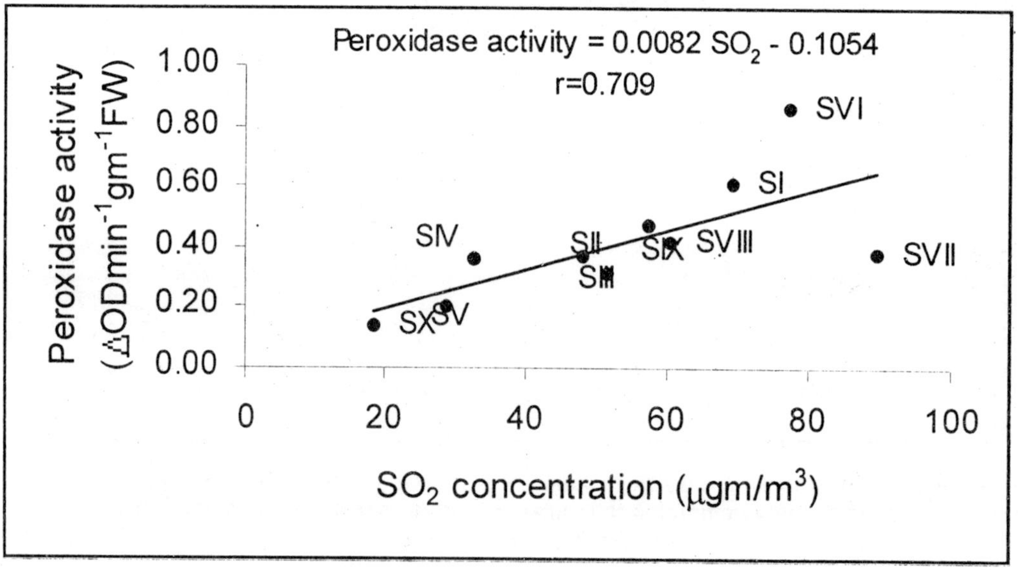

Figure 13.5: Correlation Between Ambient SO_2 Concentration (µgm/m^3) and Peroxidase Activity (Δ OD min.$^{-1}$ gm^{-1} FW) in *Azadiracta indica* at Different Sampling Sites

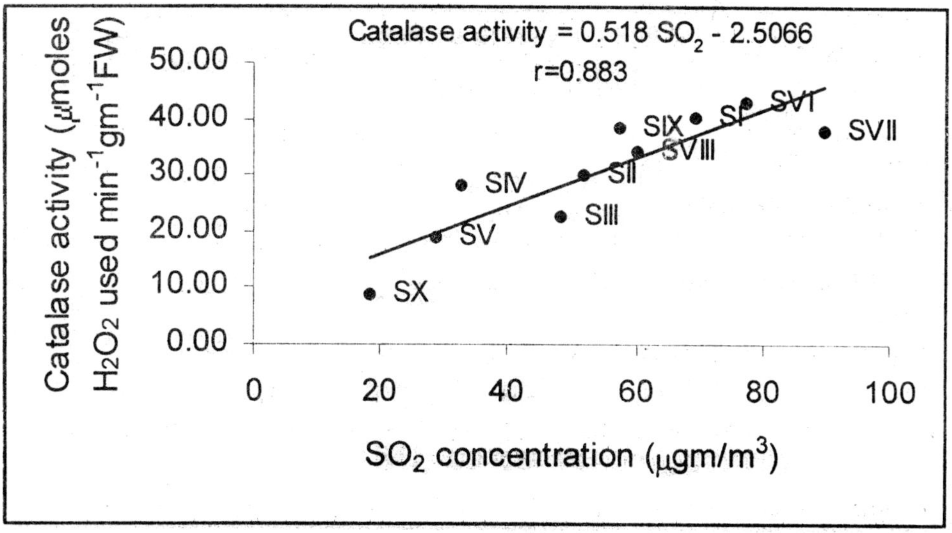

Figure 13.6: Correlation Between Ambient SO_2 Concentration (μgm/m³) and Catalase Activity (μ moles H_2O_2 used min.$^{-1}$gm^{-1} FW) in *Azadiracta indica* at Different Sampling Sites

with SO_2 (Malhotra and Khan, 1984; Horsman and Wellburn, 1975) could be the result of either cellular activity to metabolize H_2O_2 produced by a free radical mechanism or the oxidation of absorbed SO_2. Hydrogen peroxide is not the final product in the series of reactions involved in the scavenging of ROS. It is further reduced to H_2O by catalases in peroxisomes and by ascorbate peroxidase in the chloroplasts and cytosols (Asada and Takahashi, 1987).

Conclusion

The present study revealed that the plants have acclimatized to SO_2 pollution stress. The morpho-physiological responses of plants may vary according to the nature and the dose of the pollutant and the species. However, at biochemical and molecular levels, there appears to be a similarity among different pollutants and also among most of the environmental stresses. Plants try to respond suitably by adjusting their metabolism so that minimum damage is done due to air pollutants. Broadly, two types of protective responses are recorded at molecular level: (i) Increase in antioxidant enzymes and metabolites and (ii) Induction of protection-related secondary metabolite genes. If the plants are able to express these responses adequately, pollution-induced 'visible' or 'hidden' damages do not occur. However, if these protective responses are inadequate and are unable to cope with the incidence and the dose of the pollutant, the injury occurs.

References

Asada, K. and Takahashi, M., 1987. *Photoinhibition*, (Eds.) Kyle, D., Osmond, C.B. and Arntzen, C. Elsevier Science Publishers, Amsterdam, pp. 227–287.

Barber, J.M., 1980. *Z. Pflazen Physiol.* 97: 135.

Garrido, L.M., 1964. Determination of sulphur in plant materials. *Analyst*, 89: 61–66.

Gavali, J.G., Saha, D. and Krishnayya, N.S.R., 2002. Difference in sulphur accumulation in eleven tropical tree spp. growing in polluted environment. *Indian J. Environ. Hlth.*, 44(2): 88–91.

Horsman, D.C. and Wellburn, A.R., 1975. Synergistic effect of SO_2^- and NO_2^- polluted air upon enzyme activity in pea seedlings. *Environ. Pollut.*, 8: 123–133.

Jackson, M.M., 2005. Roadside concentration of gaseous and particulate matter pollutants and risk assessment in Dar-Es-Salaam, Tanzania. *Env. Moni. and Assess.*, 104: 385–407.

Joshi, G., 1998. Ambient air quality at roadside of an urban area with special reference to respirable dust and total suspended particulate matter. *Poll. Res.*, 17: 79–81.

Larcher, W., 1995. Plants under stress. In: *Physiological Plant Ecology*. Pub. Springer-Verlag, New York. pp. 321–433.

Malhotra, S.S. and Khan, A.A., 1984. Biochemical and physiological impact of major pollutants. In: *Air Pollution and Plant Life*, (Ed.) M. Treshow. John Wiley and Sons Ltd., U.K., pp. 113–157.

Putter, J., 1974. In: *Methods of Enzymatic Analysis*, 2nd ed. Bergmeyer, Academic Press, New York, pp. 685.

Raitio, H., Tuovinen, J.P. and Anttila, P., 1995. Relation between sulphur concentrations in the Scots pine needles and the air in Northern most Europe. *Water, Air and Soil Pollut.*, 85: 1361–1366.

Rangarajan, T.N., Arjunan, M.C. and Ponnammal, N.R., 1995. Effect of automobile pollution on few ornamental plants. *Ecol. Environ. Conser.* 1: 1–4.

Richardson, C.J., Di Giulio, R.T. and Tandy, N.E., 1989. Free-radical mediated processes as markers of air pollution stress in trees. In: *Biologic Markers of Air Pollution Stress and Damage in Forests.* pp. 251–260.

Saxena, M.M., 1990. *Environmental Analysis: Water, Soil and Air.* Agro-Botanical Publisher, Bikaner, India.

Shankar, N. Kamakshi, Saxena, A. and Saxena, D.K., 2000. *Physiol. Mol. Biol. Plants*, 6: 89–91.

Srivastava, H.S., 1975. Distribution of nitrate reductase ageing bean seedlings. *Plants and Cell Physiology*, 16: 195–999.

Srivastava, H.S., 1998. Biochemical defense mechanisms of plants to increased levels of ozone and other atmospheric pollutants. *Current Science*, 76(4): 525–533.

Thimmaiah, S.R., 1999. *Standard Methods of Biochemical Analysis.* Kalyani Publishers, New Delhi, India.

Van Assche, F. and Clijsters, 1990. Effects of metals on enzyme activity in plants. *Plants Cell Environ.*, 19: 195–206.

Verma, A. and Singh, S.N., 2004. Air quality status of central and southern regions of Lucknow city, India. *Bull. Environ. Contam. Toxicol.*, 73: 497–505.

West, P.D. and Gaeke, G.C., 1956. Fixation of sulfur dioxide as sulfitomercurate(II) and subsequent colorimetric estimation. *Anal. Chem.*, 28: 1816–1819.

Medicinal Plants: Conservation, Cultivation and Utilization (2007) *Pages 101–106*
Editors: A.K. Chopra, D.R. Khanna, G. Prasad, D.S. Malik and R. Bhutiani
Published by: DAYA PUBLISHING HOUSE

Chapter 14

Distribution Patterns of Coccinellids and Their Role in Biological Control of Mustard Aphids

Pushpa Singh and Sachin Srivastava
Department of Animal Science, Faculty of Applied Sciences, M.J.P. Rohilkhand University, Bareilly – 243 006, U.P. India

ABSTRACT

Four Coccinellid predators *viz., Coccinella septempunctata, Cheilomenes sexmaculata, Coccinella transversalis, Propylea dissecta* and two aphid species *viz., Lipaphis erysimi* and *Myzus persicae* were recorded from different experimental sites of Bareilly region in Uttar Pradesh as a result of an extensive survey of rape-crop during crop season from December 2004 to April 2005. The ladybeetle *Coccinella septempunctatii* Linn. (Coleoptera : Coccinellidae) was recorded as the most common predator associated with the aphids. Besides this, *Cheilomenes sexmaculata* and *Coccinella transversalis* were also found to be the potential predators of aphids. On the other hand, *Propylea dissecta* was rarely found (only when aphid density was maximum).

Keywords: Aphid, Coccinellid predators, Rape-crop, Biological control.

Introduction

The predaceous Coccinellids are linked to Biological control of mustard aphids more often than any other taxa of predatory organisms. The beneficial status of these organism has a rich history that is recognized by the general Public, formers and biological control practitioners (Obrycki and King, 1998). Both the larvae and adult voraceously feed on aphids it is therefore, they can play an important role in biological control programming of the polyphagous, aphid pest of our crops (Omkar and Bind, 1993). They may thus be effectively employed as an important component in the integrated management schedules of pest of our agricultural crops.

Materials and Methods

An extensive survey of rape crop (*Brassica napus*) was conducted at different experimental sites of Bareilly at fortnightly intervals during crop-season from December 2004 to April 2005. The aphids were collected by cutting the upper parts (leaf, stem, inflorescence separately) of the plants and placing them in plastic bags. These plastic bags were tied with a rubberband and brought to the Laboratory for counting and taxonomic identification as per methods of Ghosh (1970), Raychaudhuri (1980), Martin (1983), Omkar and Bind (1993) and Omkar and Bind (1995) and Bakhetia and Sachan (1997) for aphids and Omkar and Bind (1993), Agarwala and Yasuda (2000) and Omkar and James (2001) for Coccinellids. Coccinellids were collected by the hand picking from the plant. The aphids were counted manually with the help of camel hair brush. The field record of the colour of the specimen, locality and date of collection were also made. After that, specimens were transferred to the glass vials (4 × 0.5 cm) containing 70 per cent Ethyl alcohol and glycerol (5 : 1) for taxonomical studies.

Results and Discussions

The cumulative species composition of Coccinellids in rape-crop (*Brassica napus*) included *Coccinella septempunctata, Cheilomenes sexmaculata, Coccinella transversalis, Propylea dissecta* and the aphid species were *Lipaphis erysimi* and *Myzus-persicae.* The average aphid as well as Coccinellid population estimated on the plants of different localities at different period of crop growth are given in the graphs (Figure 14.1 and 14.2).

Seasonal Incidence of the Aphids

The result showed that the general trend of aphid population was the same on all the sites, showing first a period of slow increase followed by a more rapid increase leading to a peak and then a sudden and steep decline. These observations are in conformity with those of Barbagallo Inserra and Fostel (1972) and Roy (1975). The peak in the aphid population remained in the last fortnight of February (*L. erysimi* = 412.33, *M. persicae* = 349.66 aphids/plant at Bilwa, *L. erysimi* = 755.33, *M. persicae* = 509.00 aphids/plant at Bitherichainpur, *L. erysimi* = 622.33, *M. persicae* = 440.00 aphids/plant at Lal Phatak area). The result also showed that the population of *L. erysimi* was always higher (except Lal Phatak on 12-01-05 there was no *L. erysimi* and Bithrichainpur on 27-12-04 *L. erysimi* were 34.33 and *M. persicae* were 52.22 aphids/plant. *M. persicae* was higher than *L. erysimi*) then *M. persicae,* indicating that *L. erysimi* is the most common insect pest of mustard crop in India as reported by Bakhetia *et al.* (1989).

Seasonal Incidence of the Coccinellid Predators

Coccinella septempunctata

The findings of present study indicated that it was the most commonly occurring predator of aphids as also been suggested by Omkar and Bind, 1993. It remained active from February to the middle of the April. The result showed that it was found in maximum number in all the experimental sites. It was regularly found from first appearance till to the crop harvesting. It feed on both the aphid species, *Lipaphis erysimi* and *Myzus persicae* so it play very important role in the biological control programming of the aphids.

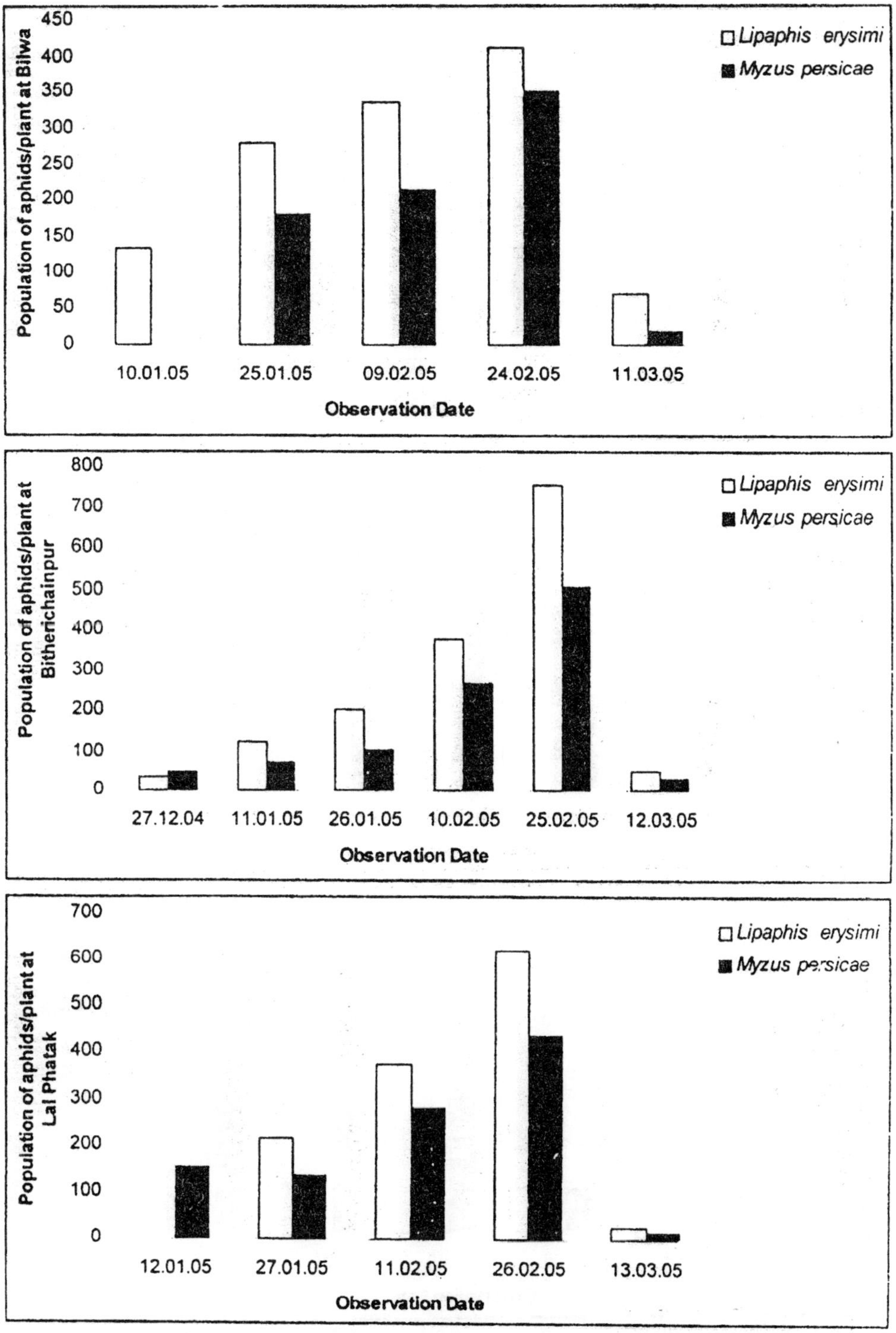

Figure 14.1: Population of Aphids at Different Experimental Sites of Bareilly

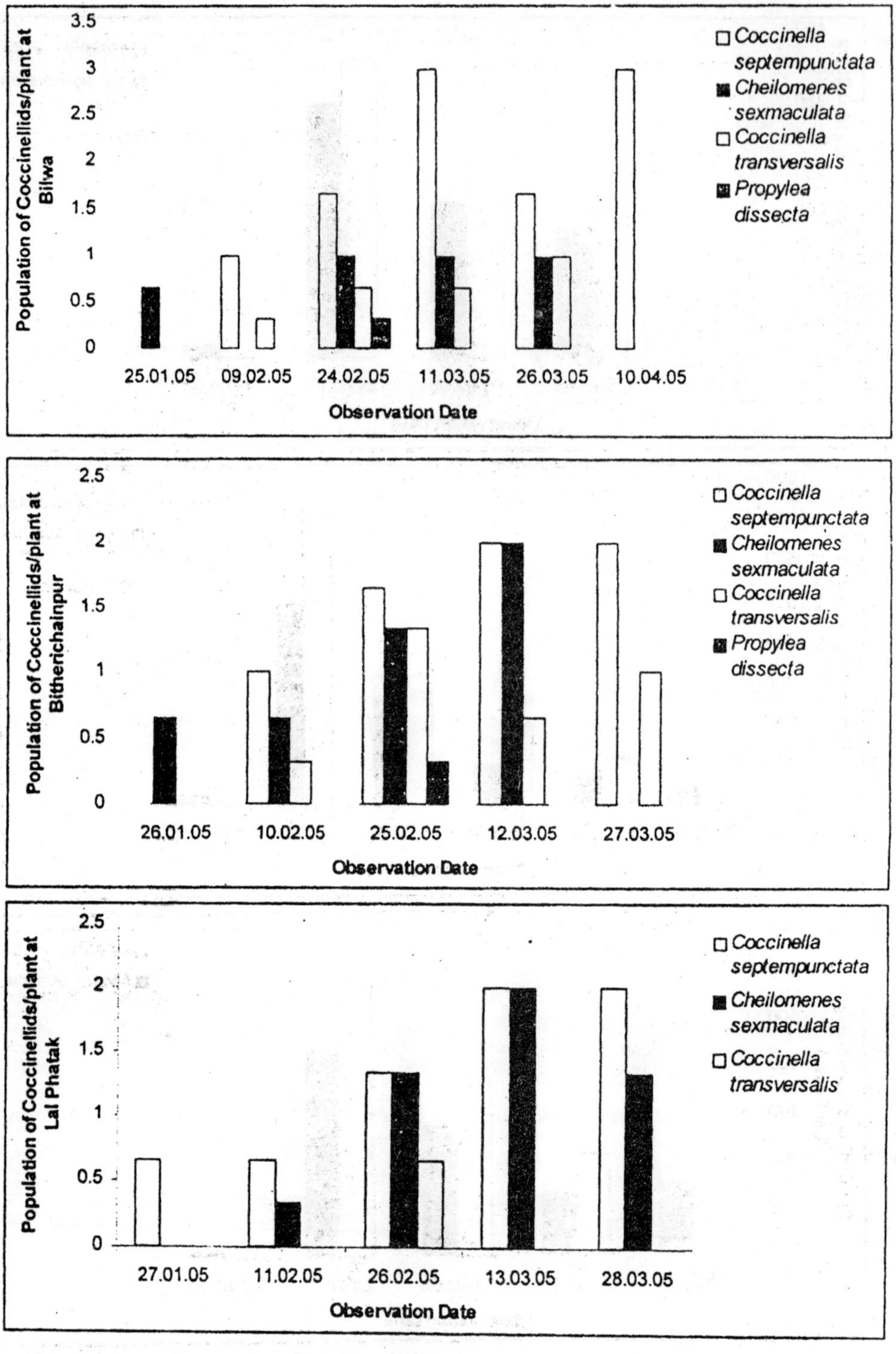

Figure 14.2: Population of Coccinellids at Different Experimental Sites of Bareilly

The grub of the beetle consume more aphid than adults (Hamalainen, 1977) and have been reported to play an important role in regulating the aphid population.

Cheilomenes sexmaculata

It was another very common species of Coccinellids but less common then *Coccinella septempunctata*. It also feed on both the aphids and remained active from February to the last fortnight of the March, therefore, it also play an important role in the biological control of aphids. It is known to have a prey range of 57 species of aphids (Agarwala and Yasuda, 2000).

Coccinella transversalis

It also feed on both the aphid species, but was sporadically found. It also remain active fromed February to the last fortnight of the March. It is also helpful in aphid bio control. Both the larvae and adults were collected from mustard fields.

Propylea dissecta

It was rarely found in the last fortnight of February when the aphid density was maximum. Although, it was not commonly found but helpful in biological control of aphids.

It was observed from the study when the population of aphid increased, the population of ladybeetles were also increased rapidly in February and play an important role in supressing and regulating the aphid population. During the field collection it was experienced that Coccinellids were present in the fields even in the absence of the aphids as observed by Sinha *et al.* (1982). It is because in the absence or scarcity of aphids these ladybeetles survive longer by eating eggs of their own species (Agarwala, 1991; Agarwala and Bardhanroy 1997; Agarwala *et al.*, 1997 and Agarwala and Yasuda, 2000).

Acknowledgements

The authors are thankful to Dr. N.B. Singh, Professor and Head, Department of Animal Science, M.J.P. Rohilkhand University, Bareilly (U.P) for providing worthy guidance and necessary laboratory facilities for this work.

References

Agarwala, B.K., 1991. Why do ladybirds (Coleoptera : Coccinellidae) canllibalize? *J. Bio. Sci.*, 16(3): 103–109.

Agarwala, B.K. and Bardhanroy, P., 1997. Oviposition behaviour and reproduction efficiency in ladybird beetles (Coccinellidae : Coleoptera): A case study of *Menochilus sexmaculatus* (Fabr.). *J. Aphidol.*, 11(1): 49–59.

Agarwala, B.K., Bhattacharya, S. and Bardhanroy, P., 1997. Cluster laying of eggs does not increase the rise of cannibalism by first instar larvae in ladybird beetles. In: *Proc. Indian Nat. Sci. Acad.*, 863(1 and 2): 1–10.

Agarwala, B.K. and Yasuda, H., 2000. Competitive ability of ladybird predators of aphids: A review of *Cheilomenes sexmaculata* (Fabr.) (Coleoptera : Coccinellidae) with a world wide checklist of Preys. *J. Aphidol.*, 14(1 and 2): 1–20.

Bakhetia, D.R.C. and Ghorbandi, A.W., 1989. Relationship between the parameters of aphid population per plant and percentage of plants infested by *Lipaphis erysimi* (Kaltenbach) in Indian mustard crop. *J. Aphidology*, 3: 119–124.

Bakhetia, D.R.C. and Sachan, G.C., 1997. A bulletin on identification and management strategies for insect pest of rape seed and mustard, pp. 10–13.

Barbagallo, S., Inserra, R. and Foster, G.N., 1972. Population dynamics of *Myzus persicae* (sulzer) on Potato in sicily (Silicia, Italy) (Homoptera : Ahididae), *Entomologica*, 8 : 21–23.

Ghosh, L.K., 1970. A notes on the preliminary survey of aphids from Bihar, India. *Sci. and Cult.*, 36: 419–420.

Himalainen, M., 1977. Control of aphids on sweet peppers, *Chrysanthamums* and roses in small green houses using the ladybeetles *Coccinella septempunctata* and *Adalia bipunctata* (Col., Coccinellidae). *Ann. agric. Ferul.*, 16: 117–131.

John, J. Obrycki and Timothy J. Kring, 1998. Predaceous Coccinellidae in Biological control. *Annu. Rev. Entomol.*, 43: 295–321.

Martin, J.H., 1983. The identification of common aphid pests of tropical agriculture. *Tropical Pest Management*, 29(4): 351–411.

Omkar and Bind, R.B., 1993. Records of aphid natural enemies complex of Uttar Pradesh. II. The Coccinellids. *J. Adv. Zool.*, 14(2): 96–99.

Omkar and Bind, R.B., 1995. Records of aphid natural enemies complex of Uttar Pradesh. I. The aphids. *Indian J. Agric. Res.*, 29(4): 215–218.

Omkar and James, B.E., 2001. Searching and feeding efficacy of *Coccinella transversalis* Fabricius on brinjal aphid, *Aphis gossipii* Glover. *Boil. Mem.*, 27(1): 20–26.

Roy, P., 1975. Population dynamics of mustard aphid *Lipaphis erysimi* (Kaltenbach) (Aphidedae : Hemiptera) in West Bengal. *India J. Ent.*, 37(3): 318–321.

Raychaudhuri, D.N., 1980. *Aphids of North-east India and Bhutan*, pp. 1–521.

Sinha, T.B. Ranjan, K. Pandey, Rajendra Sing, C.P.M. Tripathi and Arvind Kumar, 1982. The functional response of *Coccinella septempunctata* Linn., A Coccinellid predator of mustard aphid *Lipaphys erysimi* Kalt. *Entomon.*, 7(1): 7–10.

Medicinal Plants: Conservation, Cultivation and Utilization (2007) *Pages* **107–111**
Editors: A.K. Chopra, D.R. Khanna, G. Prasad, D.S. Malik and R. Bhutiani
Published by: DAYA PUBLISHING HOUSE

Chapter 15

Pharmaceutical Products and Anti-microbial Activity of Bryophytes: Uses of "Green Brain"

Kajal Srivastava* and Shivom Singh
P.G. Environmental Management, Department of Botany, Bareilly College, Bareilly – 243 005, (U.P.) India

ABSTRACT

The bryophytes are a diverse group of lower plants. It is among ancient amphibious plants and considered as the first green plant to develop during the evolutionary process. Bryophytes have enormous properties as they are used in pharmaceutical product, horticulture, household purpose and biological technique beside that they have high tolerance potential for biomonitoring as bioindicators. They are studied for purpose ranging from pollution monitoring to their use in folk medicines. Because of their multifarious uses and application bryophytes are known as "Green Brain".

Bryophytes are one of the least investigated groups of plants for bioactive molecules. So, it is an attempt to briefly examine some of the uses and application of this primitive group of lower plants.

Keywords: Bryophytes, pharmaceuticals, folk medicine, antibiotic, antifeedent, genomic.

About Bryophytes

Bryophytes are autotrophic plants with some 23,000 described species world wide, making it the largest group of land plants. The group includes three quite distinct lineages: the mosses, hornworts

* E-mail: kajalkaju_18@rediffmail.com.

and liverworts. The bryophytes are generally considered as "Key" group (Mishier and Norris, 2004). The first bryophytes appear in fossils from the Devonian era about 350 million years ago. Liverworts are bilaterally symmetric and may be strap shaped or thalloid, a growth also seen in hornworts. Hornworts are quite distinct group differ microscopically from thalloid liverworts in the presence of single chloroplast in each cell.

Bryophytes tend to be shade loving plants and are most abundant and conspicuous in moist, humid habitat but are also found in grassland and deserts, where they endure prolonged dry periods. Bryophytes have successfully exploited many environments, perhaps partly because they are rarely in direct competition with higher plants (Anderson, 1980). They are vital plants and have indirect use in the formation of soil and rocks in vegetation covers and soil conservation and act as a pioneer plant in plant succession. Moss and liverworts provide sustainable substrate for fixation of nitrogen in association with Cynobacteria and also contribute in carbon gain. Though mosses appear all year round, their maturity is specifically limited from the end of October to February during which they develop spores for reproductive purpose.

Bryophytes play a major role in maintaining the ecosystem's humidity level, by their ability to absorb and retain water (Anderson *et al.*, 1990). Mosses (bryophytes) have potential in the biomapping of atmospheric precipitations; they can survive in stress conditions as they have surprisingly high tolerance capacity. Present use of bryophytes includes ecology, horticulture, fuel production, household uses, medicines and even in food. These small plants have immense value for sustainable development. Due to these utility and their primitiveness bryophytes festinate botanist.

Medicinal Plants Resources Base

Medicinal value of plants are increasing day by day and of mosses has been judged to the high level. All world is emphasizing on medicinal value of plants and India is one of them. India is richest in this field and has rich plant diversity of Himalaya–over 8000 angiosperms, 44 gymnosperms, 600 pteridophytes, 1737 bryophytes, 1159 lichens and 6900 fungi etc. Indian Himalayas are largely a rugged, mountainous region where altitude varies. This altitude variation has resulted in a complex diversity in topography, metrology, flora and fauna (Gaur; *et al.*, 1984). Medicinal plants are viewed as a possible bridge between sustainable economic development, affordable health care and conservation of vital diversity. As mentioned by several workers that Indian Himalayas are rich in bryoflora therefore India is one of the major raw material producing nation of South Asia and with in the country and is known as treasure house of medicine. The Himalaya supports a large number of bryo-species, which were extensively traditionally and now is being used by the pharmaceutical industry for preparation of drugs used in Indian System of Medicines (Sharma *et al.*, 1997).

Medicinal Uses of Bryophytes

More than 70 per cent of all medicinal compounds have derived from a small fraction of the world's biodiversity. There is great potential to exploit further world's genetic resources by exploring the huge chemical diversity present in plants. This group is least investigated among plants for bioactive molecules. Yet in nature they appears to be well protected against grazing and pathogens by there chemical constitutes. Some bryophytes such as the bog-moss *Sphagnum* have well known antibiotic properties. Because of its absorbent and antiseptic properties it was used for dressing during World War I to make pillows for resting of wounded members for soldiers transported to hospitals from battlefields (Glime ans Saxena, 1990). Irish moss is a very useful herb as it has high content of nutrients.

It contains vitamins A, D, E, F, and K. It has high content of iodine, calcium and sodium, which contributes in glandular system. It has high mucilage content, which makes it soothing to inflamed tissues and lungs and kidney problems (Blockeel *et al.*, 1998). Irish moss has been used externally to soften skin and prevent wrinkles. It purifies and strengthens the cellular structure and vital fluids of the system.

Bryophytes have various therapeutic applications, which are currently used in the treatment. Liverworts do have champions, including herb list that value it for purported medicinal uses (Banerjee and Sen, 1979). "Wort" means "Herb" and it is called the Herb of the liver because of an old belief, that it could cure liver disease and hydrophobia (rabies). Along this they have many diversified uses. There extract is not only a potent fungicide and bactericide, but also a weak biocide (stomach pest) against animal pests (Saxena and Hareinder, 2004). A chemical analysis of the moss *Rhodobryum gigantenum* indicates that it contains volatile oils, lactones and amino acids, which increase the rate of blood flow in aorta by 30 per cent (3 year collaborative project between RBGE, SCRI and SIDR).

Bryophytes in Folk Medicines

Folk medicine is a part of traditional culture in most of world heritage. It contains information not only about illness but also methods of healing, how to avoid illness and protects health. In India the burned ash of mosses mixed with fat and honey is used as an ointment for cuts, burns and wounds in the Himalayan region (Dickinson, 1995). *Riccia* species are used as an external application to cure ringworm and the paste made from fresh thalli of Patharshali (*Plagiochasma sp.*) is used in blisters on the body and also applied for the treatment of skin eruption caused by hot sunlight in summers. Sphangnol (pit tar) from *Sphagnum* moss has also high treatment value for skin diseases (Nirmala Pradhan, 2005). Chinese traditional medicine name 40 kinds of bryophytes that have been used to treat illness of the cardio vascular system, nervous prostration, tonsillitis, bronchitis, cystitis, yellow jaundice as well as skin disease and burns. New Zealand treated veneric diseases with a paste and applied as poultice (Higuchi *et al.*, 2000). *Marchantia*, a common liverwort, has the chemical constituents to cure pulmonary tuberculosis and also ailment for liver diseases. It has been tested well that the tea prepared from common hair cap moss helps to dissolve stones in kidney and gall bladder. It is also a good medicine to prevent common cold.

Anti-Microbial Activity/Antifeedents

Liverworts are not susceptible to fungal diseases and anti-microbial activity has been seen in extracts of *Reboulia* and *Pallaviciania* possibly due to lunularic acid. The anti-microbial effects explain the successful uses *e.g.* peat mosses as surgical dressing. The mosses could not only soak up four times as much liquid as cotton but also inhibit infections because of the anti-microbial effects. All bryophytes contain cocktails of different active compounds, mainly terpenoids, to protect themselves against infections of fungi and bacteria, with which they live in direct contact (source: Frahm@uni-bonn.de). These effects of bryoflora were thus not developed by chance but are a necessity for their survival. The anti-microbial effects of bryophytes go back on an inhibition of cell division, not only of bacteria and fungi but also of mammal cells. Other effects include anti-feeding effects against beetles, slug and snail or fish killing effects. Several insect anti-feedents have now been found in diverse bryophytes making this group of plants a useful source of insecticides and insect repellant.

Antibiotics

Bryophytes also act as antibiotic agent. Mc Cleary and Walkington in 1966 found eighteen mosses that showed strong inhibition to gram-positive and gram-negative organisms because of its antibiotic properties. They also suggest that presence of non-ionized organic acids with low pH and phenolic compounds, which may be probably responsible for their antibiotic effects.

Some other scientists also studied the utility of bryophytes in antibiotics, Gupta and Singh in 1971 found that petroleum ether extracts of *Barbula* and *Timmiella* species were active against gram-positive and gram-negative bacteria, the highest occurrence of antibacterial activity was found in the extract of *Barbula* species. Prenylbenzyl from *Radula* species inhibits the growth of *Staphylococcus aureus* (Asakawa *et al.*, 1982b).

Anti-Tumour Activity

Anti-tumour properties were also reported from compounds of bryophytes. A new enteudesmanolide, diplophyllin, was isolated from *Diplophyllin albicans* and *D.taxifolium* having an alpha methylene lactone unit, showed significant activity (ED50 4-6mg/ml) against human epidermoid carcinoma (KBcell culture). It's optical enantiomer, derived chemically from the compound isoanantolactone, exhibited anticancer activity (ED50 20-37 μg/ml) (Ohta *et al.*, 1983). Compounds from *Plagiochila fasciculate* seemed to inhibit P388 cells (leukaemia). The sesquiterpenoides, which showed a reproducible inhibitory activity against the cell culture of human carcinoma of the nasopharynx, was isolated from leafy liverworts (Asakawa, 1981). They have great potential for anti-leukemia activity. Recent research suggests that moss also slows the growth of cancer cells in culture. (Hallingback and Hodgetts, 2000).

Production of Biopharmaceuticals in Bryophytes

Bryophytes has been recently recognized as an ideal producer of recombinant proteins with respect to glycosylation, due to the elaborated post-translational capability of moss cells, the glycosylation patterns have been manipulated to obtain similar proteins to those found in animal cells. Gilbert Gorr from Germany is currently working on the application of bryophytes for production of recombinant pharmaceuticals.

The moss bioreactor is based on the cultivation of transgenic moss tissues as suspension cultures under contained conditions (Decker, 2004). The recombinant protein of interest is targeted to the secretary pathway and accumulates in the simple medium, which greatly facilitates the purification process. Moreover, bryophytes like *Physcomitrella patens* as the mainly used moss have a favorable safety profile *e.g.* absence of human pathogens (Koprivova *et al.*, 2004).

Conclusion

From the above discussion it is concluded that bryophytes is representing an economic development point in the province and possessing distinctive characteristics of its own. Due to mentioned utility bryophytes are named as "Green Brain". Use of bryophytes in biomedicine and pharmaceutical industry give priority to the development of natural medicines with high added value for export and further increase the series of new products. They bear great potential for the production of biopharmaceuticals with comparability to animal cell culture derived products, which would be more economic and viable solution. But all this requires nations to protect the traditional knowledge and customary practices related to the use of biological resources despite this many beneficial mosses can still be explored in various parts of the earth. This is the consequence of our least knowledge about natural resources utility.

References

Anderson, L.E., 1980. Cytology and reproductive biology of mosses. In: *The Mosses of North America*, (Eds.) R.J. Taylor and A.E. Leviton. Pacific Division of the American Association for the Advancement of Science, San Francisco, p. 37–76.

Anderson, L.E., Crum, H.A. and Buck, W.R., 1990. List of the mosses of North American north of Mexico. *Bryologist*, 93: 448–499.

Asakawa, Y., 1981. Biologically active substances obtained from bryophytes. *J. Hattori Bot. Lab.*, 50: 123–142.

Askawa, Y., 1982. Chemical constituents of the Hepaticae. *Prog. Chem. Org. Natur. Prod.*, 42: 1–285.

Banerjee, R.D. and Sen, S.P., 1979. Antibiotic activity of bryophytes. *Bryologist*, 82: 141–153.

Blockeel, T.L. and Long, D.G., 1998. A checklist and census catalogue of British and Irish Bryophytes. *Cardiff: British Bryology Society.*

Dickson, C., 1995. The pharmacy in the forest. *Mother Earth News*, p. 40–45.

Decker, E.L. and Reski, R., 2004. The moss bioreactor. *Curr. Opin. Plan. Biol.*, 7: 166–170.

Glime, J.M. and Saxena, D.K., 1990. *Uses of Bryophytes.* Today and Tommorow Printers and publishers, New Delhi, India.

Gaur, R.D., Semwal, J.K. and Tiwari, J.K., 1984. A survey of high altitude medicinal plants of Garhwal Himalaya. *Bull. Med. Ethnobot. Res.*, 4(3–4): 102–116.

Gupta, K.G. and Singh, B., 1971. Occurrence of antibacterial activity in moss extracts. *Res. Bull. Punjab Univ. Sci.*, 22: 237–239.

Hallingback, T. and Hodgetts, N., 2000. *Mosses, Liverworts and Hornworts: Status Survey and Conservation Action Plan for Bryophytes.* IUCN, Cambridge, U.K.

Higuchi, M., Wang, L.S. and Long, D.G., 2000. *Haplomitrium hookeri* (Sm.) Nees new to China and *Apotreubia yunnanensis* Huguchi new to Sichuan. *Bryological Research*, 7: 309–313.

Koprivova, A.C., Stemmer, F. Altmann, A. Hoffmann, S. Kopriva, G. Gorr, Reski, R. and Decker, E.L., 2004. Targeted knockouts of *Physcomitrella* lacking plant-specific immunogenic N-glycans. *Plant Biotech. J.*, 2: 517–523.

McClearly, J.A. and Walkington, D.L., 1960. Mosses as possible source of antibiotics. *Science*, 131: 108.

Mishler, B. and Norris, D., 2004. *Valley Life Sciences Building*, UC Berkeley.

Ohta, Y. Abe, S. Komura, H. and Kobayasthi, M., 1983. Prelunulario acid, a possible immediate in the prenyl-propancid-polymalonate pathway. *J. Amer. Chem. Soc.*, 105: 4480-4481.

Pradhan Nirmala, 2005. *Bryophytes: Multiple Utilities.* Nepal Sambat, Pohelaga Paru.

Saxena D.K. and Hariendar Kaur, 2004. Uses of bryophytes. *Resonance*, 9: 56–65.

Sharma, J.R., Mudgal, V. and Llajra, P.K., 1997. *Floristic Diversity and Conservation strategies in India.* Botanical Survey of India Ministry of Environment and Forest. P5. The project is a 3-year collaborative one between RBGE, Scottish Crop Research Institute (SCRI), Dundee and Strathclyde Institute of Drug Research (SIDR) located with in Strathclyde University in Glasgow.

Medicinal Plants: Conservation, Cultivation and Utilization (2007) *Pages 113–120*
Editors: A.K. Chopra, D.R. Khanna, G. Prasad, D.S. Malik and R. Bhutiani
Published by: DAYA PUBLISHING HOUSE

Chapter 16

Effect of Alcoholic Extract of Three *Adiantum* Species of Ferns Formulation for Stamina in Male and Female Albino Mice Subjected to Forced Swim Stress

D.K. Bhatia and R.K. Pande
PG Department of Zoology, DBS (PG) College, Dehradun

ABSTRACT

The antistress effect of a polyherbal formulation:"Adiantum Herbal" was studied in both male and female albino mice subjected to forced swim stress. The gum acacia 2 per cent was chosen as standard drug for comparison. The swimming endurance and haemoglobin tests indicate that the Ayurvedic herbo-formulation improved the stamina as well as haemoglobin in both sexes of mice and the effect was dose dependent. The LD_{50} of this formulation was more than 500 mg/kg. b.w. in mice, suggesting the absence of any toxicity. It can be thus concluded from this study that Ayurvedic Herbal preparation Adiantum Herbal 'could be effective for improving the stamina in female albino mice and male mice and this preparation can be used as antidepressant drug.

Keywords: Poly-herbal formulation, Swimming Endurance, Haemoglobin, Antistress

Introduction

In the 1930's Hans Selye defined stress as the reaction of an organism to various stimuli. These diverse stimuli together can be called as stressors (Selye 1956). Stress would manifest itself as physiological, biochemical and behavioural changes. Intense or chronic stress would then lead to stress related diseases such as hypertension, diabetes, stroke, cancer, depression etc (Vogel, 1993). A wide variety of stresses, both physical and emotional, act via neural pathways to the hypothalamus to increase corticotropic releasing hormone secretion (CRH) and ACTH and cortisol secretion (Vander *et al.*).

Swimming in small laboratory animals has been widely used for studying the physiological changes in the capacity of the organism, in response to stress (Tan *et al.*, 1992, Greenen *et al.*, 1988). The forced swimming test developed by (Porsolt *et al.*, 1977) has now become a widely accepted model for studying physical stress in animals. Water temperature is another important factor in the forced swimming test. By varying this temperature, (Richter, 1957) found that rats could survive as long as 80 hours in lukewarm water (36°C). Increase or decrease in the water temperature above/below this point influences the overall behaviour of the animal and changes the involvement of corticorticoids (Abel, 1991).

A number of Ayurvedic herbal formulation that claim to cure anemia, general tonic, detoxicant, Ageing (Nadkarni; and Nadkarni, 1976; Bajaj and Vohra, 1998; Satyan, 2001) have been reported. Many of such preparations in Ayurveda are called Rasayanas. It is believed to strengthen the body resistance to infections, diseases, enhance longevity and anti-fatigue. In the present study another Ayurvedic Poly-herbal preparation "Andiantum Herbal", which contains 50 per cent alcoholic extracts of three Himalayan ferns *i.e. Adiantum incisum, Andiatum capillus-veneris and Adiantum lunulatum* have been evaluated for its potential stamina boosting or anti-fatigue activity and haemoglobin enhancing properties in mice.

Materials and Methods

Animals

Healthy colony breed mice (25–30g) of both male and female were used. The animals were housed in polypropylene cages (5 in each cage) in animal house at 25 ± 2°C with relative humidity of 50-70 per cent and 12 hours dark and night cycle. Food and water was given *adlibitum*. Total of 48 healthy mice (24 males and 24 females) were randomly divided into 6 groups of 8 mice in each group.

Preparation of Herbal Formulation

A Polyherbal complex formulation 'Adiantum Herbal' is prepared in our laboratory. "Weight amount of powdered plant material *i.e. Adiatum incisum, Adiantum capillus-veneris* and *Adiantum lunulatum* is soxhleted with measured volume of 50 per cent ethanol-water solvent for such time, till no more solvent is obtained. The extract so obtained was reduced to a semi-solid state, under low temperature and reduced pressure using a rotary apparatus. This was henceforth designated as 'Alcoholic' extract". This solid alcoholic extract of different species of ferns extract were mixed with equal amount, to get a "Adiantum Herbal" formulation. Desired weight of this formulation is taken according to body weight of mice and mixed with 2 per cent gum acacia to obtain an aqueous suspension for administration in the both sexes of mice, in graded dose for varying period of treatment.

Treatment Schedule

The group 'A', 'A1' were fed with 2 per cent gum acacia powder oral suspension and served as Control while animals in group 'B', 'B1' and 'C', 'C1', were administered doses of 250mg/kg body weight and 500mg/kg body weight of the above mentioned Ayurvedic Herbal formulation for 15 days (Table 16.1).

Table 16.1: Treatment Schedule of Mice

Groups	*Dosage in mg/kg b.wt.*	*Treatment in days*
A Male	2 per cent gum acacia (Control)	30
B Male	250mg/kg b.wt.	30
C Male	500mg/kg b.wt.	30
A1 female	2 per cent gum acacia (Control)	30
B1 female	250mg/kg b.wt.	30
C1 female	500mg/kg b.wt.	30

All value is mean ± SE of 8 mice.

Force Swimming Test

This test was based on the method described by Sharma *et al.* (1995) and Nagaraja (1999). The mice were forced to swim in the bucket water till they just started drowning and were unable to sustain themselves, so rescued at that stage. Actual time of swimming for individual animals was recorded. The animals were killed by cervical dislocation and blood was collected from heart immediately for haemoglobin estimations (Dacie, 1968).

Statistical Analysis

The data were expressed as mean difference ± SE and analysed using student's 't' test and 'p' value less then 0.05 were regarded as statistically significant (Snedacor and Cochran).

Results

Effect of formulation on body weights: The data in table 2 reveals that there were no significant changes in body weight of both male and female mice as a result of the treatment in all the groups (Table 16.2 and Figure 16.1).

Table 16.2: Average Body Weight of Albino Mice after Treatment with the Formulation

Group	*Dose mg/kg b.w.*	*Initial b.w. (gms)*	*Final b.w. (gms)*
A male	Control	27.5 ± 0.59	27.6 ± 0.59
B male	250mg/kg b.wt.	27.5 ± 0.59	27.5 ± 0.59
C male	500mg/kg b.wt.	26.25 ± 0.91	27.8 ± 0.91*
A1 female	control	25 ± 0.66	26.9 ± 0.58
B1 female	250mg/kg b.wt.	27.5 ± 0.59	27.5 ± 0.59*
C1 female	500mg/kg b.wt.	27.12 ± 0.92	27.0 ± 0.92*

All value is mean ± SE of 8 mice.

(* $P < 0.05$ Compared with control groups).

Effect of Formulation on Swimming Endurance

Ayurvedic Herbal formulation revealed interesting results in the swimming endurance in treated albino mice of both sexes. Table 16.3, indicates that the male mice are more efficient swimmers as

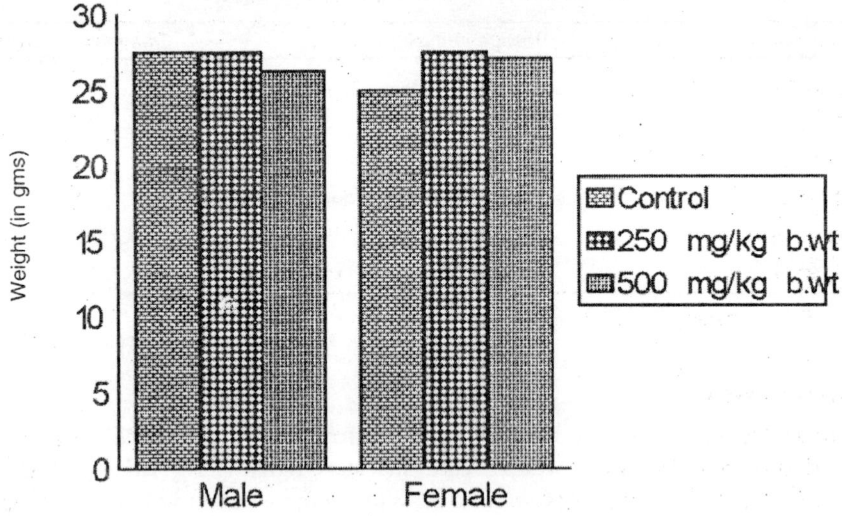

Figure 16.1: Average Body Weight of Albino Mice After Treatment with the Formulation

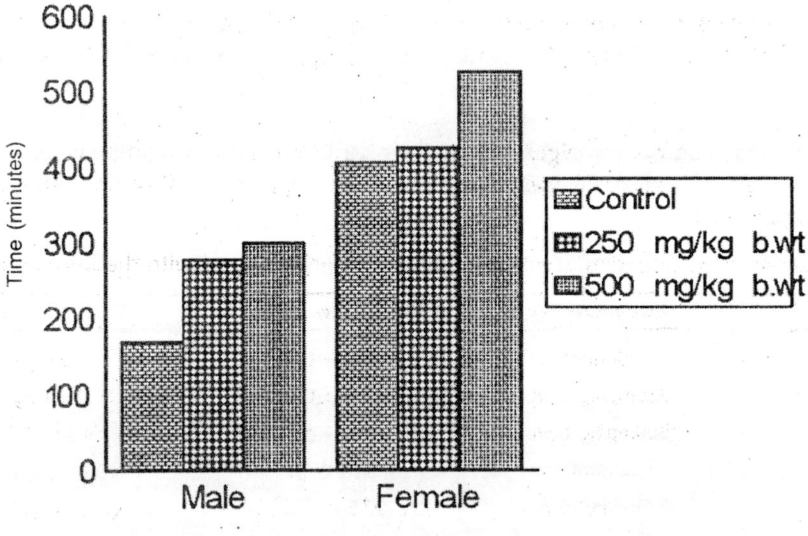

Figure 16.2: Average Swimming Endurance Times of Albino Mice After Treatment with the Formulation

compared to the female mice. Further, the formulation resulted 63.96 per cent and 76.73 per cent increase in swimming endurance in male mice over control animals at 250, 500 mg/kg b.w. dose, which was found to be statistically significant. The response was observed to be dose dependent. Similarly, the formulation resulted 4.85 per cent and 29.56 per cent increase in swimming endurance in female mice as compared to control animals at 250, 500 mg/kg b.w. dose which was found to be statistically significant. The response was observed to be dose dependent (Table 16.3 and Figure 16.2).

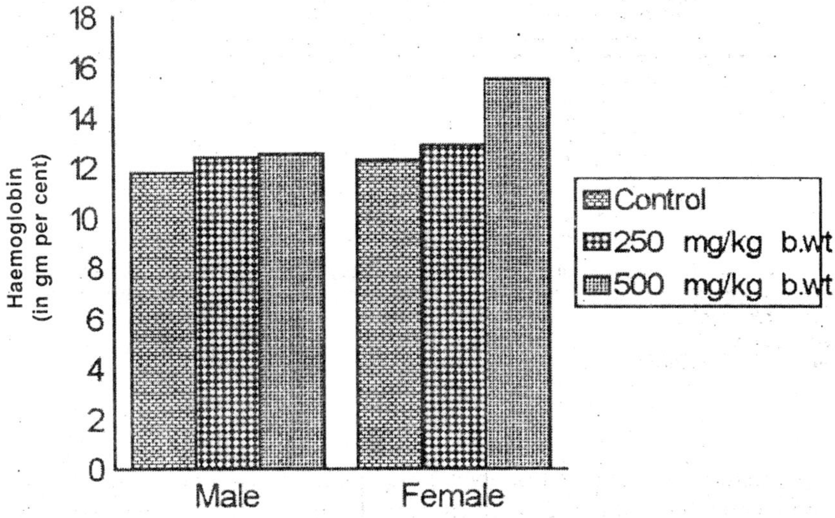

Figure 16.3: Average Haemoglobin of Male and Female Albino Mice

Table 16.3: Average Swimming Endurance Times of Albino Mice After Treatment with the Formulation

Groups	*Dose in mg/kg b.w.*	*Swimming Time in (minutes)*	*Increase in Swimming Time (per cent)*
A Male	control	169.32 ± 19.67	
B Male	250mg/kg b.wt.	277.63 ± 83.88*	63.96
C Male	500mg/kg b.wt.	299.25 ± 33.03	76.73
A1 Female	Control	405.88 ± 32.03	
B1 Female	250mg/kg b.wt	425.57 ± 6.58*	4.85
C1 Female	500mg/kg b.wt	525.85 ± 43.12*	29.56

All value are mean ± SE of 8 mice.

(*P < 0.05) compared with control groups.

Effect of Formulation on Haemoglobin

Table 16.4 indicates that the Ayurvedic Herbal formulation resulted in 5.26 per cent and 6.45 per cent increase in the haemoglobin levels of male mice compared to the control group, which was found to be statistically significant. The increase of haemoglobin level was observed to be dose dependent. Similarly some herbal formulation resulted in 4.88 per cent and 26.59 per cent increase in the haemoglobin levels of female mice compared to the control group, which was found to be statistically significant. The increase of haemoglobin levels was observed to be dose dependent (Figures 16.3, Table 16.4).

Table 16.4: Average Haemoglobin (gm per cent) of male and female albino mice

Groups	*Dose in mg/kg b.w.*	*Haemoglobin (*gm per cent)*	*Increase in Haemoglobin (%) as Compared to Control*
A Male	Control	11.77 ± 1.08	
B Male	250mg/kgb.wt.	12.39 ± 2.14*	5.26 per cent
C Male	500mg/kgb.wt.	12.53 ± 0.52*	6.45 per cent
A1 Female	Control	12.28 ± 1.00	
B1 Female	250mg/kgb.wt.	12.88 ± 1.13*	4.88 per cent
C1 Female	500mg/kg b.wt.	15.54 ± 0.98*	26.59 per cent

All value are mean ± SE of 8 mice.

(*P < 0.05) compared with control groups.

Discussion

The various formulations have been described in our ancient text of Ayurveda. These Ayurvedic formulations are believed to cure the disease from its root cause, without any side effects. They are believed to strengthen the body's resistance to infection and diseases and enhance longevity. There are various metal and non metal base herbal formulations used for treatment of diseases in human, (Satyan *et al.*, 2001) also reported that Ehb herbo-mineral formulation which contains iron; produces significantly higher and dose dependent increase in haemoglobin level in anemic rodents. Mice or rats when forced to swim in a restricted space from which they cannot escape, after an initial period of vigorous activity, adopt a characteristic immobile posture in which they remain floating in water making only these movements necessary to keep their head above water. It has been suggested that immobile posture observed may serve as screening model for antidepressant drugs (Porsolt *et al.*, 1977a; Porosolt *et al.*, 1977b). The immobility in this model is reduced by a variety of treatments which are therapeutically effective in depression (Prosolt *et al.*, 1978a; Porsolt *et al.*, 1978b)

The anemic infants and children often-impaired motor development and coordination decreased physical activity and fatigue. In male and female human being, anemia causes decreased resistance to fatigue and decreased resistance to physical work. The efficacy of Ayurvedic formulation for anti-fatigue in mice in this study has shown encouraging result. The results of the present study suggest that Ayurvedic "*Adiantum* Herbal" formulation induces significant physiological changes in the body of test animals that allow them to face the stress more efficiently. However, the mechanism of action of this formulation needs to be studied further. The increase in the haemoglobin level, after the treatment with formulations may also have enhanced the swimming capacity of the treated animals.

The swimming endurance test and haemoglobin levels, resulted in increasing the swimming efficacy and the efficacy was at its highest in the female mice fed with Ayurvedic formulation, than the male counterpart (Figures 16.2 and 16.3).

Anteddra and Dixit. 1997, found similar result when *Embica officinalis* and *Aegle marmelos* extract (1 gm/kg) was given to mice. Bopiah (2000) also reported similar finding what the present study observed. It reveals that when 50 per cent ethanol extract of the formulated Ayurvedic product is administered in the mice, it increased swimming behavior in mice, (as compared to control group). Shoji (2000) also reported that the oral administration of Kyushin to mice at 90mg/kg increased the swimming duration significantly.

It can be thus concluded from this study that Ayurvedic Herbal preparation Adiantum Herbal 'could be effective for improving the stamina in female albino mice and male mice and this preparation can be used as antidepressant drug.

References

Abel, E.L., 1991. Gradient of alarm substance in the forced swimming test. *Physiol. Behaviour*, 49: 321–323.

Atendra, R.S. and Dixit, K.S., 1997. Effects of *Emblica officinalis* and *Aegle marmelos* on swimming induced stress in mice. *Indian Journal of Physiology and Pharmacology*, 41(5): 490A.

Bajaj, S. and Vohra, S.B., 1998. Analgesic activity of gold preparation used Ayurveda and Unani Tibb. *Indian Journ. Med. Res.*, 108: 104.

Bopaiah, C.P., Pradhan, N. and Venkataram, B.S., 2000. Pharmacological study antidepresent Ayurvedic product in rat. *J. Ethanopharmacol.*, 72(3): 411–419.

Dacic, J.V., 1968. *Hematology*, 6th Edition.

Greenen, D., Buttrick, P. and Scheuer, J., 1988. Caridiovascular and hormonal responses to swimming and running in the rat. *J. Appl. Physical.*, 65: 116–123.

Nadkarni, A.K. and Nadkarni, K.M., 1976. *Indian Materia Medica*, 3rd edn. Popular Prakashan, Bombay 2: 32.

Nagaraja, H.S. and Jaganathan, 1999. Forced swimming stress induced changes in the physiological and biochemical parameters in albino rats. *Indian J. Physiol Pharmacol.*, 43(1): 53.

Porsalt, R.D., Bertin, A. and Jalfre, M., 1977a. Behavioural despair in mice: A primary screening test for antidepressant. *Arch. Int. Pharmacol.*, 229: 327–336.

Porsolt, R.D., Anton L.G., Blavent N. and Jalfre, M., 1978a. Behavioural despair: A new model sensitive to antidepressant treatment. *Eur. J. Pharmacol.*, 47: 379–391.

Porsolt, R.D., Betrin, A. and Jalfre, M., 1978b. Behavioural despair in rats and mice: strain difference and effect of imipramine. *Eur J. Pharmacol.*, 51: 291–299.

Porsolt, R.D., Le Pichnon, M. and Jalfre M., 1977b. Depression: A new animal model sensitive to antidepressant. *Nature*, 277: 730–732.

Richter, C.P., 1957. On the Phenomenon of sudden death in animals and man. *Phychosom. Med.*, 9: 191–198.

Satya, K.S., Agrawala, S.K., Chauhan, S. and Ghosal, S., 2001. Effect of herbo-minerals formulation Ehb in experimental anaemia in rodents. *Indian Journal of Experimental Biology*, 39(7): 668–672.

Selye, H., 1956. In: *Stress of Life*. McCraw Hill Book Company, London, H, Stress, p. 18–38

Sharma, A.K. *et al.*, 1995. Ethnopharmacology of *Trichopus zeylanicus* and *Travancariaus* spp.: The ginseng of Kerala, India. In: *Glimpses of Ethnopharmacology*, (Eds.) P. Pushpangadan, U. Nyman V.V. George. TBGRI, Kerala, p. 137–145.

Shoji, M., Hosada, R. and Morishita, S.I., 2000. Prolongation swimming time by 'Kyushin' a drug containing senso (Chansu) and the related natural medicines. *Natural Medicines*, 54(5): 247–252.

Snedecor, G. and Cochran, W.G. *Statistical Method*, 7th Edn. Iowa State University Press. *Ames*. (IA), pp. 258.

Tan, N., Morimoto, K., Sugiura, T., Morimoto, A. and Murakami, N., 1992. Effect of running training on the blood glucose and lactate in rats during rest and swimming. *Physical Behav.*, 43: 41–46.

Vander, A., Sherman, J.H. and Luciano, D.S. *Human Physiology*, 5th edition, Mcgraw Hill, New York, p. 274–275.

Vogel, W.H., 1993. The effect of stress on toxicological investigations. *Human and Experimental Toxicology*, 12: 265–271.

Medicinal Plants: Conservation, Cultivation and Utilization (2007) *Pages 121–126*
Editors: A.K. Chopra, D.R. Khanna, G. Prasad, D.S. Malik and R. Bhutiani
Published by: DAYA PUBLISHING HOUSE

Chapter 17

Phytochemical, Antifungal and Antibacterial Studies of *Premna cordifolia* (Stem)

J.S. Jangwan[1], N.K. Agarwal[2] and J.S. Kathait[1*]
[1]School of Natural Product, Department of Chemistry, [2]Department of Zoology. HNB Garhwal University, SRT Campus, Badshahi Thaul – 249 199, Tehri Garhwal (U.A.) India

ABSTRACT

From stem bark of *Premna cordifolia* a mixture of saturated fatty acid (C_{15}-C_{31}), a flavonoid glycoside *Viz.* apigenin-7-0-β-D-glucoside have been isolated along with β-amyrin, sitigmasterol, taraxasterol, stearic, palmitic and ligneric acids. They have been characterized by IR, ^{1}H-NMR, ^{13}C-NMR and GC/MS studies. Ethanolic extract showed antifungal and antibacterial effects on various microorganism and fungal, yeast cells.

Keywords: Premna cordifolia, verbenaceae, fatty acid, flavonoid, Antifungal and antibacterial.

Introduction

Premna cordifolia (Verbenaceae) is a Shurb. Bark dark brown (Kanjilal *et al.*, 1982). The Plant is used in fever, headache and applied externally in dropsy (Kirtikar and Basu, 1975). A survey of literature revealed that no work has been reported on this plant although various iridoid glycosides and diterpenes have been reported from different species of genus premna (Sudo *et al.*, 1997a; Sudo *et al.*, 1997b; Sudo *et al.*, 1999).

* Corresponding Author: Telephone: 0137-6236827

Experimental

General experimental procedures: The melting points are uncorrected. IR Spectra were recorded on MIDAC, M-Series, FTIR Instrument. The ^{1}H-NMR Spectra were run at 400 MHZ and ^{13}C-NMR Spectra at 100.533 MHZ in pyridine -D_5 with TMS as internal standard GC/MS were recorded on (JEOL-JMS-D_{300} Spectrometer). Column Chromatography Silica Gel (Merk 60-120 Mesh), TLC kiesel gel 60G (Merk). The Spot on TLC were visualized by Spray with 10 per cent alcoholic H_2SO_4 and alcoholic $FeCl_3$ followed by heating paper Chromatography whatmman. No. 1 Paper using by decending mode and line hydrogen phthalate as the developer. The following System were used C_6H_6-EtoAc (9:1), C_6H_6-Me_2 Co (9:1), $CHCl_3$-MeOH (95:1), $CHCl_3$-MeOH (90:10).

Plant Material

The Plant Material was collected from Painula, Tehri Garhwal, U.A. (India) in the month of September. The authentification of pant material was made by Dr. R. Dayal, Scientist Taxonomy section, FRI, Dehradun U.A. (India).

Extraction and Isolation

The air dried and powdered stem bark (2kg.) were extracted with petroleum ether followed by extraction with ethanol. A waxy substance is obtained when the petroleum ether extract is concentrated. The waxy substance was saponified with ethanolic KOH (100 per cent) and the hydrolysate so obtained was extracted with ether two part were obtained Viz (Kirtikar and Basu, 1975). Ether soluble (non-saponifiable) (Kanjilal *et al.,* 1982). Ether insoluble (Saponifiable). From saponifiable portion, the presence of methyl esters of stearic, palmitic and ligneceric acids were established by paper chromatography (Lederer and Lederer, 1957). From non saponifiable portion of the hydrolysate, solvent was removed under reduced pressure when a yellowish brown solid was obtained. The solid on chromatographic resolution over silica gel resulted isolation of four compounds 1(160mg), 2(220mg), 3 (180mg) and 4 (130mg) respectively. Ehanolic extract on concentration under reduced pressure afforded a greenish mass. This solid mass was subjected to column chromatography over silica gel (Eluent $CHCl_3$:MeOH) resulted in the isolation of two compounds 5 (480mg) and 6 (220mg) respectively.

Characterization of Compound 1

White solid (160mg), (m.p.196-198°) Found: C, 84.35; H, 11.89 per cent; Calcd for: $C_{30}H_{50}O$; C, 84.50, H, 11.73 per cent; IR ι (kBr): 3350, 2940, 2880, 1680, 1385, 1370, MS: M/Z 426 (M^+) 411, 392, 151, 257, 234, 218, 207, 203, 189, 175, 169, 147, 133.

Characterization of Compound 2

White solid (220mg) m.p. 168-169°) Found: C, 84.70, H, 11.16 per cent; Calcd for: $C_{29}H_{48}O$; C, 84.68; H, 11.17 per cent IR. ι max (kBr) 3440,2960, 1640, 1465, 1445, 1375, 1365, 1070, 990, 958, 824 cm.$^{-1}$ NMR (DCl_3) δ (ppm) 0.70 (CH_3), 0.90 (s) 0.93 (d), 0.96 (d), 1.0 (s) and 5.3 (t) for OH group mass: m/z 412 (m+), 398, 380, 3br, 271,229 and 197.

Characterization of Compound 3

White needles (180mg) (m.p.220-222°). Found; C, 84.51, H,11.73 per cent; Calcd for: $C_{30}H_{50}O$. C, 8450, H, 11.72 per cent, IR ι max (kBr) 2470, 2980, 2960, 2855, 1650, 1460, 1375, 1050, cm^{-1}

Characterization of Compound 4

White needles (150mg) (m.p. 156-157°) Found: C, 73.05; H, 7.33 per cent; Calcd for: $C_{20}H_{24}O_4$. C, 73.17, H, 7.32 per cent IR ι max (kBr) 2900, 2820, 1745, 17br, 1450, 1200 cm^{-1} NMR: ($CDCl_3$) δ (ppm). 1.8

and 1.68 doublet of methyl group 4.75 to 5.2 (2H Oleifinic); 5.64 and 6.26 (exomethyline group) 17.05 (1HBr) 2.80 and 2.85 (methyline protones).

Characterization of Compound 5

White powder (420 mg) IR: ι max (kBr) cm^{-1} 1700 (carboxylic group) (2550, 1470, 1460, 923, 920 -CH_2-) group.

Characterization of Compound 6

Yellow needles (280 mg) (m.p. 227-229°). Found C, 58.30, H, 6.70 per cent; Calcd for: $C_{21}H_{20}O_{10}$ C, 58.33; H, 4.82 per cent UV: λ max (MeOH): 269, 390nm. λ (max) MeOH + NaOMe: 27,390 nm. λ (max/ MeOH + $AlCl_3$): 300, 350, 385 nm. IR (max) kBr: 3410, 1650, 1600, 1520, 1455, 1360, 1310, 1280, 1190, 1080, 1030, 850, 735, cm^{-1}. NMR ($CDCl_3$) δ (ppm) 6.80, (s, H-3), 6.60 (d, H-6), 6.88 (d H-8), 6.90 (d, H-3', 5'), 7.88 (d, H-2', 6'), 5.10 (d, J= 6.5 Hz, M, anomeric proton of sugar), 5.70 (-s, C_4-OH), 12.90 (s, 1H, C_5–OH), exchangeable with D_2O 3.90–4.20 cm^{-1} sugar protons.

Hydrolysis of 6

Hydrolysis of 6 was done with 7 per cent H_2SO_4 in usual manner the aglycone separated by ether extraction was identified as apigenin and the sugar was identified as glucose on the basis of paper chromatography.

Antibacterial and Antifungal Studies

Antibacterial Activity

The in vitro antibacterial activity of the sample solution was studied by agar diffusion method (Kavagh, 1970; Collins and Lyne, 1970). The test organism were seeded into sterile nutrient agar medium (Hi-media) by uniformly mixing one loopful of the inoculum with 20 ml of sterile melted nutrient agar after has been cooled to 48-50°C, Poured in a sterile petridish. When agar solidified, four holes of uniform diameter (6 mm) were made using a sterile borer. Then in each cup 50 µl from different concentrations of the extract such as 1µg/ml, 100 µg/ml, 1mg/ml, 50mg/ml and 100 mg/ml solution were added after dissolving in suitable quantities of propylene glycol. Simultaneous Controls with propylene glycol were also studied. Ampicillin (1µg/ml) was used as a standard drug for comparison. The plates were incubated at 37°C for 24 h. The zone of inhibition was calculated by measuring the minimum dimension of bacteria free zone around the cup.

Antifungal and antiyeast studies: The antifungal and antiyeast activities were tested by the same procedure described for testing antibacterial activity using potato dextrose agar medium (Hi-media). The standard drug to compare the antifungal and antiyeast activities was fluconazole (5µg/ml).

Result and Discussion

Compound 1 to 4 and 6 have been identified as β–amyrin, stigmasterol, Taraxasterol, ovaloliolide and apigenin–7-0-β-D–glucose respectively on the basis of comparing their spectral data. Co-TLC. Co-IR, mixed m.p with that of authentic samples (Jones *et al.*, 1958; Dominguez and Rojas, 1973; Immer *et al.*, 1965; Phillips, 1972). The characterization of 5 as a mixture of aliphatic carboxylic acid [C_{15}-C_{31}]. The compound exhibited the present of carboxylic 1710 cm^{-1} and–CH_2–(2550, 1470, 1469, 930, and 920) groups in the IR spectrum. Based on this observation and GC/MS studies (Phillips, 1972) (CF Figure 17.1). The compound was identified as mixture of aliphatic carboxylic acids (C_{15}–C_{31}) having the general formula n–$C_n H_{2n+1}$ COOMe. The relative quantities were n–$C_{15} H_{31}$ COOMe 6.9 per cent;

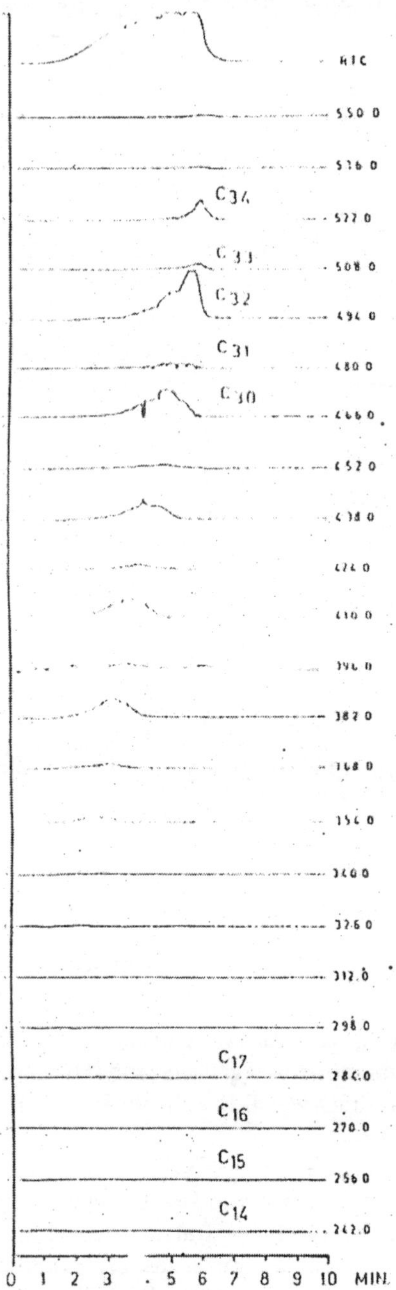

GC/MS. of mixture- of aliphatic fatty acids.

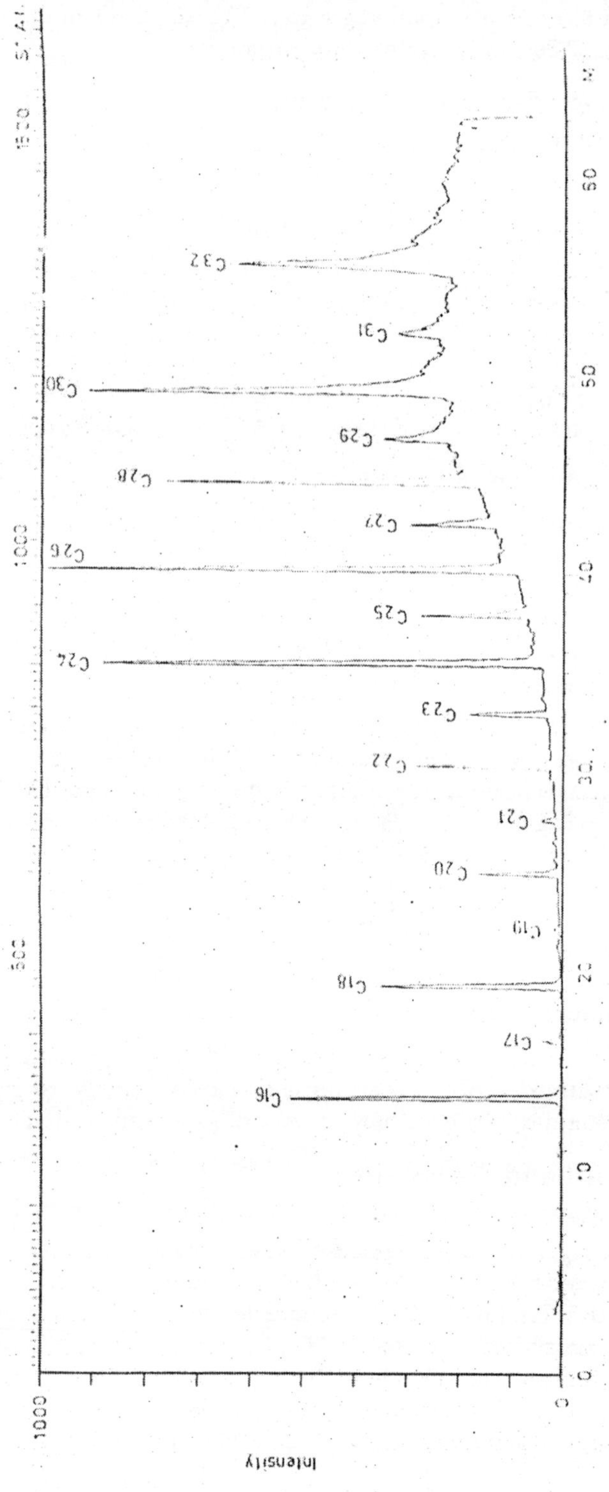

Figure 17.1: Gas Chromatography of Mixture of Aliphatic Fatty Acids

n–$C_{16}H_{31}$ COOMe 3 per cent; n–$C_{17}H_{35}$ COOMe 5.3 per cent; n–$C_{18}H_{37}$ COOMe 0.1 per cent; n–$C_{19}H_{39}$ COOMe 1.8 per cent; n–$C_{20}H_{41}$ COOMe 0.2 per cent; n–$C_{21}H_{43}$ COOMe 3.9 per cent; n–$C_{22}H_{45}$ COOMe 1.7 per cent; n–$C_{23}H_{47}$ COOMe 3.9 per cent; n–$C_{24}H_{49}$ COOMe 2.7 per cent; n–$C_{25}H_{51}$ COOMe 13.8 per cent; n–$C_{26}H_{53}$ COOMe 2.3 per cent; n–$C_{27}H_{55}$ COOMe 10.1 per cent; n–$C_{28}H_{57}$ COOMe 2.3 per cent; n–$C_{29}H_{59}$ COOMe 20.1 per cent; n–$C_{30}H_{61}$ COOMe 1.8 per cent; n–$C_{31}H_{63}$ COOMe 15.6 per cent.

Antibacterial, Antifungal/Antiyeast Activity of Alcoholic Extract of Tested Plant Sample

The zone of inhibition obtained with different concentrations of the extract and of the standard drugs were shown in Table 17.1. the alcoholic extract of *Premna cordifolia* was found to be having antimicrobial activity in a dose dependent manner (1µg/ml, 100 µg/ml, 1µg/ml, 50µg/ml and 100 µg/ml) against all the test organism. Significant activity was found with the extract at a concentration of 100 µg/ml, as compared with standard. This study provides Justification for the use of the Plant in folk medicine to treat various infectious disorders.

Table 17.1: Effect of Alcoholic Extract of *P. nepaulese* on the Selected Strains of Microorganism

Type	*Strain*	*Zone of Inhibition*				*Standard**	*Control (Propylene Glycol)*
		100 µg/ml	*1 µg/ml*	*50 µg/ml*	*100 µg/ml*		
Gram Postive Bacteria	*B. Subtils*	11	13	18	17	20	0
	B. Pumilus	07	10	13	16	18	0
	S. aureus	08	08	02	16	13	0
	M. glutamicus	09	–	15	18	19	0
Gram negative Bacteria	*P. aeroginosa*	07	10	–	18	19	0
	P. valgaris	11	13	15	10	18	0
	P. marcescens	08	11	18	12	20	0
	E. coli	09	11	12	11	16	0
Fungi	*A. niger*	07	10	03	19	16	0
	R. oryzae	08	12	16	18	17	0
	A. wentii	10	–	16	18	22	0
Yeast	*S. cerevisiae*	12	09	17	12	20	0
	C. lunata	09	08	06	13	19	0

* Standard: For antibacterial activity–ampicillin (1µg/ml); For antifungal activity-fluconazole (5µg/ml); and antiyeast.

Acknowledgement

Our thanks are due to Prof. Hideaki otsuka, department of Pharmacognosy, School of Biomedical science Kasumi, minami–ku Hiroshima, Japan for recording spectra (IR, NMR, GC/MS) and thanks are also due to Dr. Iqbal Ahmad, Asstt. Prof., Dept. of Agricultural microbiology faculty of agricultural science, Aligarh muslim University, Aligarh, U.P. (India) for performing antibacterial antifungal/ antiyeast activity.

Reference

Collins, C.H. and Lyne, P.M., 1970. *Microbial Method*. Baltimic Park Press.

Dominguez, X.A., and Rojas, P., 1973. *Phytochemistry*, 12 (1): 224.

Heilborn, I. and Bunbury, H.M., 1953. *Dictionary of Organic Compound*. Eyne and Spottis Woode, London, 1: 158.

Immer, H., Polonsky, J. and Toubiana, R., 1965. *Tetrahedron*, 21(8): 2117–2131.

Jones, R.N. *et al.*, 1958. *J. Amer. Chem. Soc.*, 80: 612.

Kanjilal, U.N., Das, A., Kanjilal, P.C. and De, R.N., 1982. *Flora of Assam*, 3: 471–472.

Kavagh, F., 1970. *Analytical Microbiology*. Academic Press, New York.

Kirtikar, K.L. and Basu, B.D., 1975. *Indian Medicinal Plants*. Periodical Experts, Delhi, 3: 1926–1931.

Lederer, E. and Lederer, M., 1957. *Chromatography*. Elsiever Publication, pp. 189.

Phillips, C.J., 1972. *Gas Chromatography*. Academic Press, New York.

Sudo, Hirokazu, Ide and Toshihori, 1997. *Phytochemistry*, 46(6): 1147–1150.

Sudo, Hirokazu, Ide and Toshihori, 1997. *Phytochemistry*, 46(7): 1231–1236.

Sudo, Hirokazu, Takushi,Anki, Hirata and Eiji, 1999. *Phytochemistry*, 51(8): 1495–1499.

Medicinal Plants: Conservation, Cultivation and Utilization (2007) *Pages 127–131*
Editors: A.K. Chopra, D.R. Khanna, G. Prasad, D.S. Malik and R. Bhutiani
Published by: DAYA PUBLISHING HOUSE

Chapter 18

Phytochemical Examination of *Pittosporum nepaulense* and its Effect on Microorganism as an Antibacterial Agent

J.S. Kathait[1*], Veena Joshi[1], N.K. Agarwal[2], J.S. Jangwan[1]
[1]School of Natural Product, [2]Department of Zoology
Department of Chemistry, H.N.B. Garhwal University,
S.R.T. Campus Badshahi Thaul – 249 199, Tehri Garhwal (U.A) India

ABSTRACT

From methanolic extract of stem bark of *Pittosporum nepaulense* gave n-Hexacosamic acid, Lupeol and ursolic acid. They have been isolated and characterized by column chromatography, Co-TLC IR, ^{1}H-NMR, ^{13}C-NMR, FAB–MS, spectroscopical studies. These compounds exhibited antibacterial activities against different microorganism.

Keywords: *Pittosporum nepaulense, Antibacterial, Microorganism Phytocompound, Inhibition zone, Acids.*

Introduction

Pittosporum Nepaulense (Pittosporaceae) is a small ever green tree, bark graynish with large warty lenticels. It is use in rheumatism, chest affection and phthisis and leprosy (Gaur, 1999; Kirtikar and Basu, 1975a). A survey of literature revealed that no wark has been reported on this plant. Although

* Corresponding Author: Phone –01376- 236827.

some terpenoid glycosides have been reported from other species (Raguse Consolacion and John, 1997; Yasioka *et al.*, 1972; Ogihawa *et al.*, 1989).

Experimental

General Experimental Procedures: The melting point are uncorrected. IR spectra were recorded on MIDAC, M-Series, FTIR instrument. The ^{1}H-NMR Spectra were run at 400 MHZ and ^{13} C–NMR Spectra at 100.533 MHZ in pyridine–d_5 with TMS as internal standard. Mass spectra (70 ev, JEOL–TMS-DX 300 spectrometer). Column chromatography silica gel (merk 60-120 mesh). TLC Kiesel gel 60 G (Merk). The spot on TLC Were visualized by spray with 10 per cent alcoholic H_2SO_4 and alcoholic $FeCl_3$ followed by heating paper Chromatography whatman No. 1 paper using by descending mode and line hydrogen phthalate as the developer. The following system were used C_6H_6-EtoAc (9:1), C_6H_6–me_2 Co–(9:1) $CHCl_3$–MeOH (95:1).

Plant Material

The plant material was collected from painula, Tehri Garhwal, U.A. (India) in the month of September. The authentification of plant material was made by Dr. R. Dayal, Scientist Taxonomy section, FRI, Dehradun U.A. India.

Extraction and Isolation

The air dried and powdered stem bark (2Kg) were extracted with petroleum ether followed by extraction with ethanol. A waxy substance was obtained when the petroleum ether extract is concentrated. The waxy substance was Saponified with ethanolic KOH (100 per cent) and the hydrolysate so obtained was extracted with ether two part were obtained *viz.* (Kirtikar and Basu, 1975b). Ether soluble (non-saponifiable) (Kanjilal *et al.*, 1982). Ether insoluble (saponifiable). From saponifiable portion the presence of methyl esters of stearic and palmitic acids were established by paper chromatography (Lederer and Lederer, 1957). From non–Saponifiable portion of the hydrolysate, solvent was removed under reduced pressure when a yellowish brown solid was obtained. The solid on chromatography resolution over silica gel resulted isolation of three compound 1 (500 mg), 2 (300 mg) and 3 (150mg) respectively.

Characterization of Compound 1

White solid (500mg), (m.p 86-87°); Found: C, 78.70; H, 13.29 per cent. Calcd for: $C_{26}H_{52}O_2$; C, 78.78; H, 13.13 per cent. IR √ max (KBr): 3226-2950, 2788, 1725, 730 and 720 Cm^{-1}. NMR: ($CDCl_3$) δ (ppm)0.85(t); 1.22(m, broad band) and 3.60 (t) MS M/Z: 396 (M^+).

Characterization of Compound 2

White solid (300mg), (m.p 215-216°); Found: C, 84.50; H,11.73 per cent. Calcd for: $C_{30}H_{50}O$; C, 84.51; H, 11.72 per cent. IR √ max (KBr): 3440, 2970, 2959, 2920, 2859, 1463, 1380, 1055 CM^{-1}.

Characterization of Compound 3

White solid (150mg), (m.p 266-267°); RF: 0.53 [α]+6° (Pyridine); Found: C= 78.72 per cent; H=10.74 per cent. Calcd for: $C_{30}H_{48}O_3$; C= 78.94 per cent; H = 10.52 per cent. Molecular Weight: 456, IR $\surd^{KBr}_{max}$ Cm^{-1}: 3400, 3140, 2930, 2880, 1680, 1450, 1390, 1325, 1300, 1250, 1190, 1070, 1030, 980, 930, 880 and 745 Cm^{-1} EIMS: m/z 456 $[m]^+$, 411, 248, 208, 203 and 190. ^{1}H-NMR: δ (ppm) 0.98, 1.74 (21H, 7x CH_3), 0.84 (d, 2x CH–CH_3), 1.0 (s, 3xC-CH_3), 1.8–2.1 (m, 23H,–CH_2 and–CH-), 3.42 (s, CH–OH); 5.5 (s, olefinic H) and 9.2 (s, 1H,–COOH).

Antibacterial Studies Against various Microorganism

The in vitro antibacterial activity of the sample solution was studied by agar diffusion method (Kavagh, 1970; Collins, and Lyne, 1970). The test organism were seeded into sterile nutrient agar medium (Hi–media) by uniformly mixing one loopful of the inoculum with 20 ml of sterile, melted nutrient agar after has been cooled to 48 –50°c, poured in a sterile petridish. When agar solidified, from holes of uniform diameter (6 mm) were made using a sterile borer. Then in each cup 50 per cent from different concentration of the extract such as 0.5 per cent, 1 per cent, 2 per cent of petroleum ether, chloroform, methanol respectively, solution were added after dissolving in suitable quantities of propylene glycol. The plates were incubated at 37°C for 24h. The Zone of inhibition was calculated by measuring the minimum dimension of bacterial free zone around the cup.

Result and Discussion

Compound 1

1 (homogeneous in TLC) was assigned molecular formula as $C_{26}H_{52}O_2$ on the basis of elemental analysis and molecular weight determination (M^+ 396). It gave effervescence in cold with a saturated solution of sodium bicarbonate, indicating the presence of free carboxylic group in compounds. It did not decolourise potassium permanganate solution or bromine in carbon tetrachloride as well as gave negative test with TNM (Ruzicka and Liebigs, 1929). All these test indicated 1 as a saturated aliphatic carboxyl acid. This has been further confirmed by infrared spectral studies where in the characteristic absorption band at ι max (KBr) 2851, 2788, 1725 (C=O stretching)1468,732 and 720 cm^{-1} were observed. The spectrum of compound also showed a broad absorption band at 1055 cm^{-1} was due to the C-O stretching vibration of carboxylic group on ethylation of compond from a methyl ester $C_{16}H_{51}OCOCH_3$ (m.p. 60-61°) which indicated the presence of one carboxylic group in the molecule.In the NMR spectrum of the compound a triple centred at δ0.85 for 3H was observed which indicated the presence of one methyl group. A large broad methyl signal at δ1.22 interesting for 46H gave the indication for the presence of twenty three methylene group $(-CH_2-)_{23}$ and a signal as triplet for 2H at δ3.60 indicated the methylene group bonded to carboxylic group. In the mass spectrum, the molecular ion peak appeared at m/z 396. The intense peak at m/z 60 resulting from the cleavage at C=O group followed by rearrangement of hydrogen confirmed its carboxylic acid nature. The other peaks which appeared at an internal of the mass units by successive loss of $-CH_2$-group confirmed its long chain nature. On the basis of above observation, the structure of 1 was confirmed as n-hexacosamic acid [CH_3 $(CH_2)COOH$] (reported, m.p. δ7.7-87.9°)[24]. It was further confirmed by its m.p. and Co-TLC, superimposable IR spectrum when compared with that of authentic sample.

Compound 2

The molecular formula of 2 (m.p. 215-216°, found homogeneous in TLC) was assigned as $C_{30}H_{50}O$ on the basis of elemental analysis and molecular weight determination (Rast method). It was easily soluble in petroleum ether, ether, benzene, chloroform and carbon tetrachloride, sparingly soluble in ethanol and methanol. Compound responded to Lebermann-Burchard test (Liebermann, 1884) (violet colour changing to blue green) and Noller's test (Noller *et al.*, 1942) (produced red colour). Those colour reaction indicated it to be a triterpenoid. Red colour with chlorosulphonic acid and violet colour in the Brieskorne test (Brieskrone and Briner, 1953) also suggested that the compound was a triterpenoid. It gave positive test with tetranitro methane (Ruzicka and Liebigs, 1929) (yellow colour), thereby indicating the presence of unsaturation in the molecule. The characteristic absorption bands as observed in the IR spectrum were at ι max (KBr) 3440 (OH), 2970, 2959, 2920, 2859 (C-H Stretching), 1463, 1380 (gem-dimethyl groups) and 1055 cm^{-1} (C-O Stretching). Compound gave monoacetate (m.p. 216°) on acetylation with the appearance of characteristic acetyl band at ι max (KBr) 1735 cm^{-1}, showing the presence of a hydroxyl group in the molecule which was further confirmed by characteristic absorption band at 3440cm^{-1} in its IR spectrum. From all the observation 2 appeared to be Lupeol (β-Viscol). It was identified by the direct comparison of mixed m.p. Co-TLC and superimposable IR with those of the authentic sample of Lupeol and also confirmed by the preparation of its acetyl derivative (reported, m.p. 216°) as described above.

Compound 3

It was crystallized from methanol as colourless flakes, m.p. 266-267°C. It gave positive test with Liebermann-Burchard (Liebermann, 1884). Nollers reagent (Noller *et al.*, 1942) and TNM (Ruzicka and Liebigs, 1929). On the basis of elemental analysis, molecular formula was established as $C_{30}H_{48}O_{3.}$ The DBE [(30 + 1)–48/2] which showed presence of 7 double bond equivalent in the compound C, the characteristic absorption band in IR at cm^{-1} 3400 (OH streething), 3140 (OH strectching of COOH group), 2930, 2880 (-CH stretching), 1680 (C=O stretching), 1450 (CH_2 deformation), 1390, 1325, 1300, 1250, (characteristic of ursane series). It formed a monoacetyl derivative (m.p. 276°C) thus indicating the presence of one OH group. In ^{1}H-NMR spectrum ($CDCl_3$ δppm TMS) the presence of 7-Methyl group for 21H was observed in the region of 0.68-1.74. Two secondary methyl groups were presented at δ0.84 (d, J=6.0 Hz). Whereas five tertiary methyl at δ1.0 (s, 5xC-CH_3). A multiplet at 1.5-3.2 with side bands indicating the presence of 23H accounting for –CH_2-and –CH-protons. The hydroxyl methine (broad triplet) was observed at δ3.42 indicating the presence of pentacylic triterpenoid, vinylic proton was observed at δ5.5 and the –COOH proton at δ9.2. Thus the nature of 48 protons of the compound was established. In the El mass spectrum the molecular ion peak of compound 3 was observed at m/z 456$(M)^+$. The base peak was observed at m/z 203. Other peaks were recorded at m/z 411 (c), 248(b), (a), 203(e), 190(d), and 133. The peaks at m/z 248, 208 and 203 confirmed the presence of hydroxyl at C-3 and carboxylic at C-17 in the compound. Thus, on the basic of aforementioned spectral data, the structure of compound 3 was assigned as 3-β-hydroxyl–Δ^{12}-Ursan-28-oic acid or ursolic acid (Ganapathy *et al.*, 1993). The identity was confirmed by comparison with an authentic sample (Co-TLC, Co-IR and mmp).

Antibacterial Studies of tested sample against various microorganism: The zones of inhibition obtained with different concentration of the plant extract and of the standard drugs were shown in Table 18.1 and 18.2. Those sample of *Pittosporum nepaulense* was found to be having anti–bacterial activity in the dose depending manner (0.5 per cent, 1.0 per cent, 2.0 per cent) against all the test organism. All the fraction of *Pittosporum nepaulense* (stem and leaf) showed significant activity against the tested organism. This study provides justification for the use of the plant in folk medicine to treat various infectious disorders.

Table 18.1: Antibacterial Activity of Stem Extract* of *Pittosporum nepaulense*

Microorganism	*Zone of inhibition in m.m.*								
	Petroleum Ether			*Chloroform*			*Methanol*		
	0.5%	*1%*	*2 %*	*0.5%*	*1%*	*2%*	*0.5%*	*1%*	*2%*
Salmonella typhii	1	3	–	16	2	14	18	3	1
Aromonas hydrophilla	6	12	3	8	12	15	–	–	13
Escherichia coli	2	1	2	6	2	3	6	12	16
Strptomycin	1	7	7	12	18	17	4	–	3
Amplicillin	8	5	12	5	1	3	1	3	1

* Value of the mean of three replicates.

–: No inhibition.

Table 18.2: Antibacterial Activity of Leaf Extract* of *Pittosporum nepaulense*

Microorganism	*Zone of inhibition in m.m.*								
	Petroleum Ether			*Chloroform*			*Methanol*		
	0.5%	*1%*	*2 %*	*0.5%*	*1%*	*2%*	*0.5%*	*1%*	*2%*
Salmonella typhii	4	2	6	1	3	8	2	6	1
Aromonas hydrophilla	2	1	2	–	–	5	–	17	2
Escherichia coli	1	3	4	2	4	7	3	16	1
Strptomycin	7	9	15	1	12	15	1	6	12
Amplicillin	5	7	13	3	6	9	14	9	16

* Value of the mean of three replicates.

–: No inhibition.

Acknowledgement

Our thanks are due to Prof. Hideaki otsuka, Department of Pharmacognosy, School of Biomedical Science Kasumi, Minami-Ku, Hiroshima, Japan, For recording spectra (IR, UV, NMR, FABMS, FD/MS) and thanks are also due to Dr. Iqbal Ahmad, Asstt. Prof. Department of Agricultural microbiology, Faculty of agricultural sciences, Aligarh Muslim University, Aligarh, U.P. (India) for performing antibacterial activity.

References

Brieskrone, C.H. and Briner, M., 1953. *Pharm. Act. Melv.*, 28: 139.

Collins, C.H. and Lyne, P.M., 1970. *Microbial Methods*. Baltimac Park Press.

Ganapathy, S., and D. Venkata Rao, 1993. *Fitoterapia*, 54: 13.

Gaur, R.D., 1999. *Flora of the District Garhwal North-West Himalaya*. Transmedia, Srinagar Garhwal. pp. 211.

Kanjilal, U.N., Das, A., Kanjilal, P.C. and De, R.N., 1982. *Flora of Assam*, 3: 471–472.

Kavagh, F., 1970. *Analytical Microbiology*. Academic Press, New York.

Kirtikar, K.L. and Basu, B.D., 1975a. *Indian Medicinal Plants*. Periodical Experts, Delhi, 1: 229.

Kirtikar, K.L. and Basu, B.D., 1975b. *Indian Medicinal Plants*. Periodical Experts, Delhi, 3: 1926–1931.

Lederer, E. and Lederer, M., 1957. *Chromatography*. Elsiever Publication, pp. 189.

Liebermann, C., 1884. *Ber. Deusch. Chem. Ges.*, pp. 1804.

Noller, C.R., Smith, R.A., Harris, G.H. and Walkar, J.N., 1942. *J.Amer. Chem. Soc.*, 44: 3047.

Ogihawa, Kazuhito, Munesada, Kiyotoka, Suya and Takayuki, 1989. *Phytochemistry*, 28(11): 3085–3091.

Raguse Consolacion, Y. and John, A., 1997. *Phytochemistry*, 53(3): 545–547.

Ruzicka, L. and Liebigs, R., 1929. *Ame. Chem.*, 25: 471.

Yasioka, Itiro, Hino, Katsuhiko, Matsuda, Akiko and Kitagawa, Isao, 1972. *Chem. Pharm. Bull.*, 20(7): 1499–506.

Medicinal Plants: Conservation, Cultivation and Utilization (2007) *Pages 133–137*
Editors: A.K. Chopra, D.R. Khanna, G. Prasad, D.S. Malik and R. Bhutiani
Published by: DAYA PUBLISHING HOUSE

Chapter 19

Isolation of Active Chemical Constituents and Study of Active Anticancer Alkaloid from the Root Extract of *Pongamia pinnata* (Vent)

Pawan Kumar Sagar
State Drug Testing Laboratory, Rishikul Government Ayurvedic Pharmacy, Haridwar, Uttaranchal

ABSTRACT

A preliminary extracted and Isolated medicinal value analysis for medicinal plant has been carried out which act against cleaning foul ulcers, flat ulcer gonorrhea, anticancer. In the first phase of spectral and structural analysis medicinal plant *Pongamia pinnata (Vent)* have been screened which are used in the treatment of various ulcer and leprosy, cancer disease. It is found that the plants contain a number of secondary metabolites and have the pharmacological actions. Isolated medicinal value analysis confirms in alkaloids and steroids with active chemical constituents of alcoholic root extract of *Pongamia pinnata* medicinal plant promote act against the treatment of Cancer, Ulcers, Gonorrhea.

Keywords: Medicinal value, Isolation, Fractionated compound, Flat ulcer, Cleaning ulcer, Anticancer alkaloid.

Introduction

The paramount impotence of naturally occurring plants extraction has been well demand. Many Herbal preparation contained mixture of natural drugs extract. Different drugs of the herbal formulation, contain the same classes of the compounds. Identification of the characteristics is usually possible. In view of the extensive work on natural product *Pongamia pinnata* (*vent*) promminative species many of which are medicinal value as contained. Aromatic and Hetrocyclic active compound. The medicinal value of the *Pongamia pinnata (Vent)* in cancer, cleaning foul ulcer, flat ulcer, gonorrhea.These contain active medicinal value constitute found to analyze of spectral and structural by H'NMR, F.T.I.R and separation technique by T.L.C, column chromatography etc[1]. Authentic Ayurvedic medicinal plant material of *Pongamia pinnata (Karanja)* was produced northern Uttaranchal and Himalaya region of India. Two types of species are found in this region: 1. *Pongamia pinnata (vent)*, 2. *Pongamia globra*. A test sample of natural product material *Pongamia pinnata* (*vent*) plant part has collected from the Gurukula Ayurvedic Medical College, G.K University Haridwar (Uttranchal). It is washed, mixed and obtained natural product plant material in the form of powder (Sivarajan and Balchandran, 1994).

Materials and Methods

The plants were collected during their flowering periods Nov-Dec to May-June and identified with the help of standard flora. Isolated medicinal value and active chemical constituents screening approach of the medicinal plant has been done. The plant has been isolated of chemical constituent and fractionated compound. The medicinal plants used against cancer (liver) were screened for the presence of anticancer alkaloids and steroids by the conventional methods proposed reference (Troup and Sanskaran, 1956-57; Bhushan and Narayanan, 1960; Patel and Yawalkar, 1963; Bhattacharya and Das, 1969). The root part of the plant was collected and freezes air-dried either by exposing to sunlight. It is than coarsely powdered and each part of the plant is then extracted with 150 ml Methanol, (95 per cent), 150 ml Ethyl Alcohol (95 per cent), 150 ml Acetone, 150 ml Benzene, 150 ml Petroleum ether and fluid for 72 hours in an air tight conical flask using soxhlet extract on assembly. The filtrates were subjected for identification as given under chemical test and separated of fractions using T.L.C, column chromatography techniques. The structural and spectral analysis has done through H'NMR, FT-IR, UV-visible spectroscopy analysis of medicinal fractionated test sample (Jai Shanker and Basu, 1961; Prasad and Kaul, 1987; Sagar and Paliwal, 2003). Extract of Herbal and Natural drug determined from Chromatography displays a large number of more or less overlapping zones (UV and Visible) so that identification and classification of the compounds present is difficult, only partly successful. In such cases it is necessary to submit the preparation to column chromatographic fractionation or other special procedures for the separation of individual classes of compounds (Jai Shanker and Basu, 1961; Prasad and Kaul, 1987; Sagar and Paliwal, 2003). If the different Herbal and Natural drugs of their formulation contain the some classes of compounds and active principles identification of the characteristics compounds is usually possible. Chromatography (T.L.C.) Detection:Useing Stationary Phase-T.L.C layer plate, 40 × 20 cm and 100 × 20 cm, Thickness of the coated plates with Si-gel range 1-2 mm, Adsorbent Silica gel-G grade (with binder), Mobile phase-(Used Solvent System)-Methanol-petroleum ether 7:1 v/v ratio, Detection Range-Visible region 400-780 nm, U.V region 200-390 nm. Column Chromatography Detection:Useing Stationary Phase-Column length-125cm, Column dia-22 cm, Adsorbent-Silica gel-H grade (without), Mobile phase, (Used Solvent system)-Methanol-petroleum ether 7:1 v/v ratio, Detection-Visible region 400-780 nm, U.V region 200-390 nm.

Extracted material were subjected to the study of R_f, valves, λ^{max}, I.R., H'NMR spectroscopy from advance techniques of active chemical constituents having medicinal value of separated fractions, which have contain anticancer alkaloid compound. Determination of active chemical constituent having medicinal value: Separated fractions, Active chemical constituents, Medicinal values are as respectively:-C-A/F-B, Paclitaxel(Anticancer Alkaloid); C-B/F-E, Fluorophenylanine (Anticancer Immune Stimulant); C-C/F-A, Vinblastin sulphate(Anticancer Alkaloid); C-D/F-A, Vincristine sulphate(Anticancer Alkaloid); C-E/F-D, Tenoporide (Anticancer Cell Cycle Regulator); C-F/F-C, Oetoposide(Anticancer Cell Cycle Regulator).

Column Chromatography Separation of Medicinal Extracts

Table 19.1: Separation of Root Extract Part (Room Temperature: 27–28°C Humidity: 46 per cent)

Sl.No.	*Separation Fraction*	*Colour Appearance of Separated Fractions*	*λ_{max} (nm)*	*R_F Value (cm)*
1.	A	Greenish Yellow	606	0.131
2.	B	Light Reddish	613	0.181
3.	C	Light Yellowish Orange	736	0.135
4.	D	Light Yellow	604	0.155

Table 19.2: Separation of Leaves Extract Part (Room Temperature: 27–28°C Humidity: 46 per cent)

Sl.No.	*Separation Fraction*	*Colour Appearance of Separated Fractions*	*λ_{max} (nm)*	*R_F Valuo (om)*
1.	A	Dark Green	613	0.103
2.	B B1	Greenish	536	0.1067
	B2	Yellowish Orange	565	0.1108
	B3	Light Green	531	0.1153
3.	C C1	Yellowish	554	0.1067
	C2	Yellowish Green	562	0.1125
	C3	Light Green	548	0.1222
4.	D	Yellow Orange	614	0.1043

Results and Discussion

In modern medicine system there are lots of uses of herbal and natural products drugs for both permanent and temporary diseases. During the course of physiological activities. Some chemicals in the form of secondary metabolites are synthesized in the medicinal plant. Most of the active chemical constituents have a very significant therapeutic action on the human health system. Keeping these things under consideration has been isolated medicinal value screened. The presence of R_f, λ^{max} I.R., H'NMR response of separated fractions and various active chemical constituents having medicinal value of anticancer alkaloid are summarized in given Figure 19.1. Some of the Anticancer alkaloids of active chemical constituents found anticancer compound such as Paclitaxel, Fluorophenylaline, Vinblastin, Vincristine (sulphate). (given in Figure 19.1, C-A/F-B, C-B/F-E, C-C/F-A, C-D/F-A." and Teniposide, Fluoxetine, Oetoposide derivative, C-E/F-C,C-G/F-D,C-G/F-D, are present in root extract of medicinal plant *Pongamia pinnata (vent.)*. These compounds of anticancer alkaloids performed exclusive properties against cancer such as found cells cycle regulator of cancer cell and immune stimulant against cancer cell cure of patients. The present investigation is the obvious lines of feature research find out the active chemical constituents principles of biochemical analysis of natural product, which act against cancer (Sagar and Paliwal, 2003).

Figure 19.1 (With Fraction Coding)

C-A/F-B

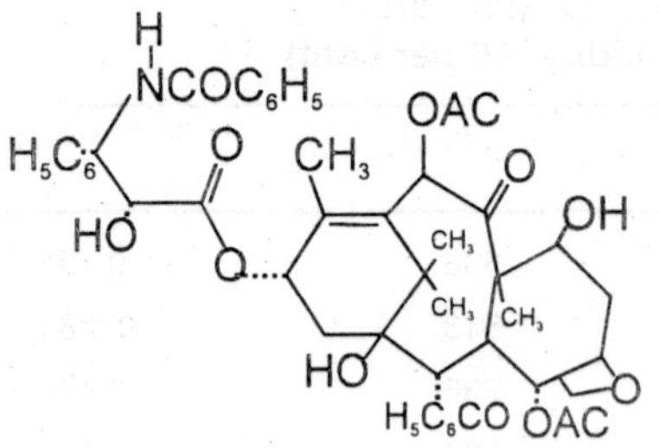

Paclitaxel

C-B/F-E

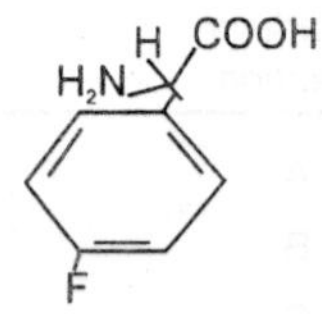

Fluorophenylalanine

C-C/F–A

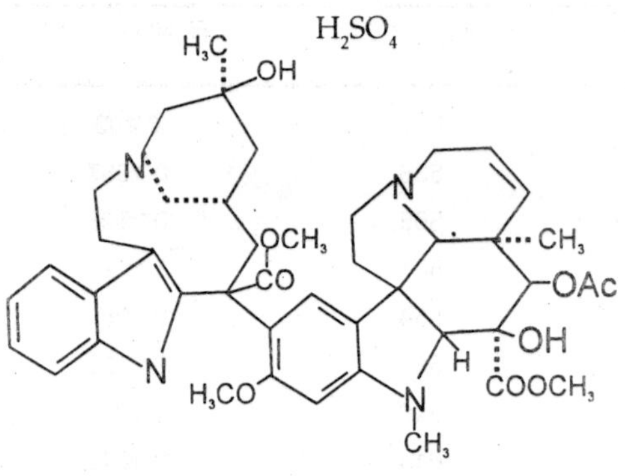

Vinblastine Sulphate

C-D/F–A

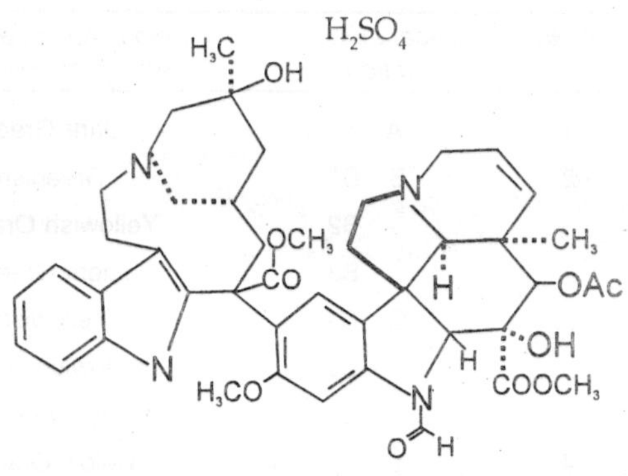

Vincristine Sulphate

C-E/F-D

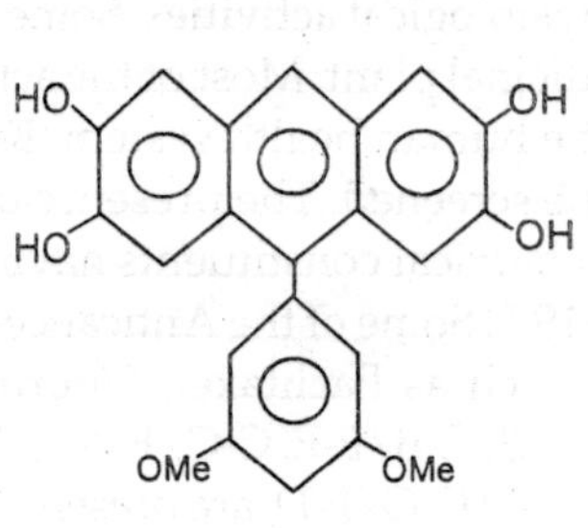

Teniposide

C-F/F-C

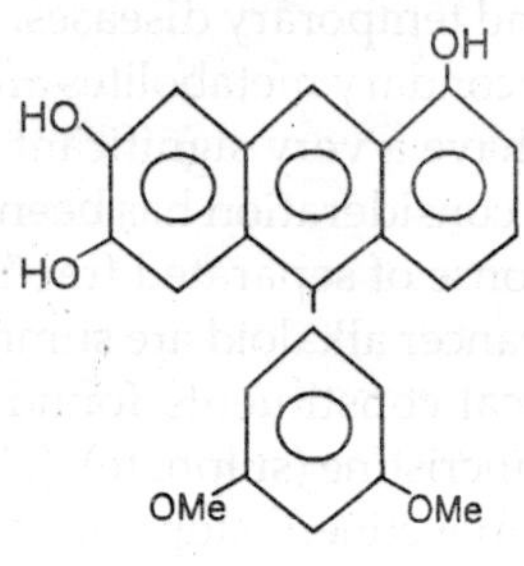

Oetoposide

Acknowledgement

Grateful thanks are due to Dr. R.K Paliwal (Former), Prof. and Head of Department of chemistry, Gurukul Kangri University Haridwar, Uttaranchal, Dr. Navneet Kumar Department of Microbiology, Gurukul Kangri University Haridwar, Uttranchal. Extends the sincere thanks to Dr. Raj kumar (scientist) I.N.M.A.S, D.R.D.O, New Delhi,for providing advance research study.

References

Bhattacharya, A.K. and Das, A.K., 1969. *Quart. J. Crude Drugs Res.*, 9: 1408.

Bhushan and Narayanan, *ibid.*, 1960. 4, 30, 93, Patelan 179.

Jai Shanker and Basu, N.K., 1961. Separation of Kurchi alkaloids by paper chromatography. In: *Proc. Rajasthan Acad. Scie.* 8: 88.

Patel and Yawalkar, *ibid.*, 1963. pp. 7.

Prasad, S. and Kaul, P.N., 1987. Seasonal variation in the alkaloidal content kurchi bark. *Indian J. Pharma.*, 19: 131.

Ruyter, Carl Michael and Mahmood, Akram, 1991. Investigation of the alkaloidal content of *Rauwalfia serpentina* root. *Planta Med.*, 57(4): 328–330.

Sagar, P.K. and Paliwal, R.K., 2003. Isolation and Study of active material having medicinal value present in *Pongamia pinnata (vent.)*, p. 103–106.

Siphahi, B.D., Malani, A.T. and Heble, M.R., 1990. Growth and alkaloid production in different cell lines of *Catharanthus roseus* (L) G.Don. *Ind. J. Exp. Biol.*, 28(6): 516–518.

Sivarajan, V.V. and Balchandran Indira, 1994. *Ayurvedic Drugs and their Plant Sources*, pp. 215.

Smith, J.L., Smart, N.J., Kurz, W.G.W. and Misawa, 1987. The use of organic and Inorganic compounds to increase the accumulation of indole alkaloids in *Catharanthus roseus* (L) G.Don cell suspension culture. *J. Exp. Bot.*, 38(194): 1501–1506.

Troup, I. and Sanskaran, 1956–57. *Indian Oil seeds J.*, pp. 331, 224, 347.

Troup, I. and Sanskaran, 1959. *Indian Oil seeds J.*, pp. 3, 179.

Medicinal Plants: Conservation, Cultivation and Utilization (2007) *Pages 139–146*
Editors: A.K. Chopra, D.R. Khanna, G. Prasad, D.S. Malik and R. Bhutiani
Published by: DAYA PUBLISHING HOUSE

Chapter 20

Antibacterial Activity of Medicinal Plants Against Dental Infections

Prabhat and Navneet
Department of Botany and Microbiology, Gurukul Kangri University, Hardwar – 249 404

ABSTRACT

The extracts of six medicinal plants *i.e. Terminalia chebula, Mimusops elengi, Achyranthes aspera, Acacia catechu, A. arabica* and *Glycyrrhiza glabra* were prepared in four different solvents *i.e.* petroleum ether, acetone, methanol and water. Each extract was tested for their antibacterial activity against five dental infection bacteria *(Staphylococcus aureus,Streptococcus mutans, S.salivarius, S.sanguis* and *Lactobacillus acidophillus)* by well diffusion method. All the plants showed significant activity against all pathogens, but the methanolic extract of *T.chebula* showed maximum zone of inhibition against *S.aureus* (27 mm) and the minimum zone of inhibition was determined in petroleum ether extract of *M.elengi* and *A.aspera* against *S.mutans* and *S.aureus i.e.* 9mm. Methanolic and aqueous extracts showed greater activity than petroleum ether and acetone extracts. Phytochemical analysis of these medicinal plants showed the presence of many biologically active constitutents of plant which might have exerted synergistic antimicrobial effect.

Keywords: Phytochemical, Dental caries, Antibacterial activity.

Introduction

Certain bacteria, viruses and fungi produce diseases which are manifested in or about the oral cavity. Some of these diseases or lesions are of a specific nature and are produced by a specific contribution to the problem of caries etiology (William *et al.*, 1994). The highest caries susceptibility is in the age group of 20-40 years, also the females are more susceptible to dental caries as compared to males (Nigam and Srivastawa, 1990). Dental decay is a chemico parasitic process consisting of two stages, the decalcification of enamel or its total destruction and the decalcification of dentine (dissolution of the softened residue) (Marsh, 1992). The cariogenic Streptococci is critical to the development of pathogenic plaque. A large number of *Streptococcus spp, Actinomyces* spp. and *Lactobacillus* spp. are involved in root caries and periodontal diseases (Schiipach *et al.*, 1995, Slots and Rams, 1992).

Antibiotic resistance has increased substantially in the recent years and is posing an ever increasing therapeutic problem (Guillemot,1999, Jones, 1988, Austin *et al.*, 1999) One of the method to reduce the resistance to antibiotics is by using antibiotic resistance inhibitors from plants (Kim *et al.*, 1995).

Plants are known to produce a variety of compounds to protect themselves against a variety of pathogens. It is expected that plant extracts showing target sites other than those used by antibiotics will be active against drug resistant pathogens. However, very little information is available on such activity of medicinal plants (Ahmad and Beg, 2001).

In the present study we have selected 6 medicinal plants against dental infection bacteria, including *Staphylococcus aureus, Streptococcus mutans, S.sanguis, S.salivarius* and *Lactobacillus acidophillus*. The selection of medicinal plants were based on their ancient or vedic uses, the phytochemical analysis were carried out of potentially strong active plant extracts.

Materials and Methods

Plant samples were collected locally from Shivalik range of Himalayas in Hardwar. All the plants were identified at Botanical Survey of India, Dehradun Uttaranchal. The plant parts were shade dried at room temperature and powdered by using blender. The plant extract was prepared by using soxlet assembly in four different solvents *i.e.* petroleum ether, acetone, methanol and water. The polarity of solvents leached out compounds soluble in the particular solvents The extracts were concentrated by using vacuum evaporator. Muller Hinton agar (Himedia No 173) media was used to test the antimicrobial activity against *S. aureus, Streptococcus mutans, S.sanguis S.salivarius* and *L. acidophillus*, by well diffusion method (Ahmad *et al.*, 1998) The pathogens were isolated from dental infection patients from the Aggarwal Dental Clinic at Royal Plaza, B.H.E.L. More, Haridwar and identified by using specific biochemical test with compared MTCC culture No. 890,1144, 1938, 447.

8 mm. diameter wells were punched in the agar and filled with extracts and respective solvents for negative control and antibiotic ampicillin (100 µg/ml) was used as positive control. The plants were incubated at 37°C for 18–24 hours. The antimicrobial activity was evaluated by measuring the diameter of inhibition zone in mm.

Phytochemical analysis of plant extracts for their major group of phytoconstituents and the active group of certain extracts was under taken using standard qualitative method (Scalbert, 1991, Chukwuran, 1997 and Ahmad, 1999).

Results

The botanical name family, common name, vedic name, part used, chemical phytoconstituents and the traditional uses of all the six plants are given in Table 20.1. Each of the six plants were prepared in extracts of four different forms, namely petroleum ether, acetone, methanol and aqueous extracts and tested against dental infection pathogens. Table 20.2 represents the summary of the antibacterial activities of the various extracts with respect to each of the test organism at concentration of 200mg/ml. Antibacterial activity was found in all the 24 plant extracts of different plant parts. *Terminalia chebula* (fruits), *Glycyrrhiza glabra* (roots) and *Acacia arabica* (bark and fruits) exhibited significant antibacterial activity with maximum zone of inhibition in methanolic extract. The antibacterial activity of active extracts were observed in the increasing order–*A. aspera* < *M. elengi* < *A. catechu* < *A. arabica* < *G. glabra* < *T. chebula*. The maximum zone of inhibition against *S.aureus i.e.* 27mm was observed in methanolic extract of *T. chebula* and the minimum zone of inhibition in petroleum ether extract of *A. aspera* against *S. aureus i.e.* 9mm. Similarly methanolic extracts of *T. chebula* showed *maximum antibacterial* activity against *S. mutans* (23mm), *S. salivarius* (26mm) and *L. acidophillus* (24mm), while *G. glabra* is effective against *S. sanguis* (20mm). The phytochemical analysis of these six plants showed the presence of many biologically active plant constituents as depicted in Table 20.3. Glycosides, flavonoids, alkaloids and saponins were detected in *A. aspera, A. arabica* and *Mimusops elengi. Tannins,* were detected in all extracts, saponins were not found in *T. chebula A. catechu* and *G. glabra.*

Table 20.1: The Ethnobotanical and Phytochemical Data of Six Indian Vedic Medicinal Plants

Specimen No.	*Botanical Name Family*	*Common and Vedic Name*	*Part Used*	*Known Phytoconstituents*	*Traditional Use*
1.	*Terminalia chebula* (Combretaceae)	Harar (Haritiki)	*Fruit*	Chebulic, tannic acid Anthroquinone, Chebuligic acid, Coritagit, (Harborne and Baxter, 1995)	Laxative, ulcers teeth, piles
2.	*Mimusops elengi* (Sapotaceae)	Moulshri Bakul	Bark Fruit	Saponin, pentacyclic triterpens mimusopgenonre steroidal glycosides (Shaha *et al.*, 2001)	Diarrhoea, dysentery, astringent, Gum diseases
3.	*Achyranthes aspera* (Amaranthaccae)	Chirchita (Apamarga)	Whole Plant	Achyranthin, ecdysterone, stigmasterol, sitosterol Triterpenoides, rhamnose glycosides 17 pentatriacontanol (Mishra *et al.*, 1993)	Cough asthma, bronchitis snake bite, anemia, dropsy, leprosy, teeth (Gokhale *et al.*, 2002)
4.	*Acacia catechu* (Mimosaceae)	Khair (Khadhira)	Stem	Quercetin, poriferasterol, B-D glucoside, tannicacid, catechuic acid, or catechin flavone glycoside (5,7,3,4, tetrahydroxy 3-methoxy flavene (Sharma *et al.*, 1997 and Yadava, 2002	Ulcers, urinary discharges, strengthens, the teeth, diarrhoea, and tonsils (Nadakarni, 1976)
5.	*A.arabica* (Mimosaceae)	Babool (Baboola)	Bark Fruits	Galacto araban Arabic acid	Astringent, cough, leucoderma, gumdiseases gonorrhoea, diarrohoea, Mouth and teeths, skin disease.
6.	*G.glabra* (Leguminaceae)	Mulahathi	Roots, Rhizomes	Phenolic Compounds. Glycosides Cinnamic acid, Isobatin, Liquirstin asparagive, liquirtin Coumarin and tannin (Bhardwaj *et al.*)	Rheumatoid, arthiritis, Tonsil Expectorent, antitissuessive cough, antiinflammatory, laxative

Discussion

The diseases produced by a number of microorganisms are manifested in or about the oral cavity. Some of these diseases are of a specific nature and are produced by a specific microorganism while

Table 20.2: The Antibacterial Activity of Medicinal Plant Extracts

Pathogens	Plants																							
	A. aspera				*A. arabica*				*A. catechu*				*T. chebula*				*M. elengi*				*G. glabra*			
	Pt. Ether	Acetone	Methanol	Water	Pt. Ether	Acetone	Methanol	Water	Pt. Ether	Acetone	Methanol	Water	Pt. Ether	Acetone	Methanol	Water	Pt. Ether	Acetone	Methanol	Water	Pt. Ether	Acetone	Methanol	Water
Staphylococcus aureus	9	10	12	11	19	20	22	21	12	14	14	13	25	26	27	26	14	15	16	16	20	22	23	24
Streptococcus mutans	10	12	12	11	15	16	17	17	15	15	16	17	22	22	23	22	9	12	16	14	19	18	20	21
S. sanguis	10	12	13	11	15	16	17	14	15	15	16	14	17	18	19	17	10	11	13	12	17	18	20	19
S. salivarius	10	11	12	10	16	17	17	16	13	12	15	14	22	23	26	25	10	13	15	14	18	18	19	18
Lactobacillus acidophillus	12	13	16	14	18	19	21	20	18	19	20	19	20	22	24	22	12	13	15	14	17	18	19	18

others are clinically specific and may be caused by any of a broad group of microorganisms. This microbial specificity or nonspecificity is characteristic of disease wherever they may occur in the body.

Table 20.3: The Phytochemical Screening of Methanolic Extracts

Seril No.	*Plant Extracts*	*Plant Compounds*					
		Glycosides	*Alkaloids*	*Flavonoids*	*Phenols*	*Tannins*	*Saponin*
1.	*Terminalia chebula*	+	+	+	+	+	–
2.	*Acacia arabica*	+	+	+	+	+	+
3.	*Acacia catechu*	+	+	–	+	+	–
4.	*Glycyrrhiza glabra*	+	+	+	+	+	–
5.	*Mimusops elengi*	+	+	–	+	+	+
6.	*Achyranthes aspera*	+	+	+	+	+	+

+: Present; –: Absent.

Dental caries is caused by infection with streptococcal, staphylococcal and *Lactobacillus* spp. The streptococcal and staphylococcal organisms of the beta hemolytic type that elaborate an erythrogenic toxin in the early stages of the disease,are the causal organisms of dental diseases. *S. mutans* is the main causative agent of dental caries. *Streptococcus mutans*, fermented sugars (Yamada *et al.*, 1980) and produced acids. The acids which affects this primary decalcification of enamel leads to its total destruction and the decalcification of dentin. The acids derived from the fermentation of starches and sugar lodged in the retaining centers of teeth. All pathogens isolated during present investigation are acidogenic.The streptococci ferment glucose, lactose, sucrose and maltose. The major end product of fermentation is lactic acid, dextrans and levans. These compounds showed to make dental caries (Lehner *et al.*, 1976). The enzyme fructosyltransferase and glycosylsucrose (Hoojo *et al.*, 1987, Walker *et al.*, 1983) are considered to be of special importance in the establishments of *S. mutans, S. salivarius,S. sanguis* and *L.acidophillus* in the dental plaque. These have the ability to metabolize dietary sucrose and synthesize glucan. Glucan is an insoluble, sticky or slimy gel, relatively inert and resistant to bacterial hydrolytic enzymes which cause plaque (Yamada *et al.*, 1985). The Staphylococci and Streptococci are involved in periodontal diseases normally *S.aureus* produce a light golden pigment and ferment mannitol and produce coagulase enzyme (the enzyme inducing the cloting of plasma) Streptococcal species does not ferment mannitol and coagulase enzyme. The disease produced by *S. aureus* depends upon their resistance to phagocytosis and their production of extracellular toxins and enzyme (Fast *et al.*, 1989).These microorganisms demineralized the calcified stuctures (enamel, dentin) and dissolution of the organic matrix. *S.mutans, S.sanguis S.salivarius* and *Lactobacillus acidophillus* play a major role in dental plaque formation. *Staphylococcus* spp. also ferment many sugars and sugar components that are part of dental plaque or caries (Kornman and Robertson, 1985). The causative agents of dental caries and dental plaque were isolated and identified. The morphological and biochemical tests were performed and compared with MTCC cultures.

The present study has shown that these plants are potentialy a rich source of antibacterial agents. This demonstrates their importance in traditional remedies in the rural populations. The 24 plant extracts tested, inhibited the growth of all pathogens but *T.chebula, A.arabica and G.glabra* are more effective. Our results showed more antibacterial activity of *G.glabra* against *S.aureus* as reported earlier by Nimri *et al.*, 1999.

The crude extracts (200 mg/ml) of each plant were used for determination of their potency against pathogens and compared with antibiotic (200 mg/ml). The extent of antimicrobial activity of the extracts based on inhibition zone diameter has been described as low (12-18 mm), moderate (19-22 mm) and strong activity (23-38 mm) by Ahmad *et al.* (1999). In our studies the crude extracts of *T. chebula* showed strong activity while all other plants showed moderate antibacterial activity against the pathogens.

The methanolic extract is highly effective against all pathogens because more organic compounds were leached in this solvent. Although water is reported by the traditional healers and herbalists to be the most commonly used solvent for extracting the active compounds due to its easy availability. Ahmad *et al.* (1998) screened medicinal plants to detect antimicrobial activity and clearly demonstrated that alcohol is a better solvent as compared to aqueous and hexane. Similarly water was not found to be the most effective solvent for extracting the active compounds from plants as compared to hexane and methane (Shale *et al.*, 1999).

The difference in results obtained could be due to the difference in concentrations and methods used in each study (Kumar *et al.*, 1997).

Tannins were found to be a component of plants that showed antibacterial activity. It could be one of the components responsible for the antibacterial activity since it was reported by Al Genaidy, 1993. The diameter of inhibition zone around the most active extracts are comparable with those of the standard antibiotics used as positive control.

This study is a preliminary evaluation of antimicrobial activity of the plants. It indicates that plants have the potential to generate herbal metabolites. The crude extracts demonstrating antidental caries activity could result in the discovery of new chemical classes of antibiotics that could serve as selective agents for the maintenance of animal or human health and provide biochemical tools for the study of infectious diseases. Further phytochemical studies are required to establish the types of compounds responsible for the antimicrobial effects of these medicinal plants.

References

Ahmad, I. and Beg, A.Z., 2001. Antimicrobial and phytochemical studies on 45 Indian medicinal plants against multi-drug resistant human pathogens. *Journal of Ethnopharmacology*, 74: 113–123.

Ahmad, I., Mehmood, Z. and Mohammad, F., 1998. Screening of some Indian medicinal plants for their antimicrobial properties. *Journal of Ethnopharmacology*, 62: 183–193.

Ahmad, I., Zaiba, Beg, A.Z. and Mehmood, Z., 1999. Antimicrbial potency of selected medicinal plants with special interest in activity against phytopathogenic fungi. *Indian Vet. med. Jour.*, 23: 299–306.

Al Genaidy, M., 1993. *Jordon Wild Plants and their Uses*. Amman Jordan, al Aseel Publications, pp. 198.

Austin, D.J., Kristinsson, K.G. and Anderson, R.M., 1999. The relationship between the volume of antimicrobial consumption in human communities and the frequency of resistance. *Proceeding of the National Academy of Sciences*, USA, 96: 1152–1156.

Fast, D.J., Schlievert, P.M. and Nelson, R.D., 1989 Toxic shoce syndrome associated Staphylococcal, Streptococcal pyrogenic toxins are potent inducers of tumornecrosis factor production. *Infection Immunology*, 57: 291–305.

Gokhale, A.B., Damre, A.S., Kulkarni, K.R. and Sarof, M.N., 2002. Preliminary evaluation of antinflamatory and antiarthritic activity of *S. lappa, A. speciosa,* and *A. aspera, Phytomedicine,* 9: 433–437.

Guillemot, D., 1999. Antibiotic use in humans and bacterial resistance. *Current Opinion in Microbiology,* 2: 494–498.

Harborne, S.B. and Baxter, H., 1995. *Phytochemical Dictionary: A Handbook of Bioactive Compounds from Plants.* Taylor and Francis, London.

Hojo, S., Mistsutomi, M. and Yamada, J., 1987. Metabolism of Glycosylsucrase by oral microorganisms and its Hydrolysis by *S. salivarius* fructosyltransferase. *Infection and Immunity,* 3: 698–703.

Jones, R.N., 1998. Important and emerging beta lactamase mediated resistance in hospital pathogens the ampcenzymes diagnostic. *Mircobiology and Infectious Diseases,* 31: 461–466.

Kim, H., Park.S.W.,Park J.M., Moon, K.H. and Lee, C.K., 1995. Screening and isolation of antibiotic resistance inhibitors from herb material Resistant Inhibition of 21 Korean plants. *Natural Product Science,* 1: 50–54.

Kornman, K.S. and Robertson, W.J., 1985 Clinical and microbiological evaluation of therapy for *Juvenila periodontitis. Journal of Periodontology,* 56: 443–456.

Kumar, S., Bagchi, G.D. and Darokar, M.P., 1997 Antibacterial activity observed in the seeds of some coprophilus plant. *Int. J. Pharmcog.,* 35: 179–184.

Lehner, T. Challambe, S.J. and Coldwell, J., 1976. Immunologic basis for vaccination against dental caries in monkeys. *Journal of Dental Res.,* 55: 166–169.

Marsh, P.D., 1992. Microbiological aspects of the chemical control of plaque and gingivitis. *Journal of Dental Resistance,* 71: 1431–1438.

Mishra, T.N., Singh, R.S., Pandey, H.S. Prasad, C. and Singh, B.P., 1993. Two long chain compounds from *Achyranthes aspera. Phytochemistry,* 33(1): 221–223.

Moranانan, M.M., Moreir, B., Boyle-vavra, S. and Daum, R.S., 1997. Antimicrobial resistance in *Staphylococcus* infection. *Disease of Clinical North America ,* 11: 813–817.

Nadakarni, A.K., 1976. *Indian Materia Medica.* Popular Prakashan, Bombay.

Nigam, P. and Srivastava, A.B., 1990. Betel chewing and dental decay. *Fed. Oper. Dent.,* 1(1): 36–44.

Nimri, L.F., Meqdam, M.M. and Alkofahi, 1999. Antibacterial activity of Jordanian medicinal plants. *Pharmaceutical Biology,* 37(3): 196–201.

Sachipach, P., Osterkwalder, V. and Guggenheim, B., 1995. Human root caries microbiota in plaque covering sound carious and arrested carious root surfaces. *Caries Res.,* 29: 382–395.

Sahu, N.P., Mandal, N.B., Banerjee, S. and Siddique, K.A.I., 2001. Chemistry and biology of triterpenes and saponin from seed of *M. elengi. Journal of Herbs, Spices and Medicinal Plants,* 8: 29–33.

Sharma, P., Dyal, R. and Ayyar, K.S., 1997. Chemical constituents of *A. catechu. Journal of Indian Chemical Society,* 74: 60–64.

Slots, J. and Rams, T.E., 1992. Microbiology of periodontal disease. In: *Contemporary Oral Microbiology and Immunology,* (Eds.) J. Slots, and M.A. Taubman. Mosby Year Book, St. Louis, Mo. p. 425–443.

Tiwari, G.C. and Sharma P., 1996. Pesticide resistance problem and management in India. In: *IPM System in Agriculture,* (Eds.) Rajak, K.K.G. Mukherji and R.L. Rajak. Aditya Book Private Ltd., New Delhi, 1: 41–61.

Williams, S. and Williams, K., 1994. *Clinical Practice of Dental Hygienist*, 7th ed., Esther in W. Willikins. London.

Yadav, R.N. and Sodhi, S., 2002. A New flavone glycoside Beta,5,7,34, tetrahydroxy-3-methoxy flavone, 7.O.Beta D glactopyronosyl (1 to 4) O Beta Glucopyranoside from the stem of *A. catechu,* Wild. *Journal of Asian Natural Product Research,* 4: 11–15.

Yamada, T., Kimura, S. and Igarashi, K., 1980. Metabolism glucosylsucrose and maltosylsucrose by *S.mutans. Caries. Res.*, 14: 239–247.

Yamada, T.S., Abbe, T. and Abbe, K., 1985. Effects of oxygen on pyruvate, formate, lyase insitu and sugar metabolism of *S. mutans* and *S. sanguis. Infection and Immunity*, 14: 289–299.

Walker, G.J., Margarrt, D.H. and Morrey-Jones, J.G., 1983. Activity of fructanase in batch cultures of oral Streptococci. *Carbohydrate Resistance*, 113: 101–112.

Medicinal Plants: Conservation, Cultivation and Utilization (2007) *Pages 147–166*
Editors: A.K. Chopra, D.R. Khanna, G. Prasad, D.S. Malik and R. Bhutiani
Published by: DAYA PUBLISHING HOUSE

Chapter 21

Conservation of Some Useful Medicinal Plants of Haridwar District in Uttaranchal State

Anil Kumar Dhiman*
Information Scientist, Gurukul Kangri University, Haridwar – 249 404, Uttaranchal

ABSTRACT

Since the ancient times, the people depend upon the plants and their products for curing diseases and other purposes. The forests of district Haridwar represent a considerable amount of medicinal plants wealth. But these medicinal plants those constitute a large collection are in critical conditions due to over-exploitation and deforestation mainly due to urbanization of the area. This paper discusses ethnomedicinal uses of some of the important plants found in this area. The emphasis has also been made to lists out those plant species, which are either going to be extinct or are on the verge of the extinction.

Keywords: Conservation, Ethonomedicinal uses, Local People and Vegetation.

Introduction

Haridwar, the holy city is one of the oldest living cities mentioned in the ancient Hindu scriptures. It is mentioned as Mayapuri, Kapila, Gangeshwar and Mokshdwar in ancient scriptures and epics.

* E-mail: akvishvakarma@yahoo.com.

This is considered as the gateway of the four pilgrimages, Badrinath, Kedarnath, Gangotri and Yamnotri of Uttaranchal. This is first city where Ganga emerges out from the mountains to touch the plains. Haridwar has not only remained a preferred place of saints and sages but also served as a centre of attraction for many years for learning the arts, science and culture.

Haridwar city is situated at 28°C–10°E on the river Ganga at the foothills of Shiwaliks that constitute the outer Himalayas. It is extended in an area of 12,302 square kilometers at an altitude of 294.7 meters and possess a huge population of about 3,48,142 persons. Earlier, it was covered under district Saharanpur but in 1988 was given the status of an independent district and very recently it has been included in Uttaranchal state. The major languages spoken in the district are Hindi, English, Punjabi and Garwhali. Besides, some tribal caste like Gujjar etc who are residing in the interior forests, speak their native languages.

Botanical and Medicinal History of the Area

Like the other parts of the Indian sub-continent, European botanists, army officers and surgeons were the first to botanize in the North Western Himalayas. T. Hardwicke 1796 was the first European who collected the plants from North Western Himalayas. With the restoration of the Botanic garden at Saharanpur by Hasting in 1820, extensive explorations of the plants of the North Western Himalayas and neighboring plains were made. The accumulation of plant collection made by various explorers from different parts of India and adjacent regions and the collection of a large number of specimens by J.D. Hooker and T. Thomson during 1848-51 have led the compilation of flora of British India. The first outcome of this was 'Flora Indica' prepared by Hooker and Thompson in 1855 which was later published as 'Flora of British India' during 1875-97 in seven volumes. References to Saharanpur and other places are found in this work. The appointment of J.F. Duthie as successor to W. Jameson at Saharanpur Botanic garden in 1876 and the establishment of Forest school at Dehradun by W. Schlich and D. Brandis in 1878-81, gave a new impetus to the phytogeography of the Sub-Himalayan tracts in particular and of Northern India in general. Duthie's work was published as 'Flora of the Upper Gangetic Plain and of the Adjacent Shiwalik and Sub-Himalayan Tracts' during 1923-29. Rai Bahadur Upendranath Kanjilal in 1911 published his work under the name 'Forest Flora of the Siwalik and Jaunsar Forest Divisions of the United Provinces of Agra and Oudh' which was later, revised by B.L. Gupta in 1928 and published under its new name 'Forest Flora for the Chakrata, Dehradun and Saharanpur Forest Divisions'. It describes woody flora of the region, however, various references are found of this area in this work. After the establishment of Forest Research Institute at Dehradun, it became one of the most active centres of botanical researches in India, particularly dealing with the exploration and publication of forest floras. Raizada explored the area during 1931-58 and described the plants which were not included in Duthie's work.The establishment of Northern circle of the Botanical survey of India in 1956 at Dehradun opened a new dimension in the exploration of the plant wealth of the North Western Himalayas and the Gangetic plain. M. A. Rau, the founder of Herbarium in the Northern circle of the B.S.I. at Dehradun prepared a checklist of the 'Flora of the upper Gangetic plain' in 1969. The complete work of Raizada was published in 1976 as the Supplement to Duthie's Flora of Upper Gangetic Plain and Adjacent Shiwalik and Sub-Himalayan Tracts. The new forest flora has been explored by K.C. Sahni and his colleagues Ram Dayal, R.C. Gaur, H.B. Naithani, K.M. Vaid, K.N. Bahadur and K.M. Balapure of the Forest research institute, Dehradun. The other most important contribution is of Babu, who in 1977 published a valuable publication under the title 'Herbaceous flora of Dehradun'.

In the above works, the main emphasis was laid on the exploration of the plant species found in the forests of the areas but no particular concentration was made towards contributing the medicinal values. Only little work has been done on the medicinal parts of the plant wealth of the area. It is evident that the medicinal plants survey work was initiated only after the formation of Central council of ayurvedic research in the ministry of health (ISM) under which the survey of medicinal plants unit at Gurukul Kangri, Haridwar was established in the year 1962. Uniyal (1965), published a list of the medicinal plants under the name 'Saharanpur Van Khand Ki Vanoushdiya (1962-63)'. Later on Ahuja (1965), published a booklet on 'Medicinal Plants of Saharanpur', which listed 92 plants. Uniyal (1977), explored the neighboring Uttrakhand area medicinally and published the work under the title 'Uttrakhand Vanoushdhi Darshika', which contains information on some of the medicinal plants of this area. Other important studies on Haridwar and its adjoining area include that of Dhiman (1997), Dhiman and Kaushik (1999 and 2000) and Dhiman (2001). Some of the medicinal uses along with sacred uses of the plants are discussed by Dhiman (2003 a and b) Very recently; many plants of medicinal importance have been listed and discussed by Dhiman (2004; 2005 b and 2006) in his work `Medicinal Plants of Uttaranchal State', Wild Medicinal Plants of India and `Ayurvedic Drug Plants' in details.

Climate and Vegetation

The four distinct seasons *viz.*, autumn, winter, spring and summer can be seen here. The climate of the area is relatively temperate with an average rainfall of about 1127.2 mm which is chiefly confined to monsoon months. There exists a highest temperature of 40.9°C±15.6°C in the summer season and the lowest temperature of 16.6°C±06.0°C during the winter season.

The area is represented predominantly by evergreen forest with some deciduous species of tropical and subtropical origin. The vegetation is affected by the altitude zonation and topography. The peaks of Shiwaliks have a different type of vegetation from that of damp sheltered area of Raiwala and that of Pathri forest in South.The peaks of the Shiwaliks are characterized by the presence of *Anogeissus latifolia, Centratherum anthelminticum, Drypetes roxburghii, Embelica officinalis* and to some extent by *Terminalia chebula* and *Terminalia bellerica*. While, the damp sheltered area of Raiwala possesses characteristic vegetation of *Piper longum, Centella asiatica, Helicteres isora, Bacopa monnieri* and *Tamarix dioecia* in addition to trees like *Shorea robusta, Salix tetrasperma, Limonia elephantum* and *Ficus hispida*. The vegetation in the Southern side in Pathri forest comprises especially of *Plumbago zeylanica, Piper longum, Centella asiatica, Alangium salvifolium* ssp. *salvifolium, Lannea coromandelica and Terminalia arjuna*, of these latter is said to met wild frequently in the forest. All these species are of great medicinal value too. The vegetation of the area in general can be discussed under the following types:

Hydrophytic Vegetation

This is found in monsoonal ponds and ditches, temporary marshy depressions and swamps of the area. In ponds, *Trapa natans var. bispinosa, Eichhornia crassipes and Nelumbo nucifera* commonly can be seen. The marshy borders of the water depressions are inhabited by *Eclipta prostrata* and *Polygonum* species. With the onset of cold weather, species like, *Ranunculus sceleratus* and *Soliva anthemifolia* etc. may be seen to appear which remain till the onset of summer season. Most of these have also been noted to grow in polluted sewage, water lagoons or on banks of nallas of the domestic sewage, hence can be used as pollution tolerant plants.

Marshy depressions and swampy areas and muddy zone during the monsoon, are dominated by plant species like *Bacopa monnieri, Veronica anagalis-aquatica* and *Polygonum barbatum*. The other elements that compose the flora of these habitats include *Rorippa nasturtium-aquaticum, Salix tetrasperma, Tamarix dioecia, Ageratum conyzoides* and *Calamus tenuis*.

Deciduous Forest

This type of the vegetation comprises of trees, shrubs and herbs. The common trees are *Shorea robusta, Bombax ceiba, Dalbergia sissoo, Butea monosperma, Sygyium cumini, Bauhinia variegata, Aegle marmelos, Cassia fistula, Stereospermum chelonoides, Mangifera indica* and *Tectona grandis*. The shrubs include *Zizyphus* species, *Vitex negundo, Ipomoea carnea* ssp. *fistulosa, Justicia adhatoda, Lantana camara* and *Clereodendrum* species. Among the herbs, *Achyranthes aspera, Boerhavia diffusa, Centella asiatica, Piper longum* and *Cynodon dactylon* are commonly occurring species. Some of these are not only of medicinal importance rather bind the soil on the banks of river/canal or hilly slopes and play a wonderful role in conservation of soil. With the advancement of cold weather, *Blumea lacera* and *Desmodium gangeticum* like plant species begin to appear. Besides, parasitic plant species like *Cuscuta reflexa* and *Dendrophthoe falcata* are also found.

Vegetation of villages, waste places, road-sides and forest clearings comprises of *Holarrhena antidysenterica, Holoptelia integrifolia, Mangifera indica, Tectona grandis, Terminalia arjuna* (Common on Haridwar–Roorkee road near Bahadrabad), *Cordia dichotoma, Dalbergia sissoo* and *Bauhinia variegata. Malvastrum coromandelianum, Sida rhombifolia, Sida cordata* and *Clerodendrum* species constitute herbaceous type vegetation. The indigenous weed flora comprises of *Sida* species, *Solanum villosum, Cleome gynandra, Cleome icosandra, Boerhavia diffusa, Triumfetta rhomboidea, Physalis minima, Dactyloctenium aegypticum, Cyperus rotundus* and *Anisomeles indica* etc. The herbaceous climbers are represented by *Tricosanthes cucumerina* and *Momordica charantia* etc. The exotic weed flora constitutes of *Gomphrena celosioides, Cassia tora, Ageratum conyzoides, Scoparia dulcis, Coronopus didymus* and *Lantana camara*.

Cutigens

Capsicum annum, Coriandrum sativum, Cicer arietinum, Oryza sativa, Zea mays, Triticum aestivum, Sorghum bicolor, Pennisetum typhoides, Brassica species and *Abelmoschus esculentus* are predominantly cultivated in the neigbouring villages. Among vegetable crops, *Luffa aegyptica, Cucurbita pepo, Colocasia esculenta, Spinacia oleracea, Daucus carota, Raphanus sativus, Allium cepa, Allium sativum, Brassica oleracea* and *Solanum melongena* are commonly cultivated in fields and gardens.

The fruit trees cultivated comprise of *Psidium guajava, Litchi chinensis, Pyrus communis, Prunus persica, Prunus domestica, Mangifera indica* and *Citrus* species. *Delonix regia, Millingtonia hortensis, Sarca asoca, Polyalthia longifolia, Azadirachta indica, Cassia fistula, Kigelia africana* and *Grevillea robusta* are common avenue trees met in the area. The ornamentals include *Cestrum nocturnum, Quisqualis indica, Tagetes erecta, Helianthus annuus* and *Clerodendrum indicum*.

Methodology

The present account is based on the survey of the area made during 1993-97 for Ph. D. work by the author. The information on ethnomedicinal uses was gathered through personal interview with the inhabitating villagers, vaidyas and local medical practitioners. Later some surveys were also made to update the information. The tribal inhabitants and practitioners have been heavily exploiting the area from generation to generation. It has been observed that the commonly available plants are hardly available now at approachable places due to over-exploitation and eradication of the commonly used plant species.

Enumeration

The information on ethnomedicinal uses of some of the plant species, which are generally used by the local people in Haridwar district, is given below. The plants are arranged alphabetically according to their botanical names. Besides, their local names and family names and information on local distribution are also provided.

Acacia catechu (Linn.) Willd. (Fabaceae)

Local name(s): Khair.

Distribution: Common at beds of Suswa river in Raiwala and in forests of Pathri and Chandi range near Kangri.

Parts used: Bark and heartwood.

Ethnomedicinal uses: Its resinous extract in powder form is used for drying wounds by the local people.

Acacia nilotica Delile ssp. _indica_ (Benth.) Brenan (Fabaceae) (Syn. _A. arabica_ (Lamk.) Willd.var. _indica_ Benth.; _A. nilotica_ var _indica_ (Benth.) Mill _A. arabica_ sensu Baker)

Local name(s): Kikar.

Distribution: Cultivated and also found wild in forest near Kangri village.

.*Parts used*: Bark, pods, leaves and gum.

Ethnomedicinal uses: Locally, the twigs of the plants are used as *datun* (natural tooth brush) to strengthen the gums and teeth.

Achyranthes aspera Linn. (Amranthaceae)

Local name(s): Chirchita, Lathjira.

Distribution: Common every where, usually in dry places and along the road sides.

Parts used: Whole plant.

Ethnomedicinal uses: The dried leaves of the plant are smoked in asthma and the roots are used in toothache. In malarial fever, the root is tied to the ear for remedy.

Aegle marmelos Correa ex Roxb. (Rutaceae)

Local name(s): Bel.

Distribution: Common in the forests area and also cultivated for its fruits in the gardens and as a sacred tree near temples.

Parts used: Fruits, seeds, flowers, leaves, bark and roots.

Ethnomedicinal uses: According to a legend of the "'Sakandh Puran', the Goddess Parvati meditated under this tree for many years. The place now has been styled as Bilkeshwar, westwards to the railway line near T.B. Hospital at Hardwar. Locally, the pulp of the ripe fruits is used for the preparation of a tasteful aromatic *sharbat*, which is a popular drink throughout India in hot weather. The fresh leaves are also chewed by the diabetic patients to control blood sugar.

Alstonia scholaris (Linn.) R. Br. (Apocynaceae)

Local name(s): Saptaparna, Saptaparni.

Distribution: Not very common, but can be seen on the Jwalapur-Rishikesh road from Kankhal to Chandi bridge and at Gurukul Kangri Vishwavidyalaya campus at Haridwar.

Parts used: Leaves, bark and wood.

Ethnomedicinal uses: Locally, the bark is crushed into a dilute paste and is applied externally in thoracic pain.

Azadirachta indica A. Juss. (Meliaceae) (Syn. _Melia azadirachta_ Linn.)

Local name(s): Nim, Nimb.

Distribution: Cultivated for shade and as ornamental tree in villages and sometimes along the road-sides.

Parts used: Fruits, seeds, flowers, twigs, bark and gum.

Ethnomedicinal uses: Its branches along with the leaves are kept on the door frame in the houses, where the persons are suffering from measles and small pox. The twigs are frequently used as '*Datun*' by the people for strengthening their teeth and gums. Young apical leaves after crushing and mixing with butter are given to the young ones of animals (calves) to cure diarrhoea.

Boerhavaia diffusa Linn. (Nyctaginaceae) (Syn. _B. repens_ Linn.)

Local name(s): Punarnava.

Distribution: Common weed found everywhere in waste places.

Parts used: Whole plant.

Ethnomedicinal uses: Locally, a paste of roots is taken two times a day on empty stomach to cure blood dysentery and in piles. Besides, the whole plant is cooked and eaten as vegetable in anaemia and piles.

Bombax ceiba Linn. (Bombacaceae) (Syn. _B. malabaricum_ DC.; _Salmalia malabarica_ (DC.) Schott and Endl.)

Local name(s): Semul, Simbhal.

Distribution: Planted along road-sides and also met in the forest near Kangri and Raiwala.

Parts used: Flowers, leaves, root, bark, seeds and young fruits.

Ethnomedicinal uses: Semul is a vedic plant and is frequently mentioned in the vedic literatures. It is known as Yamadrunaa, or tree of Yama, the god of death. Locally, about 1-2 teaspoonful powder of its roots is taken on empty stomach daily with honey or 'khand' as an aphrodisiac.

Butea monosperma (Lamk.) Taub. (Fabaceae) (Syn. _B. frondosa_ Koen. ex Roxb.; _Erythrina monosperma_ Lamk.)

Local name(s): Dhak, Palsh.

Distribution: Commonly found in the forests; also occurs along the road-sides on Haridwar-Roorkee bypass road and very common on Haridwar-Laksar road and also industrial area bypass road.

Parts used: Seeds, flowers, bark, roots and leaves.

Ethnomedicinal uses: The dried flowers are warmed and are tied over abdomen and swellings of testicles.

Caesalpinia bonduc **(Linn.) Roxb. (Fabaceae) (Syn.** ***C. crista*** **Linn.;** ***C. bonducella*** **(Linn.) Fleming;** ***Guilandina bonduc*** **Linn.)**

Local name(s): Karanj, Latakaranj, Putikaranaj.

Distribution: Found in the deciduous forests of the area concerned and also cultivated as hedge plant in villages like Kangri and Pili etc. can be seen also wild in nearby areas of Gurukul Kangri Vishwavidyalaya, Haridwar.

Parts used: Seeds.

Ethnomedicinal uses: A paste of its seed-kernels is applied in scorpion stings and as a poultice on hydrocele.

Callicarpa nudiflora **Hook. and A. (Verbenaceae) (Syn.** ***C. acuminata*** **Roxb.;** ***C. reevesii*** **Wall. ex Schauer;** ***C. macrophylla*** **var.** ***sinensis*** **Cl.)**

Local name(s): Priyangu.

Distribution: Found wild in the forests of Raiwala and in Chilla near Bairaz; also along road sides as shrubberies.

Parts used: Leaves and roots.

Ethnomedicinal uses: Locally, the fruits are eaten and a paste of its roots and fruits is applied to treat mouth and tongue sores.

Calotropis procera **(Ait.) Ait. f. Ssp.** ***hamiltonii*** **(W.) Ali (Asclepiadaceae) (Syn.** ***C. hamiltonii*** **W.;** ***C. procera*** **auct. non (Ait.) f.)**

Local name(s): Aak, Aakada, Aakha.

Distribution: Common in waste places, river-beds, roadsides and forest clearings.

Parts used: Flowers, leaves, latex and root-bark.

Ethnomedicinal uses: The fresh leaves of the plant are warmed and are applied as poultice in rheumatism, gout and to relieve pains. Besides, the plant is also used for miracle purpose, for which the whole plant is eradicated at any of the occasion but treated by mantra in the night of lunar junction at 12 pm. Then, the plant is burnt with *Butea monosperma* and the smoke is given in the effects of ghosts and conjuration.

Cannabis sativa **Linn. (Cannabinaceae)**

Local name(s): Bhanga, Ganjika.

Distribution: Found in waste places, along road-sides and in moist places.

Parts used: Leaves and flowering tops.

Ethnomedicinal uses: Its leaves are bruished and smoked by the people very much. Besides, the female flowering tops of the plant are used for the treatment of hydrocele and prolapse of uterus. In case of prolapse of uterus, the leaf-paste is put in soft muslin cloth and kept inside the vagina at bed time by the women. This treatment is seen very effective in the initial stages of uterus prolapse.

Celastrus paniculatus Willd. (Celastraceae)

Local name(s): Malkangni.

Distribution: Found wild in the forest in Raiwala and Chandi range near Kangri and Sidhashrota.

Parts used: Seeds, bark, leaves and roots.

Ethnomedicinal uses: Locally, the people apply a poultice of the paste of its leaves and roots in headache.

Centella asiatica (Linn.) Urban (Apiaceae) (Syn. *Hydrocotyle asiatica* Linn.)

Local name(s): Brahmi.

Distribution: Common at moist places throughout the region, chiefly in Pathri and Raiwala.

Parts used: Whole plant.

Ethnomedicinal uses: Locally, a syrup is prepared from the herb and is given to children for increasing memory and also used as a local remedies for diarrhoea of children. The entire plant is boiled in water and their decoction is given in treatment of leprosy.

Cissampelos pareiera Linn. (Menispermaceae)

Local name(s): Patha.

Distribution: Commonly found along hedges, forest edges, forest clearings and scrub jungles.

Parts used: Leaves and roots.

Ethnomedicinal uses: The powder of its roots along with two grains of *Hordeum vulgare* is given thrice a day to cure malarial, typhoid and general fever. The juice of its leaves mixed with the powder of black pepper is given in diphtheria.

Cleome gynandra Linn. (Cleomaceae) (Syn. *Gynandropsis pentaphylla* (Linn.) DC.; *G. gynandra* Briq.)

Local name(s): Hulhul, Jakhya.

Distribution: Common in waste places, road-sides and sandy river bands.

Parts used: Leaves, seeds and roots.

Ethnomedicinal uses: It has long been known domestic remedy of the Hindus. Locally, the native people use its seeds as a spice and their leaves are cooked and eaten as vegetable. Besides, a half teacup decoction of its seeds and leaves, is taken daily in typhus fever and the leaves are applied externally to boils to prevent pus formation.

Cleome icosandra Linn. (Cleomaceae) (Syn. *C. viscosa* Linn.)

Local name(s): Hulhul, Safed hulhul.

Distribution: Common in agricultural fields, waste places and along road-sides.

Parts used: Seeds and leaves.

Ethnomedicinal uses: Locally, the people uses its seeds as a spice. Besides, the leaves are cooked as vegetable and given to the patients suffering from oedema.

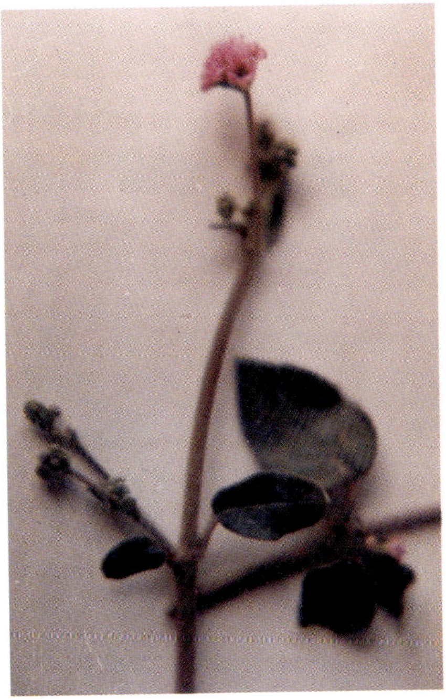

Figure 21.1: *Boerhavia diffusa*

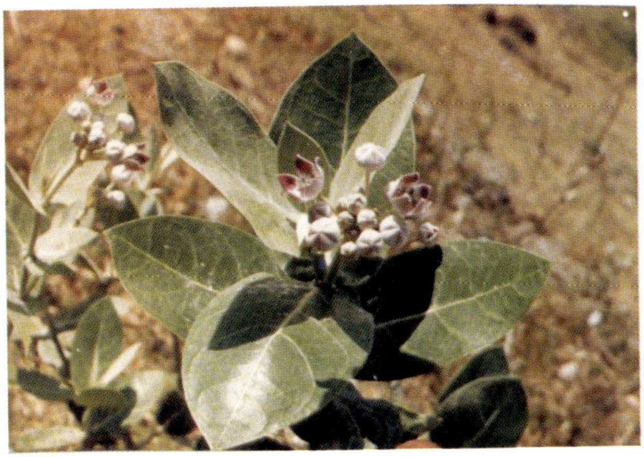

Figure 21.2: *Calotropis proceaa*

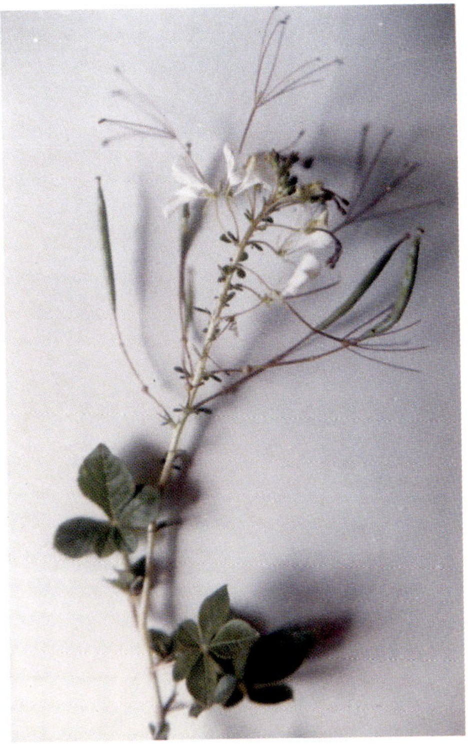

Figure 21.3: *Cleome gynandra*

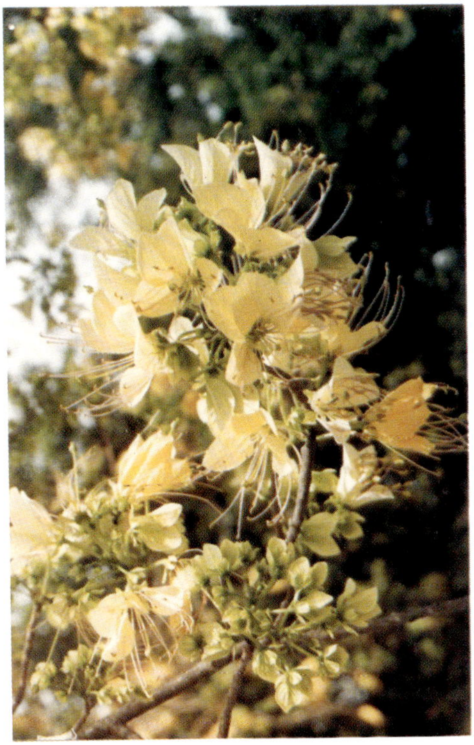

Figure 21.4: *Crateva magna*

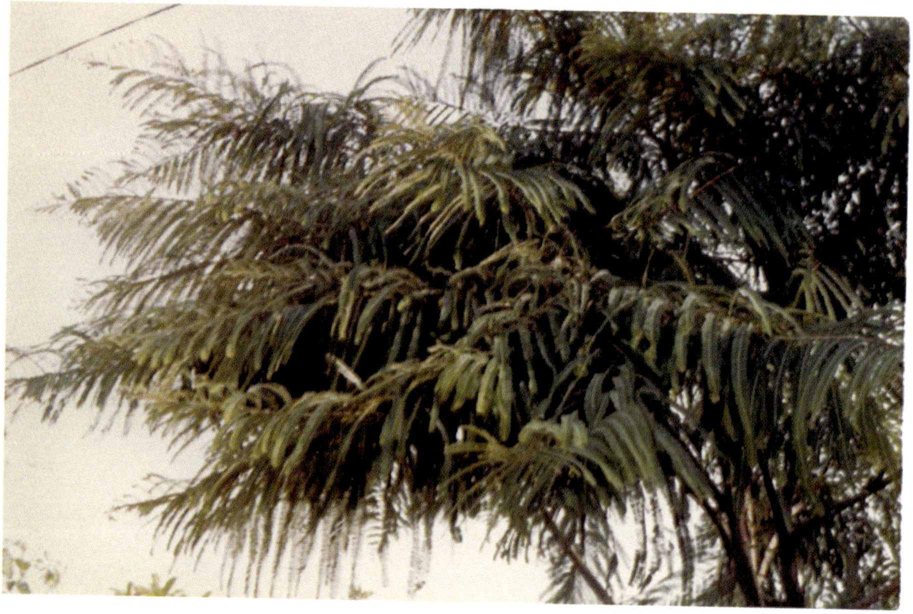

Figure 21.5: *Embelica officinalis*

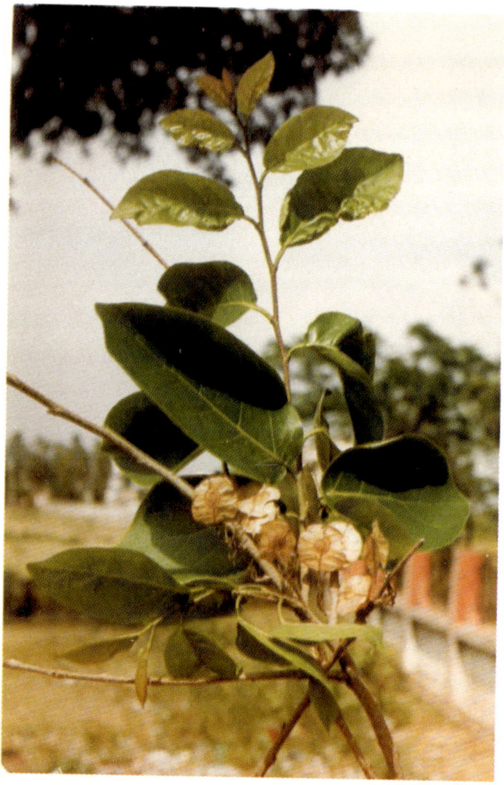

Figure 21.6: *Holoptelea integrifolia*

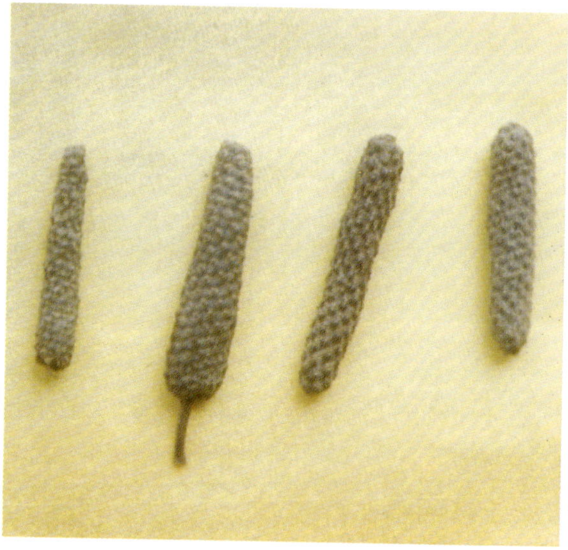

Figure 21.7: Fruits of *Piper longum*

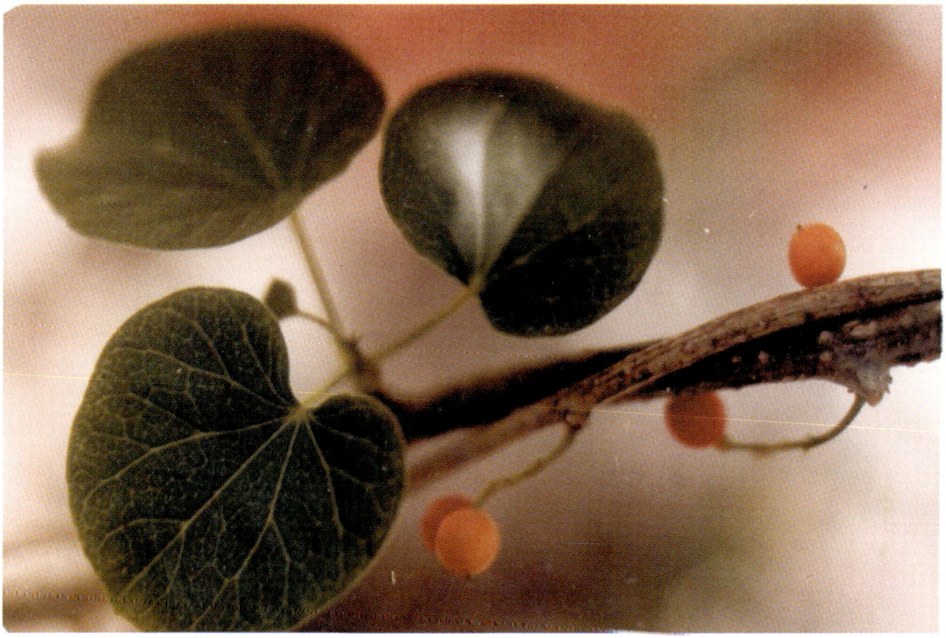

Figure 21.8: *Tinospora cordifolia*

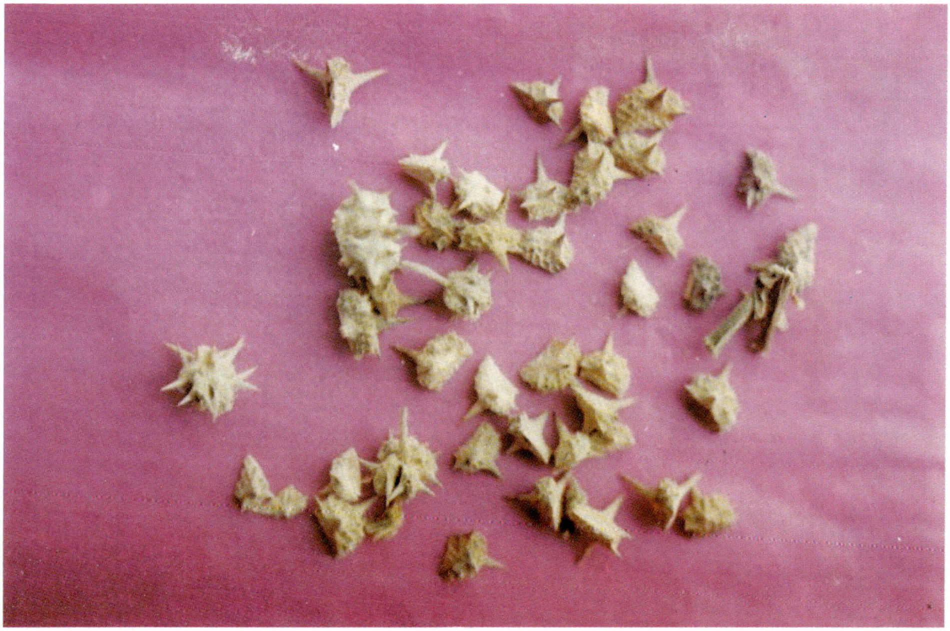

Figure 21.9: Fruits of *Tribulus terrestris*

Clerodendrum indicum (Linn.) O. Kuntze (Verbenaceae) (Syn. _C. siphonanthus_ R. Br.; _Siphonanthus indica_ Linn.)

Local name(s): Chingari.

Distribution: Cultivated in gardens for its flowers and sometimes as a hedge plant.

Parts used: Leaves and roots.

Ethnomedicinal uses: The juice of its leaves mixed with butter is applied externally to herpetic eruptions.

Cordia dichotoma Forst. (Ehertiaceae) (Syn. _C. myxa_ sensu Cl.; _C. lowriana_ Brandis)

Local name(s): Lassora, Lissora.

Distribution: Common in Motichur-Lachhiwala range and Neel parvat forest near Kangri; also found planted along road-sides on Haridwar–Roorkee road near Ranipur-mode river bridge.

Parts used: Fruits, seeds, leaves and bark.

Ethnomedicinal uses: The ripe fruits of the plant are eaten by the natives in spermatorrhoea. The dried flowers after heating are applied over abnormal testicles in swellings. Besides, a paste of the fruits also is applied externally in headache.

Crateva magna (Lour.) DC. (Capparidaceae) (Syn. _C. religiosa_ var. _nurvala_ (Buch.–Ham.) Hook. f. and Thoms.; _C. lophosperma_ Kurz; _C. nurvala_ Buch.–Ham.; _Capparis magna_ Lour.)

Local name(s): Barna, Varun.

Distribution: Found cultivated as well as in wild forms in forest of Neel parvat near Kangri village and in Raiwala.

Parts used: Leaves, stem-bark and root-bark.

Ethnomedicinal uses: A couple of buds pounded with the salt is taken before meals to promote appetite and a decoction of its bark to remove calculi.

Cuscuta reflexa Roxb. (Cuscutaceae)

Local name(s): Akashbel.

Distribution: Very common in forests over the shrubs or trees as parasite and also on the hedges. Common host plants of 'Amarbela' in this region are *Justicia adhatoda, Zizyphus mauritiana, Clerodendrum* spp., *Cassia* spp., *Acacia* spp., *Melia azadirachta, Mangifera indica* and *Ficus* species.

Parts used: Whole plant.

Ethnomedicinal uses: The juice of stem is applied to kill lice and about 2 teaspoonful juice is taken thrice a day in haematuria by the people.

Cyperus rotundus Linn. (Cyperaceae)

Local name(s): Motha.

Distribution: Very abundant in gardens, along roadsides, agricultural fields, grassy localities and vacant plots; also being grown at Shantikunj and its sister concern Brahamvarchas at Haridwar.

Parts used: Tubers.

Ethnomedicinal uses: Its roots combined with other aromatics are used in indigestion of children. The fresh tubers are applied over breast in the form of 'lep' (malagma) as galactagogue. Besides, its stem and leaves are crushed and are applied for jaundice, disorders of stomach and irritation of bowels and also to heal wounds by the inhabitants.

Datura metal **Linn. (Solanaceae) (Syn.** ***D. fastuosa*** **Linn.;** ***D. fastuosa*** **Linn. var.** ***alba*** **(Nees) Cl.;** ***D. alba*** **Nees)**

Local name(s): Dhatura.

Distribution: Commonly along roadsides and on waste places in villages; also found to be grown near Shiva temples as the plants are considered sacred and its fruits and flowers are used for worship.

Parts used: Seeds, leaves and roots.

Ethnomedicinal uses: The plant is considered sacred and its flowers and fruits are used for the worship of God Shiva. Besides, to tighten flabby breast of women, four or five leaves are heated over open fire after smearing them with mustard oil and are tied over breast once a day for 8-10 consecutive days.

Datura stramonium **Linn. (Solanaceae) (Syn.** ***D. stramonium*** **var.** ***tatula*** **(Linn.) Cl.)**

Local name(s): Kala dhatura, Shyam dhatura.

Distribution: In waste places, riverbeds and along road sides, but not so commonly and sometimes also grown in gardens.

Parts used: Fruits, seeds, flowers and leaves.

Ethnomedicinal uses: The plant like that *D. metal* is a sacred plant and its leaves and flowers are used for the worship of God Shiva. Its leaves are smoked like cigarettes for narcotic effects and also in asthma by the local people. Besides, a paste of its fruits with turmeric is used to check inflammation of the breast.

Drypetes roxburghii **(Wall.) Hurusawa (Aspicliaceae) (Syn.** ***Putranjiva roxburghii*** **Wall.)**

Local name(s): Jiyapota, Putranjivi.

Distribution: Found in Raiwala and Chandi Devi forests.

Parts used: Leaves, seeds and fruits.

Ethnomedicinal uses: The nuts of this plant are strung up in rosaries by those women whose male child die immediately after birth. Besides, the leaves after crushing are applied to swollen throats of cattle.

Eclipta prostrata **(Linn.) Linn. (Asteraceae) (Syn.** ***E. alba*** **(Linn.) Hassk.;** ***Verbesina prostrata*** **Linn.)**

Local name(s): Bhangra, Bhringraj.

Distribution: Common in watersides, fields, road-sides, waste places and grassy humid localities.

Parts used: Whole plant.

Ethnomedicinal uses: The decoction of the plant is given in uterine haemorrhages. The juice of the plant in combination with 'ajwain' seeds as tonic and deobstruent and two drops of this juice along with eight drops of honey are given to newly born children suffering from catarrh. Besides, the bruised herb is also applied on hairs externally to dye them.

Emblica officinalis Gaertn. (Euphorbiaceae) (Syn. _Phyllanthus emblica_ Linn.; _Cicca emblica_ Kurz.)

Local name(s): Amla, Anvla.

Distribution: It is seen in forests of the area; also grown in gardens for its edible fruits.

Parts used: Fruits.

Ethnomedicinal uses: Its dried fruits are immersed in water in a new earthen vessel for a whole night to yield a decoction which is used as a collyrium in opthalmia. A *sherbat* prepared from its fresh fruits with or without raisins and honey is drunk as a cooling drink. This *sherbat* with lemon juice is also taken for bacillary dysentery. Besides, it's a paste of its fruits and leaves is given orally about 100 gm thrice daily for 5 days in Sun stroke.

Ficus bengalensis Linn. (Moraceae)

Local name (s): Bar, Bargad

Distribution: Cultivated in avenues; also in villages for shade and met wild in the forests.

Parts used: Seeds, latex, bark and tender ends of the aerial roots.

Ethnomedicinal uses: The plant is considered as a sacred tree and it is a common belief that Brahma was transformed into Vata tree. Locally, a small quantity of its milky juice dropped in 'batasha' is taken daily as aphrodisiac and alone also in dysentery and this juice is also applied on cracked heels. The tender ends of hanging roots are given for obstinate vomiting.

Ficus racemosa Linn. (Moraceae) (Syn. _F. gloomerata_ Roxb.)

Local name(s): Goolar, Gular, Udumbar.

Distribution: Generally grown in gardens and villages; also found wild.

Parts used: Leaves, fruits, latex, bark and roots.

Ethnomedicinal uses: The leaves and bark of this plant are used as poultice for eczema. The small blister-like 'galls' common on the leaves are soaked in milk and mixed with honey are given to prevent pitting in small pox. From the roots, a fluid is obtained by making an incision in the root and this is taken as a powerful tonic. Besides, the bark grounds with onions, cumin and coconut spathes and mixed with vinegar is given to cattle suffering from rinder-pest.

Gloriosa superba Linn. (Liliaceae)

Local name(s): Languli.

Distribution: Along forest edges, in forest clearings, scrub jungles and on the hedges.

Parts used: Whole plant.

Ethnomedicinal uses: Its root stocks are cut into pieces, meshed and boiled in sesamum oil for about half an hour, then the oil is filtered and applied twice a day followed by massage on painful joints.

Helicteres isora Linn. (Sterculiaceae)

Local name(s): Marorphali.

Distribution: Gregariously in the dry deciduous forest of Raiwala.

Parts used: Fruits, seeds, bark and roots.

Ethnomedicinal uses: About 20-25 gm of seed powder of the plant is used thrice a day for one week in the treatment of dysentery and stomach pain.

Holarrhena antidysenterica (Linn.) Wall. (Apocynaceae)

Local name(s): Chirabilva, Papri.

Distribution: It is seen in the forests in Raiwala and Chandi range near Kangri. Also found planted along road-sides near Kangri and Shyampur on Haridwar-Najibabad road.

Parts used: Seeds.

Ethnomedicinal uses: A combination of the seeds, old cotton and honey is used by the natives as a local application to the *os uteri* in cases of the inflammation of the uterus.

Holoptelea integrifolia Planch. (Ulmaceae)

Local name(s): Chirabilva, Papri.

Distribution: Commonly in the forests of Haridwar near BHEL and Kangri; also found planted along road-sides.

Parts used: Bark and seeds.

Ethnomedicinal uses: Its fruits are eaten locally and a leaf-paste is applied externally in the treatment of skin diseases like ringworm and itches.

Ipomoea carnea ssp. _fistulosa_ (Mart. ex Choisy) Austin (Apocynaceae) (Syn. _I. fistulosa_ Mart. ex Choisy; _I. crassicaulis_ (Benth.) Robinson; _Batatas crassicaulis_ Benth.)

Local name(s): Hakim, Sada suhagan.

Distribution: Very commonly in the watersides of streams and canals; often cultivated as a hedge plant.

Parts used: Seeds and flowers.

Ethnomedicinal uses: Locally, the leaves are warmed and are tied over the affected area in sprains and swellings.

Justicia adhatoda Linn. (Acanthaceae) (Syn. _Adhatoda vasica_ Nees; _A zeylanica_ Med.)

Local name(s): Bansa, Kalabansa.

Distribution: It is found in waste places, scrub jungles, forest edges, forest clearings and along road-sides. Often planted as hedge plant, as cattle do not browse it.

Parts used: Leaves and wood-ashes.

Ethnomedicinal uses: Locally, the leaves are applied as a poultice on skin affections. Its leaves and wood-ashes mixed with honey are used for cough and asthma and the dried leaves alone are smoked for rapid recovery from asthma.

Mucuna pruriens (Linn.) DC. (Fabaceae) (Syn. _M. prurita_ Hook.; _Dolichos pruriens_ Linn.; _Stizolobium pruriens_ (Linn.) Medicus)

Local name(s): Kaunch.

Distribution: Common in scrub jungles, forest clearings and on hedges in the villages.

Parts used: Pods, seeds, roots, and leaves.

Ethnomedicinal uses: A piece of its roots is tied over wrist in dropsy and seeds are applied over scorpion stings. Besides, a piece of cloth dipped in the decoction of its roots is inserted in vagina as *'Yoni Sanchochan Yog'* to make vagina contractive. The powder of its seeds is also taken as aphrodisiac.

Murraya koenigii (Linn.) Spreng (Rutaceae)

Local name(s): Curry nim, Meetha nim.

Distribution: Found in ravines and on waste lands along the road-sides; also cultivated in gardens for its fresh leaves which give agreeable flavour to curries.

Parts used: Whole plant.

Ethnomedicinal uses: Locally, the leaves are cooked as vegetable and chewed by the children to cure mouth sores and to stop vomiting. The leaves either fresh or dried are used to flavour curry. Besides, its fruits are also eaten by the local people.

Phyllanthus fraternus Webster (Euphorbiaceae) (Syn _P. niruri_ sensu Hook. f.)

Local name(s): Bhuian anvala.

Distribution: Very common is gardens, field, waste places and along road-sides.

Parts used: Whole plant.

Ethnomedicinal uses: The decoction of the plant is given in jaundice and the latex from the plant is applied on the sores locally.

Piper longum Linn. (Piperaceae)

Local name(s): Pippali.

Distribution: In shady localities; abundantly in Pathri forest and Raiwala.

Parts used: Fruits and roots.

Ethnomedicinal uses: The powder of its fruits mixed with honey is given in cold, cough, asthma and hiccough locally. This is also given in combination of *Aswagandha* root–powder after boiling it in milk in cold.

Rauvolfia serpentina Benth. ex Kurz (Apocynaceae)

Local name(s): Sarpgandha.

Distribution: In waste places and in shady localities; can be seen in somewhat bulk in Pathari forests and in Ranipur range but in past, it is seen that its growth has been checked due over eradication of the plants for medicinal purposes by the local people.

Parts used: Leaves and roots.

Ethnomedicinal uses: Its roots are still used today, mainly in insanity as 'pagal ki dava' and in high blood pressure. Besides, local working women in interior parts, smear their breast with its root-paste and put their crying babies to suck on them for sleep.

Ricinus communis Linn. (Euphorbiaceae)

Local name(s): Arand, Arandi.

Distribution: Wild in waste places and as a hedge plant in villages.

Parts used: Seeds, leaves and root-bark.

Ethnomedicinal uses: Locally, the leaves of the plant are applied as a poultice over the breast to bring on copious discharge of milk and heated leaves as a lactagogue. The warm leaves are also tied over the effected parts of the body in sprains. Besides, a paste of its leaves is made with luke warm ghee and is applied on the swollen joints.

Terminalia arjuna (Roxb.) W. and A. (Combretaceae)

Local name(s): Arjun.

Distribution: Found planted on Haridwar-Roorkee and Haridwar-Rishikesh road and also planted as an ornamental tree in the avenues. Besides, can be seen wild in Pathri forest.

Parts used: Fruits, leaves and bark.

Ethnomedicinal uses: The powder of its bark boiled in milk is taken as a cardiotonic locally. Besides, its twigs are also used as *datun* to clean mouth and teeth and also to remove mouth sores.

Terminalia bellirica (Gaertn.) Roxb. (Combretaceae) (Syn. *T. bellirica* var. *laurinoides* Cl.; *Myrobalanus bellirica* Gaertn.)

Local name(s): Bahera.

Distribution: In the deciduous forests of this area but not so common.

Parts used: Fruits, bark and gum.

Ethnomedicinal uses: Locally, its fruits are used in coughs, hoarseness, sore throat and dyspepsia. It is an ingredient of *triphala*, which is taken for constipation by the local people daily. Besides, a peel of its fruits with a little pulp is given to children to chew in coughs and colds.

Terminalia chebula Retz. (Combretaceae)

Local name(s): Harad.

Distribution: Common in the deciduous forests of the region; rarely met at the peaks of Shiwaliks in this area, but not so common in Raiwala.

Parts used: Fruits, bark, gum and leaves.

Ethnomedicinal uses: The plant is supposed to be originated, when Indra was drinking nectar in heaven, a drop of the fluid fell on the earth and produced the Haritaki plant. Its myrobalans are safe and effective purgative and form an ingredient of triphala, which is used for constipation locally. It is a common belief that by merely holding of its fruits of certain varieties removes constipation.

Tinospora cordifolia **(Willd.) Miers ex Hook.f. and Thoms. ((Menispermaceae)**

Local name(s): Giloe, Gugunchi.

Distribution: Commonly found on the hedges in this area.

Parts used: Leaves, stem, roots and fruits.

Ethnomedicinal uses: The herb is often bruised and put into water, the liquid thus formed being drunk by the Brahmins at some of the religious ceremonies. Besides, a necklace of small pieces of the stem known as 'kamlani-mala' is also worn as a cure for jaundice.

Tribulus terrestris **Linn. (Zygophyllaceae)**

Local name(s): Gokhru.

Distribution: It is met as a common weed in the fields and waste places.

Parts used: Entire plant.

Ethnomedicinal uses: A decoction of entire plant or of its fruits is drunk locally to remove the gravels, especially of urinary tracts.

Withania somnifera **Dunal (Solanaceae)**

Local name(s): Ashgandh, Ashwagandha.

Distribution: As weed in waste places but not so common in the area.

Parts used: Fruits, seeds, leaves and roots.

Ethnomedicinal uses: Locally, an infusion of its leaves is taken in fever by the local people. The powder of its root is taken alone with milk for general weakness and debility. Besides, the powder of the roots along with that of *Piper longum* fruits after boiling in milk and added with sugar is taken in cold.

Conclusion

A brief study of the vegetation shows that due to urbanization of the area and over exploitation of the natural resources, of plant wealth in particular the environment is becoming polluted and there is a great decrease in the plant vegetation. The following medicinal plants were recorded to be on the verge of sharp decline in their population.

1. *Acacia nilotica* ssp. *indica*
2. *Aegle marmelos*
3. *Azadirachta indica*
4. *Barleria prionitis*
5. *Butea monosperma*
6. *Caselalpinia bonduc*
7. *Cannabis sativa*
8. *Centella asiatica*
9. *Crateva magna*
10. *Embelica officinalis*
11. *Holarrhena antidysenterica*

12. *Justicia adhatoda*
13. *Ocimum sanctum*
14. *Piper longum*
15. *Rauvolfia serpentiana*
16. *Solanum surrattense*
17. *Stereospermum chelonoides*
18. *Terminalia bellirica*
19. *Tribulus languinosus*
20. *Withania somnifera*

It has also been observed that the community residing in interior or the remote areas, collect herbal plants from these areas and sell the plants or plant parts in the market to earn their livelihood. Many of the traditional healers, Vaidyas also collect the medicinal plants for the treatment of various diseases. In the process, they unearth the roots, rhizomes, bulbs, tubers and plucky flowers, fruits and other important parts of the plants for extracting drugs. Besides, the area is over-exploited for the other purposes like food, fuel and as a fodder. If this situation continues for next coming few years then many of the plants will be endangered and loss will be irreparable.

So, efforts should be made to conserve them in *in situ* and *ex-situ* conditions so that the maximum benefits can be made out of the God gifted herbal vegetation. The knowledgeable local person from the tribal areas, the NGO's, volunteer organizations, as suggested by Dhiman (2005, a) and also the semi-government institutions should be involved and properly trained for the purpose. Many other plant species of medicinal importance have been listed by Kaushik and Dhiman (2000), they can also be planted to enrich medicinal plant wealth in this area.

References

Ahuja, B.S., 1965. *Medicinal Plants of Saharanpur*. Survey of Medicinal Plants, G.K.V., Hardwar.

Babu, C.R., 1977. *Herbaceous Flora of Dehradun*. Publications and Information Directorate, C.S.I.R., New Delhi.

Dhiman, A.K., 1997. A survey of medicinal plants of Haridwar and adjoining area vis-a-vis the taw plant drugs being sold in local market. *Ph.D. Thesis*, Gurukul Kangri Universitiy, Haridwar.

Dhiman, A.K. and Kaushik, P., 1999. Avenue trees for conservation of environment at Haridwar. In: *Sustainable Ecosystem and Environment*, (Eds.) D.R. Khanna, Ashutosh Gautam and Aditya Gautam. Action for Sustainable Development and Awareness (ASEA), Rishikesh, pp. 85–89.

Dhiman, A.K. and Kaushik, P., 2000. Occurrence of pollution tolerant plant species at Haridwar. In: *Environmental Protection*, (Eds.) A.K. Thukral and G.S. Virk. Scientific Publishers, Jodhpur, pp. 352–359.

Dhiman, A.K., 2001. Medicinal plants wealth of Haridwar and adjacent area. *Sachitra Ayurved*, 53(12): 914–925.

Dhiman, A.K., 2003a. *Sacred Plants and their Medicinal Uses*. Daya Publishing House, New Delhi.

Dhiman, A.K., 2003b. Sacred plants of Haridwar (Uttaranchal) and their medicinal uses. In: *Advances in Plant Sciences*, 16(11): 377–384.

Dhiman, A.K., 2004. *Medicinal Plants of Uttaranchal State*. Chowkhamba Sanskrit Series Office, Varanasi.

Dhiman, A.K., 2005 a. Problems of medicinal plant wealth upon the phytogeography of Uttaranchal. *Advances in Plant Sciences*, 18(11): 615–623.

Dhiman, A.K., 2005b. *Wild Medicinal Plants of India*. Bishen Singh Mahendra Pal Singh, Dehradun.

Dhiman, A.K., 2006. *Ayurvedic Drug Plants*. Daya Publishing House, New Delhi.

Duthie, J.F., 1923–29. *Flora of Upper Gangetic Plain and Adjacent Shiwalik and Sub Himalayan Tracts*, Vols. 1 and 2. Bishen Singh Mahendra Pal Singh, Dehradun.

Gupta, B.L., 1928. *Forest Flora of the Chakrata, Dehradun and Saharanpur Forest Divisions, Uttar Pradesh*. International Book Distributors, Dehradun.

Kanjilal, U.N., 1911. *Forest Flora of the Siwalik and Jaunsar Forest Divisions of the United Provinces of Agra and Oudh*. Government Printing Press, Calcutta, India.

Hooker, J.D., 1875–1897. *The Flora of British India*, Vols. I–VII. L. Reeve and Co. Ltd., Kent, England.

Kaushik, P. and Dhiman, A.K., 2000. *Medicinal Plants and Raw Drugs of India*. Bishen Singh Mahendra Pal Singh, Dehradun.

Raizada, M.B., 1976. *Supplement to Duthie's Flora of Upper Gangetic Plain and Adjacent Siwalik and Sub Himalayan Tracts*. Bishen Singh Mahendra Pal Singh, Dehradun.

Uniyal, M.R., 1965. Saharanpur van khand ki vanoushdhi 1962-63. *Sachitra Ayurved*, 18(1): 39–44.

Uniyal, M.R., 1977. *Uttrakhand Vanousdhi Darshika*. Central Council of Research in Indian Medicine and Homeopathy, Delhi.

Medicinal Plants: Conservation, Cultivation and Utilization (2007) *Pages 167–178*
Editors: A.K. Chopra, D.R. Khanna, G. Prasad, D.S. Malik and R. Bhutiani
Published by: DAYA PUBLISHING HOUSE

Chapter 22

Medicinal Plant Diversity in Pindari Glacier Area of Nanda Devi Biosphere Reserve (NDBR), Uttaranchal

Laxmi Rawat, H.B. Vashistha, Deepak Kholiya and S.K. Kamboj
Forest Ecology and Environment Division,
Forest Research Institute, Dehradun, Uttaranchal, India

ABSTRACT

The Pindari Glacier is located in the Pinder Valley between longitudes 79° 13′–80° 2′E and latitudes 30° 15′N, and occupies an area of 339.39 sq kms. It lies between the Nanda Devi and Nandakote peaks and terminates at an altitude of 3627 m. Pindari's rugged beauty offers a breathtaking sight, especially for the trekker who are in love with nature in all its pristine glory.

The geographical location, climate and topography of the area have contributed to the characteristic vegetation/flora and fauna of the area. Due to relative non-interference of human activities there are still patches of virgin forests throughout the glacier area. However, the stratification is not clearly distinguishable as the topography is irregular and intercepted by valleys and plateaus of various extents.

Most of the medicinal plants of this area are found at high altitude in Bugyals, composed of *Saxifraga, Sedum, Cotoneaster, Tanacetum, Aster* and *Potentilla* herbs sp. Some of the plants of medicinal value found in this region are *Nardostachys grandiflora*, a highly valued herb for its aroma and stimulating properties and *Picrorhiza scrophulariflora*, locally called 'Katugi'–the tonic prepared out of whose root is said to have cooling effect. The broad-leaved *Rheum moorcroftianum* whose red fleshy petioles are said to be edible. Other medicinal plants of the area include *Lycopodium clavatum, Asplenium* spp. and *Equisetum* spp. etc.

The present paper describes the details of medicinal plants present in Pindari Glacier area along their ethnobotanical recordings and their IUCN status like rare, endangered and vulnerable etc.

Keywords: NDBR, Pindari Glacier, Medicinal plant diversity, Ethnobotanical, IUCN status etc.

Introduction

The basic objectives of the Biosphere reserves are to conserve the diversity and integrity of biotic communities of plants and animals within natural and semi natural ecosystems for present and future use; to safeguard the genetic diversity on which their evolution depends and to provide area and facilities for ecological and environmental research, education and training.

Over the years the guidelines for the planning and management of the Biosphere Reserves have been explained to make them more relevant to human needs and economically and socially acceptable to the population concerned. Despite various lacunae and imperfections in the realization of these objectives, the primary functions of a Biosphere Reserve remains to facilitate *in situ* conservation to all forms of life along with its support systems in its totality, so that it could serve as a referral system for monitoring and evaluating changes in natural ecosystems. The Nanda Devi Biosphere Reserve (NDBR), which came into existence on 1st January, 1988, is one of them.

In the present paper an attempt has been made to document the medicinal plant wealth of the Pindari Glacier area along with their ethnobotanical recordings and IUCN status like rare, endangered, vulnerable etc.

The Study Site

Pindari is an important tourist place of NDBR in Uttaranchal state, where number of tourists visit for different purposes like trekking, mountaineering etc. The Pindari area or Pinder valley is situated in the northern most interior part of Bageshwar district, in the Kumaun Himalayas. This area is well known for the famous *"Pindari Glacier"*. It is one of the most easily accessible of all the Himalayan glaciers and has lured mountaineers and trekkers since the last century. The Pindari Glacier is located in the Pinder Valley between Longitudes 79° 13'–80° 2'E and Latitudes 30° 15'N and occupies an area of 339.39 sq.km. It lies between the Nanda Devi and Nandakote peaks and terminates at an altitude of 3627 m. The altitudinal range of Biosphere ranges from 1,000 m to 7,816 m. The Glacier is 5 km long, the snout is about 6m high and 2.5m wide and above the snout the glacier extends for about 3 km in length and 300-400 m in width, between an altitudinal ranges of about 3600m to 5000m. Pindari's rugged beauty offers a breathtaking sight, especially for the trekker who is in love with nature in all its pristine glory.

The valley is drained by the Pinder river that emerges from the Pindari Glacier. The Pindari valley is inhabited by about 14–15 villages. The people are by and large poor and lead to very simple life. The villagers practice marginal subsistence agriculture, rear cattle for milk and sheep/goat for wool and ponies for tourists. There are many routes for trekking to Pindari Glacier as can be seen in the map given (Figure 22.1). The popular/commonest route starts from Loharkhet (1750m) to Dhakuri (2683m) then to Khati (2210m) to Dwali (2734m) to Phurkia (3210m), then to last Pindari "O' point at (3862m).

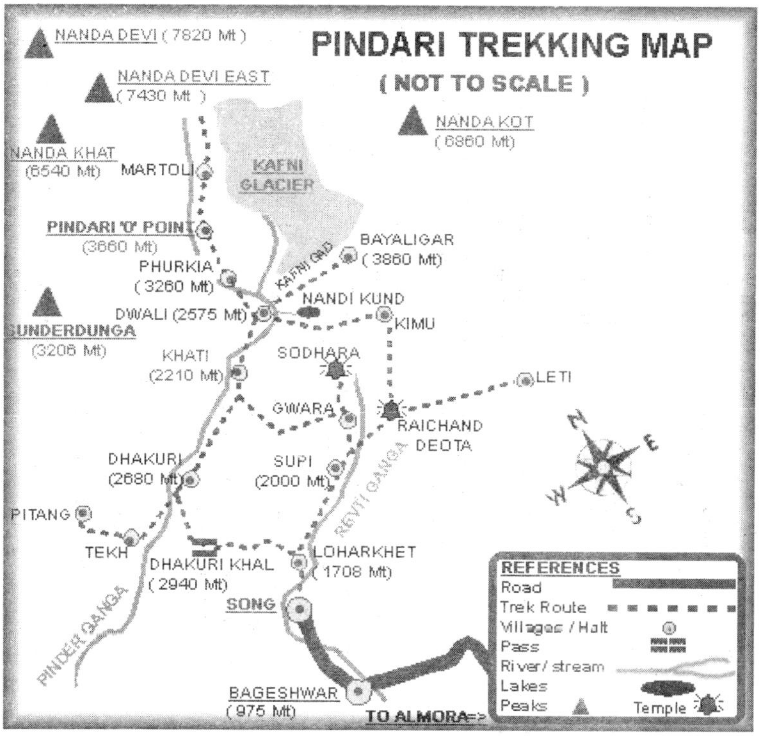

Figure 22.1: Study Area

Medicinal Plant Diversity

The Pindari valley supports attitudinally distributed vegetation, dense in growth and diverse in rich species diversity. The geographical location, climate and topography all have contributed to the characteristic vegetation and fauna of the area. Due to relative non-interference of the forest by human beings, there are still many virgin primary forest patches throughout the glacier. The temperate forests of broad leaves and conifers are present in the area. The forests of the valley are moist and have an admixture of spruce, fir, maples, horse chest nut, walnut, oaks, Rhododendrons etc. Stratifications of the forest communities along the trekking route and altitudinal gradient have been done by Rawat *et al.* (2005). However, the stratification is not clearly distinguishable as the topography is irregular and intercepted by valley and plateaus of various extents. Some other reports on medicinal plants of Uttaranchal and NDBR by Pangtey *et al.* (1994), Samant and Pal (2003), Adhikari *et al.* (2003) and Hajra and Balodi (1995) etc. have also worked out on floral composition of the area.

Beyond Phurkia, up to the foot of the Glacier, the flora is very distinct and covered with variegated graceful herbs of bright colours. Plant of tree habit are not seen in the valley. They are replaced by woody, semi-erect or prostrate plants like *Juniperus recurva, Salix elegans, Rhododendron lepidotum. R. anthopogon* and *R. campanulatum.* Another common woody prostrate shrub of wide distribution is *Cotoneaster microphyllus*. This plant is remarkable for its mat-forming habit and appears first to colonize the rocks free from snow or ice. (Hajra and Balodi, 1995). Plants of tufted habit are *Cassiope fastigiata,*

Table 22.1

Plants Botanical Name	*Local Name*	*Family*	*IUCN Status*	*Plant Parts Used/Edible*	*Medicinal Uses*
A. heterophyllum Wallich ex Royle	Mithu or Atish	"	CE	Whole plant	Used in fever and various pains, also used as tonic, less poisonous
Aconitum balfouri Stapf.	Bish	Ranunculaceae	CE	Tuberous rots	Used in fever and various pains, highly poisonous
Allium humile Kunth, *A. stracheyii* Baker	Jimbo	Lilaceae		Aromatic leaves are used as condiment	
Artemisia martima L.	Safed Purcha	Asteraceae	EN	Leaves	Leaves are used in worship.
Berberis aristata (Roxb.) DC. *B.* (Roxb.)ex DC. *B.* Lindl.	Kingor	Berberidaceae	EN, VU, R&E	Fruits and roots. Fruits are eaten raw or mixed with mustered oil.	Roots are used in various eye diseases and in diarrhoea. Extract of root is used in making dye.
Bergenia ciliata (Haw.) Sternb.	Pasanbhed or Silphori	Saxifragaceae	VU, R&E	Thick root stocks	Extract of roots used as cooling agent, tonic and in fever
Betula utilis D. Don	Bhoj or Bhojpatra	Betulaceae	EN.	Dried cell sap (Betula gum) is used as substitute of tea	The Bhoj tea is said to give a very good healing effect
Cannabis sativa L.	Bhang	Cannabinaceae		Leaves, Inflorescence and seeds. Seeds are eaten raw and are used as spices. The leaves are dried to obtain BHANG from the glandular leaves and from inflorescence (female one) GANJA is prepared. Both these have psychoactive activity	The leaves and seeds are supposed to be good healing agent. The drug obtained from leaves and inflorescence is intoxicating and analgesic, also used n stomachache. The stem are shacked in water and thrashed to get good quality fiber.
Cirsium wallichii DC.	Kandaya	"		Pith of stem is taken raw and is said to be good in thirst	
Corylus jacquemontii Decne.	Bhoti Badam or Kabasi	Corylaceae		Seeds are roasted and eaten	
Cupressus torulosa D.Don	Surai	Cupressaceae		Leaves	The leaves are used in preparing "BALMA" used in preparing local drinks (DARU)

Contd...

Plants Botanical Name	Local Name	Family	IUCN Status	Plant Parts Used/Edible	Medicinal Uses
Fagopyrum dibotrys (D. Don) Hara	Ban, Ogal	Polygonaceae		Leaves are cooked as vegetables	These are said to have heating effect.
Gerbera gossypina (Royle) Beauv.	Kapasi	"		Leaves	The wool of leaves is used to get fire by friction between a piece of stone and iron.
Hippophe salicifolia D. Don.	Sankutarwa or Tarwa	Elaeagnaceae	LR-NT	Fruits are eaten raw and are used in making pickles and "Chatni"	
Nardostachys grandiflora DC.	Masi or Jatamasi	Valerianaceae	CE, NE, CR, VU	Roots	The fragrant root stocks used as cooling agent and as tonic, also used in various heart problems
Paeonia emodi Walich ex Royle	Hadgans or Gandrain	Paeoniaceae	VU	"	Used in various urinary diseases
Picrorhiza scrophulariiflora Pennell	Katki	Scrophulariaceae	EN, VU	Seeds and roots	They are used in fever, as purgative and as tonic
Podophyllum hexandrum Royle	Papra or Charpu	Podophyllaceae	CE, EN	Fruit	Good in fever, also used as tonic and in cancerous diseases
Polygonatum verticillatum (L.) All.	Salam or Salam Mishri	"	VU, EN	Tubers	The tubers are used as tonic and in fever
Prinsepia utilis Royle	Bhekal	Rosaceae		Fruits are crushed and edible oil is extracted	
Rhododendron anthopogon D. Don	Kodya	Ericaceae	VU	Leaves are used as substitute of tea	
Rubus foliolosus D. Don, *R. niveus* Thunb.	Kali, Hisalu	"		"	The fruits are said to be good in constipation
Rhododendron lepidotum Wallich ex G. Don	Taghishya or Takkar	"	VU	"	
Rosa sericea Lindl.	Shyapla	"		"	"
Rheum. webbiana Wallich ex Royle	"	"	VU	"	
Rheum moorcroftianum Royle	"	"	VU	Roots and Leaves	Thick root stock are used as healing agent
Rhododendron arboreum Sm.	Burans		VU	The squash is prepared from the flower	The juice of flower is said to be cooling agent in diarrhoea

Contd...

Table 22.1–Comtd...

Plants Botanical Name	Local Name	Family	IUCN Status	Plant Parts Used/Edible	Medicinal Uses
Rhus parviflora Roxb.	Tungla	Anacardiaceae	VU	Fruits and leaves. Fruits are used raw	The smoke of leaves have psychoactive effect
Ribes alpester Wallich,					
R. himalense Royle ex D. Don	Darbag	Grossulariaceae		Ripe fruits are eaten raw and are used in pickles	
Rosa anserinaefolia Boiss.	Gorshyapla	Rosaceae		Fruit and roots. Fruit are eaten raw	Roots are crushed and used in various urinary diseases
Rubus ellipticus Sm,	Hisalu	"	VU, EN	Fruits are eaten raw	
Rumex hastatus D. Don	Kilmor	"		Leaves are crushed with spices to make "Chatni"	
Saussurea obvallata (DC.) Edgew.	Brahmkamal	"	CR, NE, VU, EN	Flowers	Flowers are used in worship.
Stephania glabra (Roxb.) Miers fever and bronchitis.	Ghindharu	Menispermaceae		Tuberous roots	Said to be good in various blood problems,
Taxus wallichiana Zucc.	Thuner	Taxaceae	G, CE.	Stem bark is used as substitute of tea	The tea of *Taxus* bark is said to have a great healing effect, also used in fever
Thalictrum foliolosum DC.	Ubyakoti or Mamiri	"	VU, EN	Roots	Used in various urinary and eye diseases, also used as blood purifier and as tonic
Urtica dioica L.	Kandali	Urticaceae		Leaves are cooked as vegetable	The cooked leaves are said to be very good in certain feminine diseases. The leaves are also applied in artherites. The stems are soaked in water and then thrashed to obtain fiber
Verbascum thapsus L.	Akulbir	"		Entire plant	This plant is used in certain "Jadu Tona"
Viburnum continifolium D. Don	Genu	Caprifoliaceae		Fruit and seeds. Seeds are crushed and edible oil is extracted, fruits are eaten raw	

IUCN (Red Data Book) Plants Status: CR: Critically Endangered, EN: Endangered, NE: Near Endangered, VU: Vulnerable, LR-NT: Low risk-Near Threatened, LR-LC: Low risk-Least concern, G: Indicates globally threatened species as these are endemic to India and deserve higher conservation priority, R: Rare, E: Endemic.

Table 22.2: Community Knowledge (Ethnobotanical Recording) of Some Common Medicinal and Aromatic Herbs Identified

Common/Botanical Name	*IUCN Status*	*Habit*	*Family*	*Parts Used*	*Occurrence (m)*	*Chemical Constituents*	*Uses*
(a) Medicinal Plants							
Kutki/*Picrorhiza Kurrooa*	EN, VU	Herb	Scrophulariaceae	Roots Whole plant	2745–4575	Glycoside 26. 6%	Cathartic, Stomachic, Fever, Dyspepsia, Purgative
Jatamansi/*Nardostachys Jatamansi*	CE, NE, CR, VU	Herb	Valerianaceae	Roots	3200–4575	Volatile oil 3–4%	Purgative Tonic, Antiseptic, Epilepsy, Hysteria
Atees/*Aconitum heterophyllum*	CE	Herb	Ranunculaceae	Tubers, Roots	2440–4200	Alkaloid atisine 0.4%	Tonic, Diarrhoea, Dyspepsia, Cough
Gobriya/Bish/*Aconitum balfouril*	CE	Herb	Ranunculaceae	Roots, Tubers	2440–4575	Total alkaloid 1.2% of which Pseudo-aconitine 0.4%	Leprosy, Fever, Cholera, (Poisonous) Rheumatism
Salampanja/*Orchis latifolia*		Herb	Orchidaceae	Tubers	2440–4270	Glucoside Loroglossin 0.0055%	Expectorant, Astringent
Bhutkeshi/*Corydalis govaniana*		Herb	Papaveraceae	Roots	–do–	Alkaloid protonic cholone Corlumino bisculine isocorydine	Antiperiodic Diuretic, Alterative syphilis scrofula
Bankakari/*Podophyllum hexandrum*	CE, CN	Herb	Berberidaceae	Roots	2282–4000	Podophyllotoxin (3-4%) Quercetin (8%) Essential oil (3.7%)	Purgative Alterative, Bitter tonic
Somlata/*Ephedra geradiana*		Herb		Stem	2130–4800	Total alkaloids (0.28%–2.79%) alkaloid ephedrine and pseudoephedrine	Asthmatic, Cardiac Circulatory Rheumatism, Syphilis
Nirbishi/*Delphinium elatum*	CE	Herb	Ranunculaceae	Seed	3060–4270	Total Alkaloids (1.7%). Delatine, Delpheline, Methylaconitine	Itch, Skin eruptions, Eye sores
Rewand chini/ *Rheum emodi*	VU	Herb	Polygonaceae	Root/ Rhizome	2745–4270	Various anthraquinones derivatives	Purgative, Astringent, Stimulant
Talispatra/*Taxus baccata*	CE, G	Tree	Taxaceae	Leaves/ fruits	1825–3355	Alkaloid Taxine Taxol	Sedative Antiseptic, Asthma, Bronchitis, Epilespy, Indigestion
Chirata/*Swertia Chirata*	G, CE, EN, VU	Herb	Gentianaceae	Whole Plant	1220–3050	Chiratin, Ophetic acid	Bitter tonic, Stomachic Laxative
Daruharidra/*Berberis Aristata*	EN, VU, R&E	Shrub	Berberidaceae	Root Bark, wood	1825–3050	Berberine (2.23%), Hydro sulphate (3%), Palmatine chloride	Alterative, Fever, Skin disease Jaundice, Ophthalmia

Contd...

Table 22.2–Contd...

Common/Botanical Name	*IUCN Status*	*Habit*	*Family*	*Parts Used*	*Occurrence (m)*	*Chemical Constituents*	*Uses*
Kilmora/*Berberis asiatica*	EN, VU, R&E	Shrub	Berberidaceae	Root, Bark wood	762–2130	Total alkaloid 4%–roots 1.95%–stem. Berberine, 2-09% roots, 1.29% stem	Ophthalmia Fever, Jaundice, Teucorrhoea
Padam/*Prunus cerasoides*		Tree	Rosaceae	Small branches, Bark kernel	610–2282	Glucosides	Kernel-stone/glands, Bark-check abortion
Banapsa/*Viola odorata*				Whole plant	1525–1820	Glucosides Violaquor, Citrin, Dythyl salicylate	Antipyretic, Febrifuge, Bile and Lungs troubles
Samewa/*Valeriana wallichii*	G, CR, CE	Herb	Valerianaceae	Root	1220–3660	Volatile oil (12%) Tartaric, Citric Melic, Succinic acids	Carminative Antispasmodic, Hysteria, Epilepsy Cholera, Neurosis.
Pilijari/Mamiri/*Thalictrum foliolosum*	VU, EN	Herb	Ranunculaceae	Root	1530–2440	Alkaloid Barberine 0.3%, Thalictrine	Atonic Dyspepsia, ophthalmia, Purgative, Febrifuge, Convalescence
Kapoor kachri/ *Hedychium spicatum*	VU	Herb.	Zingiberaceae	Root stock	1525–2282	Essential oil, starch 52%, Organic acid (resinic acid) 4.6%	Stomachic, Carminative, Expectorant, Bowel complaints, Vomiting, Diarrhoea
Pasanved/*Berginia ligulata*	VU, R&E	Herb	Saxifragaceae	Root	1977	Galic acid, Tenic acid (14.2%), Glucose (5.6%) Mucilage, Bergenin	Fever, Diarrhoea, Pulmonary aflictions, Antiscorbatic, Boils, Opthalmia, Kidney stones
Tejpat/*Cinnamomum tamala*				Leaves	1915	Essential oil (0.9–1.4%) in leaves, Essential oil from bark contains 70–85% cinnamic aldehyde	Stimulant, Carminative, Rheumatism, Colic diarrhoea, Scorpion sting
(b) Essential Oil Yielding Plants							
Bach/*Acorus calamus*				Rhizome	Upto 2440	1.5–3.5%	Perfumery (medicinal and flavouring, also stimulant)
Tejpat/*Cinnamomum tamala*				Leaves	1915	0.8–1.4%	Stimulant, Flavouring of Sweets/ confectionery
Jatamansi/*Nardostachys jatamansi*	CE, NE, CR, VU	Herb	Valerianaceae	Roots	3202, 4575	0.3–0.4%	Disease of respiratory and digestive organs, jaundice, Leprosy
Nairpati/*Skimmia laurelo*		Shrub	Rutaceae	Leaves	1825, 3050	0.5–0.8%	Source of linalyl, Acceptable perfumery
Timur/*Zanthoxylum armetum*		Shrub		Fruit	Upto 1825	1.5–2.3%	Soap, Dental Preparation

Contd...

Table 22.2–Contd...

Common/Botanical Name	*IUCN Status*	*Habit*	*Family*	*Parts Used*	*Occurrence (m)*	*Chemical Constituents*	*Uses*
Kapoor Kachri/*Hedychium spicafum*	VU	Herb	Zingiberaceae	Root	1526, 2282	4. 0%	Perfume, soap, Hair oil, Face powder
Banajwain/*Thymus serphyllum*		Herb	Lamiaceae	Leaves/foral Tip	1525	0.5–1.0%	Cheap, flavoring agent, Ingredient of hair and scalp lotion
Jhora/*Juniperus communis*		Tree	Cupressaceae	Fruit	2130, 4270	0.8–1.6%	Stimulant, Diuretic in chronic genitourinary infections, Flavoring liquors
Billa/Dhup/*Juniperus macropoda*		Tree	Cupressaceae	Fruit	2130–4270	0.6–1.68%	Substitute for juniper oil
Samewa/Tagar/ *Valeriana wallichii*	G, CR, CE	Herb	Valerianaceae	Rhizomes	1220–2050	0.3–1.0%	Flavouring tobacco and honey, for blending in high grade perfumes as a fixative
Chora/*Angelica glauca*	CE	Herb	Umbelliferae/ Apiaceae	Root	2440	1.3%	Cordial and stimulant, Flavouring agent
Pudina/*Mentha sylvestris*		Herb		Leaves/twigs	1200	1.2%	Flavour
Devdar/*Cedrus deodara*		Tree		Wood	1200–3050	2.5%	Soap, perfumery, Antiseptic
Chir/*Pinus roxburghii*		Tree		Oleoresin	610–2280	14.20%	Varnish, Lacquers, Disinfectant
Kuth/*Saussurea lappa*	CR, NE, VU, EN, CE, E	Herb	Asteraceae/ Cardueae	Root	2500	0.6–2. 6%	High class perfumery, Cosmetics (Blending)
Bantulsi/*Origanum vulgare*		Herb		Plant	1500–3600	0.15–0.4%	Consmetics, Colic, Diarrhoea, Whooping cough
(c) Non-edible Oil Yielding Plants							
Akhrot/*Jugians regia*		Tree	Juglandaceae	Kernels	912–335	60–70%	Artistic ink, Colours, Printing ink, Soap
Bari/*Quercus incana*		Tree	Fagaceae	Aceorns	1000–2400	16%	
Bhang/*Cannabis sativa*		Herb	Cannabinaceae	Seed	Upto 1745	32–55%	Luminant, Paints, Varnish Soap
Bakain/*Melia Azedarach*		Tree		Seed	Upto 1675	40%	Soap, Paint, Varnish

Source: Flora and Fauna of Kumaun Himalaya by–Ajay S. Rawat (KMVN Ltd "Travelers guide book -2001"

IUCN (Red Data Book) Plants Status: CR: Critically Endangered, EN: Endangered, NE: Near Endangered, VU: Vulnerable, LR-NT: Low risk-Near Threatened, LR-LC: Low risk-Least concern, G: Indicates globally threatened species as these are endemic to India and deserve higher conservation priority, R: Rare, E: Endemic.

Rhodiola quadrifida, different species of *Astragalus*, etc. The pretty blues to red tinged fruits of prostrate *Gaultheria trichophylla* are very attractive as they form a regular carpet in the valley. The other handsome herbs of the valley are prostrate pink flowered *Thymus linearis*, white flowered woolly herb *Anaphalis nepalensis* and *A. cuneifolia*, yellow flowered herb *Potentilla argyrophylla* and dark crimson flowered *P. argyrophylla* var. *atrosanguinea*. During the ascent from Bugyal to the foot of the Pindari glacier one can experience the rich aroma of the herb *Tanacetum* with small yellow heads. This alpine herb forms a regular mat and is collected for its 'gogal', a gum resin used for incense. The Yellow flowered *Taraxacum officinale*, *Aster stracheyi*, a woolly herb *Leontopodium brachyactis* and *Senecio laetus* are the other members of Asteraceae family frequently seen in the alpine herbage.

The margins of the rivulet beds support variety of graceful herbs. The common genera are *Corydalis*, *Anemone*, *Pedicularis*, *Sedum*, *Potentilla*, *Primula*, *Androsace*, *Epilobium*, *Polygomum*, *Poa*, *Juncus* and *Carex*. The most attractive herb is the deep blue flowered *Cyananthus lobatus*.

The dominating plant all along the lateral moraine is *Cotoneaster microphyllus*. This is followed by *Cassiope fastigiata* and species of *Rhododendrons*. Amidst the big boulders one can see more or less the same alpine herbs in adjacent Bugyals also. The medial moraine flora is chiefly composed of *Saxifraga*, *Sedum*, *Cotoneaster*, *Tanacetum*, *Aster* and *Potentilla* species.

The mountains surrounding the Pindari valley are steep with boulders of varied size, and support vegetation up to 5300 m. beyond it is the zone of perpetual snow. The interesting plants of this area are *Saussurea obvallata*, (Brahma Kamal), Uttaranchal's state flower with transparent bracts, *Primula* species, *Aconitum falconeri*, *Meconopis aculeate*, *Morina longifolia*, *Swertia* species

Some of the plants of medicinal value collected in this region are *Nardostachys grandiflora*, a highly valued herb for its aroma and stimulating properties and *Picrorhiza scrophulariflora*, locally called 'Katugi'–the tonic prepared out of whose root is said to have cooling effect. The broad-leaved *Rheum moorcroftianum* whose red fleshy petioles are said to be edible, was also collected. Other interesting collections from this area include *Lycopodium clavatum*, *Asplenium* spp. and *Equisetum* spp.

Of the several glaciers in the Garhwal and Kumaun Himalayas, Pindari glacier is the most attractive and easily accessible, and as such has provided considerable attraction to naturalists. Botanically the area can be dived in three distinct vegetational zones. A sub alpine region from 3700-400 m, a moraine zone from 4000-4250m and an alpine zone from 4500 m to snow line.

The Tables 22.1 and 22.2 lists some of the medicinal plant species of the area having considerable ethnobotanical value along with their local names, part of the plant used/medicinal values and their IUCN status.

Acknowledgement

Authors are thankful to DFO Nanda Devi Biosphere Reserve, DFO Bagesbwar, Dr. Rajeev Barathari (Nodal Officer Eco-tourism). Dr. C.S. Chandola (Chief Wild Life Warden) for granting the prior permission to visit the Pindari area and help of all team members is greatly acknowledged.

Conclusions

The present study provides comprehensive information on the diversity, distribution pattern, IUCN conservation status of medicinal plants which are distributed in Pindari valley and adjoin Glacier region. Awareness generating among villagers by organizing training and extension programs about the socio-economic value and conservation and management of rare endangered and otherwise important medicinal plants can be step towards their sustainable utilization and conservation in natural habitat.

References

Adhikari, B.S., M.M. Babu, R.K. Saklani and D.S. Rawat, 2003. Medicinal trees of Uttaranchal state: Distribution, use pattern and prospects for conservation. *Indian Forester*, 129(2): 243–267.

Arya, S.C., 2004. Assessment of plant diversity and human development for the conservation of alpine meadows in Nanda Devi Biosphere Reserve, West Himalaya. Project summaries/short communications G.B. Pant Kosi Katarmal, Almora. *Himalayan Biosphere Reserve*, 6(1 and 2): 129–151.

Bagri, S.C., 1994. Strategy for sustainable tourism development for trekking tourism promotion and environment conservation in Garhwal Himalayas. *Journal of Tourism*, Vol. 2, H.N.B. Garhwal University, Srinagar-Garhwal.

Gupta, B.K., 1990. *Higher Plants of Indian Subcontinents*, Vol. 1. Bishen Singh, Mahendra Pal Singh, Shiva Offset Press, Dehradun.

Hajra, P.K. and Bipin Batodi, 1995. *Plant Wealth of Nanda Devi Biosphere Reserve*. Series 4. Flora of India, Botanical Survey of India, Howrah (Calcutta).

Hajra, P.K., 1983. *A Contribution to the Botany of Nanda Devi National Park in Uttar Pradesh, India*. Botanical Survey of India, Howrah (Koltaka/Calcutta), pp. 38.

Hajra, P.K., 1983. *Botany of Nanda Devi National Park*. POSSCEF, Botanical Survey of India, Howrah (Calcutta), pp. 30.

Jain, S.K. and Sastry, A.R.K., 1980. *Threatened Plants of India*. A state of the art report. BSI and MAB, New Delhi, pp. 19.

Jayat, N.D., 1990. Himalaya: Our Fragile Heritage. In: *The Souvenir of Institute of Mountaineering 25 Years*, N.I.M, Uttarkashi. (Ref. Source: *Indian Mountaineer*, Issue 10, 13, 16, 17, 19, 21, 23, 25. IMF Silver Jubilee Journal, pp. 61 and NIM, Uttarkashi).

Joshi, H.C., Arya, S.C. and Sammant, S.S., 1999. Diversity, distribution and indigenous uses of medicinal and edible plants in a part of Nanda Devi Biosphere Reserve I. *Himalayan Biosphere Reserve (Biannual Bulletin)* 1(1 and 2): 49–65.

Maikhuri, R.K., U. Rana, K.S. Rao and K.G. Saxena, 2000. Promoting ecotourism in the Buffer zone areas of Nanda Devi Biosphere reserve: An option to resolve people-policy conflict. *International Journal of Sustainable and World Ecology*, (7): 333–342.

Malhotra, B.N., B.S. Aswal and B.S. Bisht, 1987. *Glossary of Indian Medicinal Plants*. Bishen Singh and Mahendra Pal Singh, Shiva Offset Press, Dehradun.

Nautiyal, S., R.K. Maikhuri, K.S. Rao and K.G. Saxena, 2001. Medicinal plant resources in Nanda Devi biosphere reserve in Central Himalaya. *Journal of Herbs, Spices and Medicinal Plants*, 8(4): 47–64.

Nautiyal, S., R.K. Maikhuri, K.S. Rao and K.G. Saxena, 2003. Ethnobotany of the Tolcha Bhotiya tribe of the buffer zone in Nanda Devi Biosphere Reserve, India. In: *Ethnobotany and Medicinal Plants of India and Nepal*, Vol. 1, (Eds.) V. Singh and A.P. Singh. Scientific Publishers, Jodhpur (Rajasthan), pp. 119–142.

Nayar, M.P. and A.R.K. Sastry, 1987, 88, 90. *Red Data Book of Indian Plants*, Vols. I–III. Botanical Survey of India, Calcutta.

Pangtey, Y.P.S., S.S. Samant and R.S. Rawat, 1994. Enumeration of ferns of Pindari, Sarju and east Ramganga Valleys of Kumaun (Western Himalaya). In: *Higher Plants of Indian Subcontinent*, Vol. IV, (Ed.) B.K. Gupta. Bishen Singh, Mahendra Pal Singh, Shiva Offset Press, Dehradun, pp. 119–152.

Rawat Laxmi, H.B., Vashistha Deepak Khotiya and S.K. Kamboj, 2005. Assessment of plant diversity in the Pindari region of NDBR (Uttaranchal). In: *National Symposium of Changing Concepts of Forestry in 21st Century*. Y.P.S. Parmar University, Solan (H.P.), 21–22 October.

Samant, S.S. and Mohinder Pal, 2003. Diversity and conservation status of medicinal plants in Uttaranchal state. *Indian Forester*, 129(9): 1090–1108.

Samant, S.S., H.C. Joshi, S.C. Arya and S. Pant, 2000. Assessment of socio-economic status arid diversity of economically important plant resources using participatory approach: Case study from Pindari area of Nanda Devi Biosphere Reserve, West Himalaya. *Van Vigyan*, Journal of Society of Indian Foresters, 38(1–4): 55–81.

Sharma, B.D., 1994. Wildlife reserves of high altitude Himalaya. In: *High Altitudes of Himalayas: Biogeography, Ecology and Conservation*, (Eds.) Pangtey, Y.P.S. and Rawal, R.S., pp. 220–228.

Silori, C.S., 2004. Socioeconomic and ecological consequences of the ban on adventure tourism in Nanda Devi Biosphere Reserve, Western Himalaya. *Biodiversity and Conservation*, 13: 2237–2252.

Tak, P.C. and Kumar, G., 1987. Wildlife of Nanda Devi National Park: An update. *Indian Journal of Forestry*, 10(3): 184–190.

Medicinal Plants: Conservation, Cultivation and Utilization (2007) *Pages 179–182*
Editors: A.K. Chopra, D.R. Khanna, G. Prasad, D.S. Malik and R. Bhutiani
Published by: DAYA PUBLISHING HOUSE

Chapter 23

Effect of Three Different Boiling Times for Extraction of Aqueous Extract of Peepal Leaf on Growth of *Myrothecium roridum* Tode ex Fr.

Vishal K. Muliya* and Arun Arya
Department of Botany, Faculty of Science,
The Maharaja Sayajirao University of Baroda, Vadodara

ABSTRACT

Ficus religiosa L., commonly known as *Peepal* or *piplo,* is having latex which is used for sealing small holes in motor car tier. Hardened latex is used by artificers as a sealing wax to fill up cavities in hollow ornaments. It contains tannin, which is having astringent activity. An aqueous extract of the bark is having antibacterial activity. During extraction lot many chemicals are break down and lot many chemicals forms complexes which always affect the biological activity of the plant extract. Present paper deals with effect of different boiling times like half an hour, one hour, and one and a half hour extraction on the growth of a fungi *Myrothecium roridum* by using poisoned food technique. Cold extraction was also studied. Difference in extraction time and concentration of extract show different antifungal activity against *Myrothecium roridum* Tode ex Fr. Only half an hour extraction of peepal leaf extract showed positive antifungal activity while other treatments showed negative antifungal activity.

* E-mail: vkmuliya@yahoo.com.

Introduction

Ficus religiosa L. is commonly known as *Peepal* or *piplo.* Fresh leaves of peepal form one of the ingredients in Homeopathic formulations used to treat haemorrhages of many kinds like haemoptysis, epistaxis, haematuria, menorrhagia, metrorrhagia, blood dysentery and bleeding piles. Aqueous extract of fresh leaves and litter showed strong allelopathic potential against some crop plants (Anonymous, 2002). Leaf is having purgative effect also (Anjaria *et al.,* 2002). Leaf is containing 19.2 per cent carbohydrate, 13.55 per cent protein and 2.5 per cent lipid (Ruby *et al.,* 2000). It is having 22.75mg total carotene and amongst it presence of beta-carotene is 12.62 mg in 100 gm leaf (Rajyalaksmi *et al.,* 2001). Ethnobotanically its leaves are used in stomach pain (Muhammad *et al.,* 2003). It contains tannin, which is having astringent activity. An aqueous extract of the bark is having antibacterial activity (Farrukh and Iqbal, 2003). In this experiment an effort has been made to study the effect of different boiling times like half an hour, one hour and one and half hour extraction was made from fresh leaf. Cold extraction was also studied. Different times of boiling may release different chemicals and these shows different antifungal activity against test fungus, *Myrothecium roridum* Tode ex Fr.

M. roridum is known to produce toxins like ochratoxin A, trichothecens, 3-hydroxyroridin E, roridin A, roridin L, roridin M, isororidin A, epiroridin, 12, 13-deoxyroridin E, 14'-hydroxymytoxin B, 16-hydroxyroridin etc. These toxins are having cytotoxic and mutagenic activity also (Khisal *et al.,* 2002).

Materials and Methods

Fungi

Myrothecium roridum was isolated form a deteriorating object in Baroda museum and Picture Gallery, Vadodara (Shah and Arya, 2000); and Pure culture was identified based on microscopic characters and authenticated form IARI, Delhi. Pure culture was maintained on Potato Dextrose Agar (PDA) medium (Peeled Potato 200g, Dextrose 20g, Agar 20g, Distilled Water 1000ml) at 25±2°C temperature in BOD incubator.

Plant Extract

Peepal leaves were collected from arboretum of Botany department, The Maharaja Sayajirao University of Baroda, Vadodara, 100 g of leaves were washed and crushed in mixer for 20 min and then boiled for half an hour, one hour and one and half hour. 100 g leaves were crushed in cold water also. After boiling, the filtrate was taken and the water was added to make it 100 ml so that there will be concentration of 1g/ml.

Bioassay

Poisoned food technique (Nene and Thapliyal, 1979) was used to study antifungal activity of plant. Plant extract was added 5, 10, and 25 per cent v/v to culture medium PDA and the medium was sterilized at 15 lbs pressure, for 20 min. finally cultural medium was transferred to Petri plates and then these were inoculated and incubated at 25°C temp for 7 days and then colony diameter was measured to study the fungal growth.

Results and Discussion

It has been observed that there was maximum inhibition of fungal growth at 5 per cent concentration when half an hour boiling was done (Table 23.1). By increasing concentration of the leaf extract there was no increase in inhibitory action but a decrease was recorded 18.51, 11.26 and 4.92

per cent at 5, 10 and 25 per cent respectively, may be due to release of sugar or other nutrient during extraction. It was indicated that there were some compounds which were having effect on inhibition but effect is not depended on quantity. As the concentration is increasing there is increase in soluble sugars which may be the reason for decreasing the inhibition because sugars are known for increasing fungal growth. One hour boiling has given very contradictory results, may be due to release of tannin which is causing precipitation of proteins of potato in PDA medium. At 10 per cent concentration it gave 4.59 per cent inhibition while there was no inhibition at 5 per cent and 25 per cent concentration (Table 23.1). When one and half hour boiling treatment was given there was no inhibition, which indicates that all the compounds which can inhibit the fungi were not present in extract and there is deactivation of antifungal compound.

Table 23.1: Showing the Effect of Different Boiling Temperature Treatment of Leaf Inhibition of Fungal Growth

Treatment	*Concentration of Leaf Extract*		
	5 per cent	*10 per cent*	*25 per cent*
Cold aqueous extract	–5.22 ± 1.25	–2.29 ± 0.15	–9.01 ± 0.84
Half an Hour boiled aqueous extract	18.51 ± 1.09	11.26 ± 0.69	4.92 ± 0.60
One Hour boiled aqueous extract	–2.95 ± 0.06	–4.59 ± 0.13	–4.18 ± 0.41
One and half Hours boiled aqueous extract	–12.72 ± 0.28	–6.43 ± 0.28	–5.91 ± 0.41

Data showing per cent inhibition of *M. roridum* at three different concentration of leaf extract when different time treatment were given for boiling. Data represented as mean of three replicate ± standard deviation. Anova test is significant at $p < 0.05$ level.

Conclusion

Only half an hour of boiling with 5 per cent concentration is giving best results which indicate that there is no need to boil more than half an hour to extract antifungal compound form peepal leaves.

References

Anjaria, J., Parabia, M., Bhatt, G. and Khamar, R., 2002. *Nature Heals: A Glossary of Selected Indigenous Medicinal Plants of India*. Srishti Innovations, Ahmedabad.

Anonymous, 2002. *Wealth of India*, Vol. 3. CSIR Publication, New Delhi.

Farrukh, A. and Iqbal, A., 2003. Broad-spectrum antibacterial and antifungal properties of certain traditionally used Indian medicinal plants. *World Journal of Microbiology and Biotechnology*, 19: 653–657

Khisal, A.A., Rabenstein, J., Woodard, J., Baker, D.D., Bergthold, J.D., Lynch, J. Lieu, K.L. and Braude, I.A., 2002. 14'-Hydroxymytoxin B and 16-Hydroxyroridin E, two new cytotoxic trichothecenes from *Myrothecium roridum*. *Journal of Natural Product*, 65: 742–744.

Muhammad, Z., Bokharie, S.Y.A., Muhammad, A.T., Kamran, S. and Abida, A., 2003. Taxonomical description and ethnobotanical survey for indigenous use of some medicinal plants of Rawalpindi district. *Asian Journal of Plant Sciences*, 2(6): 475-479.

Nene, Y.L. and Thapliyal, P.N., 1979. *Fungicide in Plant Disease Control*. Oxford and IBH Pub. Co., New Delhi.

Rajyalakshmi, P., Venkatalaxmi, K., Venkatalakshamma, K., Jyothsna Y., Balachandramani K. and Suneetham V., 2001. Total carotenoid and beta-carotene contents of forest, green leafy vegetables consumed by tribals of south India. *Plant Foods for Human Nutrition*, 56: 225–238.

Ruby, J., Nathan, P.T., Balasingh, J. and Kunz, T.H., 2000. Chemical composition of fruits and leaves eaten by short-nosed fruit bat, *Cynopterus sphinx*, 26(12): 2825–2841.

Shah, N.R. and Arya, A., 2000. *Studies on Some Funal Biodeteriogens*. Bharatiya Kala Prakashan, Delhi.

Medicinal Plants: Conservation, Cultivation and Utilization (2007) *Pages* 183–187
Editors: A.K. Chopra, D.R. Khanna, G. Prasad, D.S. Malik and R. Bhutiani
Published by: DAYA PUBLISHING HOUSE

Chapter 24

Rare Medicinal Plants as Used in the Folklore of Garhwal Himalaya

P.P. Badoni[1], A.K. Dobriyal[2], P.K. Bahuguna[2] and H.K. Joshi[2] and (Late) G.S. Negi[1]
[1]Department of Chemistry, [2]Department of Zoology,
H.N.B. Garhwal University Campus, Pauri Garhwal – 246 001, Uttaranchal

ABSTRACT

Plants are used as therapeutics since ages. In Garhwal Himalaya also, the folk were highly enriched with the knowledge about use of numerous plants and their products for the treatment of various diseases. Locally they were called vaidyas. The paper deals with the vernacular and taxonomic details of some plants, which are used in ten common ailments.

Introduction

Plants are the rich source of many natural products most of which have been extensively used for human welfare and treatment of various diseases. There is a long history of traditional therapeutic use of these plants by the Vaidyas in Uttaranchal. A description of some vaidyas and their traditional knowledge on therapeutics is given by Negi (1994). The present communication deals with vernacular and taxonomic details of some medicinal plants, which are used for the cure of some common ailments like asthma, arthritis, common fever, headache, cough, piles, skin disease, leucorrhoea (white), stone and chronic constipation. The methodology of treatment as used by the vaidyas is also discussed.

Methodology

The study is based on the survey and experiences of the vaidyas in the Dogadda and Pokhra Blocks of Pauri Garhwal, Uttaranchal.

Results and Discussion

After thorough survey of vaidyas in the Pokhra and Dogadda Blocks of Garhwal District, about 49 ailments were reported to be cured by the vaidyas after using different parts of 102 medicinal plants. For present communication we have taken only ten common diseases, the methodology of treatment and vernacular and taxonomic details of used medicinal plants.

The treatment methods of selected diseases is as follows:

Asthma

1. The paste of Bharingi with honey is prepared and 3 gm of paste is taken in an interval of half an hour and should be consumed within 2–3 hours.
2. One seed of Datura per day is taken for a week and two seeds per day for second week, similarly three seeds per day for third week and four seeds per day for fourth week. It is very potent for asthma.
3. The powder of Ashwagandha is mixed with honey and cow's ghee and taken till the disease is cured.
4. The powder of Peepal leaves, Munakka, Kakarsinghi and Misri are taken in an equal amount and given with fresh water.

Arthritis

1. The paste of Indrayan root is prepared with water and applied on the affected part.
2. The roots of Bamboo are crushed and mixed with mustard oil. This preparation is used for massage on the affected part.
3. The seed oil of Malkangani is taken and used to massage on affected part.
4. The leaves of Amaltas are roasted with cows ghee and given the patient to chew it.
5. Five gm of Sounth powder is given with hot water twice a day.

Common Fever

1. The whole plant of Chiraita is grinded to powder and taken in every morning and in every evening with milk.
2. The powder of genthi is prepared and taken with cold water. It is very effective in fever.
3. One part of flowers of Adoosa is mixed with two part of Misri and kept in earthen pot for fifteen days. Ten gms of this mixture is given.

Headache

1. Equal amount of Mulathi, sounth, sendha namak, kuth, and kalimirch are taken and powdered. This powder is mixed with ghee and turned to tablets of gram size. One tablet is given to patient daily for twenty-one days.
2. The powder of Chiraita, long, Dhamasa and kalimirch (Black pepper) are prepared. This is given to patient with warm water.
3. The flowers of Mehandi are grinded to collect the juice. It is then applied over the head to cure headache.

Cough

1. The extract of the leaves of Arjuna and Adoosa are mixed together and is taken with honey, which is very effective for cough.
2. Two parts of Bharangi juice and four parts of curd are mixed together. It is given for four days.
3. The root quath of Sajji is prepared and given to drink.

Piles

1. Equal amount of bark of Pithpapra, Manjeeth, white sandal, til and Mochras are taken and turned to powder. Twelve gm of this is taken with goat milk to cure piles.
2. Chitrak, Trikut, Peepari, peepal mool, Dhania, bark of Patha, Gokhru, Bealgiri, Gajpeepari and ajwain are taken and turned to powder. This powder is taken in every morning with an empty stomach.
3. The fruit pulp of beal is cooked with gur and given to eat.
4. The seed coat of Reetha is burnt and turned to ash. This ash is taken with honey.

Skin Disease

1. The root of Sajji is grinded and applied over the affected part.
2. The bark of Peepari, seed of Panwar, and kalimirch are taken and burnt to ash. This ash is mixed with urine of cow to make a paste. This paste is then applied over the affected part.
3. The flowers of Mehandi are grinded to collect the juice. It is then applied over the head to cure headache.
4. Equal amount of Babchi, chitrak, Bhangra, Ashwagandha and Beal are taken and turned to powder. 4 gm of this powder are taken with water in morning for 21 days.

Leucorrhoea (White)

1. Five seeds of Dainkan are mixed with equal amount of Chandan and turned to powder. This powder is then given to drink with sugar to cure white leucorrhoea.
2. Equal amount of Nagarmotha, Ashwagandha, root of Satawar, Gokhru, Bansalochan and Geloi are taken and turned to powder. This is given to drink twice in a day.

Stone

1. Extract of Pittpapra plant is prepared and mixed with sour milk of cow and is taken for 14 days.
2. The fruit extract of Gokhru is prepared and 3 gm of extract is taken with equal amount of honey twice in a day (morning and evening).
3. Equal amount of Banana rhizome, Nagarmotha, Harr, leaves of Peepal are taken and mixed with double amount of Misri and Churna is prepared. Eight gm of this is taken with cold water.

Table 24.1: Vernacular and Taxonomic Details of the Plants Used for Traditional Therapy

Sl.No.	Vernacular Name	Common Name	Botanical Name	Family
1.	Ajwain	Bishop weed	*Trachyspermum ammi*	Umbelliferae
2.	Amaltas	Golden shower	*Cassia fistula*	Caesaliniaceae
3.	Amla	Emblic myrobalan	*Phyllanthus emblica*	Euphorbiaceae
4.	Amrood	Guava	*Psidium guajava*	Myrtaceae
5.	Arjuna	–	*Terminalia arjuna*	Combretacea
6.	Ashwagandha	–	*Withania somnifera*	Solanaceae
7.	Bahera	Belliric myrobalan	*Terminalia bellirica*	Combretacea
8.	Banslochan (gum of bans)	Bamboo	*Bambusa bamboos*	Graminae
9.	Bel	Bael	*Aegla marmelos*	Rutaceae
10.	Bharangee	–	*Clerodendrum indicum*	Verbenaceae
11.	Brahmi	Indian penny wort	*Centella asiatica*	Umbelliferae
12.	Chiraita	–	*Swertia chirayita*	Gentianaceae
13.	Chitrak	Ceylong-lead wort	*Plumbago zeylanica*	Plumbaginaceae
14.	Dainkan	Barbedoslilac	*Melia azedarach*	Meliaceae
15.	Dhatura	Madapple	*Datua stramonium*	Solanaceae
16.	Doob	Dub grass	*Cynodon dactylon*	Poaceae
17.	Geloi	Tinospora	*Tinospora cordifolia*	Menispermaceae
18.	Gokhru	Land caltrops	*Tribulus terrestris*	Zygophyllaceae
19.	Harr	Chebulic myrobalan	*Terminalia chebula*	Combretacea
20.	Indrayani	Bitter apple	*Citrullus colocynthis*	Cucurbitaceae
21.	Genthi (Jungli)	–	*Cuminum cyminum*	Urticaceae
22.	Kakarsinghi	–	*Pistacia khinjuk*	Anacardaceae
23.	Kalimirch	Black pepper	*Piper nigrum*	Piperaceae
24.	Kela	Banana	*Musa paradisiacal*	Scitaminaceae
25.	Malkangni	Lequorice	*Celastrus paniculatus*	Celastraceae
26.	Manjeeta	Indian madder	*Rubia manjith*	Rubiaceae
27.	Mehandi	–	*Lawsonia inermis*	Lythraceae
28.	Mulhathi	Lequorice	*Glycyrrhiza glabara*	Fabaceae
29.	Nagarmotha	–	*Cyperus rotundus*	Cyperaceae
30.	Neem	Margosa tree	*Azadirachta indica*	Meliaceae
31.	Peepal	Sacred fig	*Ficus religiosa*	Moraceae
32.	Peepari	Long pepper	*Piper longum*	Piperaceae
33.	Pithpara	Small flowered fumitory	*Fumaria indica*	Fumariaceae
34.	Reetha	Chinese soap	*Sapindus mukorosi*	Sapindaceae
35.	Satavari	Wild asparagus	*Asparagus racemosus*	Liliaceae
36.	Til	Gingelly	*Sesamum orientale*	Pedaliaceae

Constipation

1. Quath of Amaltas fruit is prepared and given to drink.
2. The ripen fruits of Guava (Amrood) are eaten.
3. Choorna of Harr, Bahera and Amla is prepared and is given to with water at night.
4. Ten gm of Beal fruits are boiled with 100 gm of cow milk and kept for cooling. It is given to drink.
5. The roots of Indrayana are rubbed with water and given to drink.

The vernacular names and taxonomic details of the plants used are presented in the Table 24.1. Garhwal Himalaya had been an abode for thousands of medicinal plants. About more than hundred years ago when there was no medical facility here, some thinkers started searching the old literature (Charak, etc.).

They tried the methods of treatment of various diseases discussed in those books and got success. Gradually they transformed their knowledge to their successors and this generated a system of Vaidyas (Traditional healers). They were treated as Gods by the society at that particular time as they were the only source of any kind of medication. Even today there are many families in villages who have preserved this traditional knowledge and serving the poor folk. Scientifically researches are still on to find out the chemistry of these plants.

A Word of Caution

We advise the people who are interested in applying this traditional therapy to contact either the vaidyas or to the first author of this manuscript before use as there are some specific methods to make use of the plants and their parts.

References

Negi, G.S., 1994. Study of the ancient traditional therapeutic wealth of Pauri and Tehri Garhwal-Part III, Pauri Garhwal. *Himalayan Chemical and Pharmaceutical Bulletin* (HCPB), 11: 7–17.

Medicinal Plants: Conservation, Cultivation and Utilization (2007) *Pages 189–191*
Editors: A.K. Chopra, D.R. Khanna, G. Prasad, D.S. Malik and R. Bhutiani
Published by: DAYA PUBLISHING HOUSE

Chapter 25

Antifeedant Activity of Neem (*Azadiracta indica* A. Juss) on *Spilosoma obliqua* Walker

Dinesh Kumar Bhardwaj[1]*, M.P. Tyagi and Ashish Panwar[2]
[1]Department of Biotechnology, Shri Ram College, Muzaffarnagar – 251 001
[2]K.V. College, Machhra, Meerut (U.P.)

ABSTRACT

Amongst various method used to evaluate antifeedant activity of neem formulation, treated larvae when fed on treated leaves showed maximum antifeedant activity. The trend of effectiveness of neem pesticides was azadirachtin 1 per cent > azadirachtin.03 per cent > azadirachtin 0.3 per cent > azadirachtin 0.15 per cent. 1st instars larvae were most responsive. Azadirachtin 1 per cent, azadirachtin 0.03 per cent and azadirachtin 0.3 per cent @ 0.4 to 0.8 per cent were best treatments to check the population of *S. obliqua*.

Keywords: Antifeedant, Spilosoma obliqua.

Introduction

Bihar hairy caterpillar, *Spilosoma obliqua* Wlk is a sporadic polyphagus pest of great economic value. It prefers to feed the castor (*Ricinus communis*) leaves which is an important oil seed crop (Nagia

* Permanent Address: *Village and Post–Khaikheri, Muzaffarnagar – 251 310.*

et al., 1991) for the control of this pest neem is also an important source of biologically active principle and has attracted the special intrest of entomologists an phytochemists world over. Preliminary study have been made for the possible control of *S. obliqua* using *neem* products (Bhathal and Singh, 1994 and Kumar *et al.*, 2000). Therefore, it was envisaged to study the bioecology digestive physiology and impact in the management of *S. obliqua*, with the hope that *neem* based pesticides be adopted as a safer alternative for the control of this pest.

Table 25.1: Antifeedant Activity of Neem Formulation Against I[st] Instar Larvae of *S. obliqua*

% Conc.	Azadiracthin 0.03%	Azadiracthin 1%	Azadiracthin 0.3%	Azadiracthin 0.15%
		Treated leaves Untreated Caterpiller		
0.8	61.24	68.7	55.03	52.43
0.4	53.67	62.23	36.61	48.36
0.2	25.54	44.41	23.39	44.18
0.1	13.67	38.42	11.12	34.92
Mean	38.53	53.44	31.54	44.97
		Treated leaves Treated Caterpiller		
0.8	66.44	73.22	60.79	58.42
0.4	57.85	65.76	50.28	51.98
0.2	39.21	47.57	32.99	46.55
0.1	19.89	41.92	23.28	18.35
Mean	45.85	57.12	41.84	43.83
		Untreated leaves Treated Caterpiller		
0.8	57.97	63.16	49.94	50.40
0.4	48.25	62.03	33.79	46.89
0.2	20.23	48.81	19.44	40.79
0.1	10.4	32.99	8.14	33.79
Mean	34.21	51.75	27.83	42.97

Materials and Methods

The antifeedant activity of neem formulation was studied by using three different methods. The castor leaf circles as mentioned for the determination LC_{50} values and *S. obliqua* larvae of different instars separated from stock culture were used. The insect larvae of each instar were released over leaf circles and sprayed with an automizer to the point of drip separately. Thus treated larvae were removed and placed in separate petridishes and provided with fresh castor leaf circles which acted as first method. The fresh untreated larvae were released over treated leaves, it served as second method. In third case the treated larvae were left feeding over treated leaves. Ten larvae per replicate were used, and the experiment was replicated thrice. Untreated larvae fed on untreated leaf circle were used as control. Observations were recorded daily upto 8th day of treatment. After 48 hours of treatment fresh food circles were provided daily in sufficient number, uniformly. The complete experiment was run at 25±1°C and 70±5 per cent RH in a B.O.D. incubator. The leaf area consumed by insect larvae was calculated as suggested by Benzamin *et al.* (1968). The percent antifeedant activity was worked out by using the following formula:

Percent feeding deterrence = Average leaf area consumed in control – Average leaf area consumed in treatment/average leaf area consumed in control × 100

Results and Discussion

When treated larvae were fed on treated leaves azadirachtin 1 per cent showed maximum antifeedant property at each larvae of concentration followed by azadirachtin 0.03 per cent. Irrespective of dosages these two formulations were promising, mean value of percent reduction in food consumption being 57.12 and 45.85, respectively. Fresh larvae fed on treated food or teated larvae fed on fresh food showed not much difference in antifeedant property.

Mohanty *et al.* (1988) reported the concentration required to give 50 percent inhibition of feeding for *Psoralea* corylifolia was lower (0.62 per cent) than for *Pongamia pinnata* (0.80 per cent) or lentil (1.50 per cent) against *S. obliqua*. Tripathi and Singh (1994) have also determined antifeedant activity of 2 per cent crude neem extract third instar larvae of *S. obliqua*. They have reported 99 per cent protection to castor leaves. The variation in antifeedant activity evaluated in the present study is due to different neem formulation and method of testing.

References

Benjamin, D.M., Freeman, G.H. and E.S. Brown, 1968. The determination of irregularly shaped area of leaves des-troyed by chewing insects. Ann. Appl. Bio. 61:13-17.

Bhathal, S.S. and Singh, D. 1994. Feeding deterrency of neemark against third instar larvae of hairy caterpillar *Spilosoma obliqua* Walker. *J. Ent. Res.* 18(4): 387-389.

Kumar, L., Parmar, B.S. and Kumar, L. 2000. Effect of emulsion size and shelf life of azadirachtin A on the bioefficacy of *neem* (*Azadirachta indica* A. Juss.). Emulsifiable Concentrates. *J. Agric. And food chemistry* 48(8): 3666-3672.

Mohanty, K. K., Chakraborty, D. P. and Roy, S. 1988. Antifeedant activity of oil fraction of seed of some leguminous plants against *Diacrisia obliqua Indian J. Agric. Sci.* 58(7): 579-580.

Nagia, D.K. Kumar, S. and Saini, M.L. 1991a. Effect of three different host plants on the biology and population multiplication potential of *Spilosoma obliqua* (Walker) (Lepidopteva: Arctiidae). *Plant prot. Bull. India* 43 (3 and 4): 6-8

Tripathi, A. K. and Singh, D. 1994. Screening of Natural products for insect antifeedant activity. Part I. Plant extracts. *Indian J. Ent.* 56(2): 129-133.

Medicinal Plants: Conservation, Cultivation and Utilization (2007) *Pages 193–197*
Editors: A.K. Chopra, D.R. Khanna, G. Prasad, D.S. Malik and R. Bhutiani
Published by: DAYA PUBLISHING HOUSE

Chapter 26

Modern Dosage Forms in Ayurveda: A Study from *Aryabhishak*

Vishal K. Muliya*
Department of Botany, Faculty of Science,
The M. S. University of Baroda, Vadodara - 390 002

ABSTRACT

Traditional dosage system as described by Vaidyas is correlated with modern ayurvedic medicine system. Since, last three thousand year, *Ayurveda*, the mainstream Indian system of medicine is in practice in Indian subcontinent. It is based on the experiences of highly scholar and dedicated *Vaidya*, who were preparing the medicines for individual by taking an account of patient's physiology, ability to digest the dose etc. therefore, the dosages were very specific formulation for that individual. Depending on the patient, preparation of dosage was designed in such a way that single herb or its part can give different actions in different formulation. Thus, these formulations were giving perfect effect of controlled release, sustained release, enteric coating to the active ingredient of that herb. Although, it is not described in ayurveda but on the basis of comparative study, it can be defined by analyzing traditional dosage system with modern pharmaceutical and modern pharmacological parameters. Present paper therefore, deals with such interpretations of ayurvedic formulations in moderns terminology of pharmaceutics and pharmacology form an old ayurvedic text "*Aryabhishak athva Hindustan no Vaidhraj*" (In Gujarati), authored by Late Shri Sankarji Pade and translated by Vyas Harikrushna Bhagwanlal.

* E-mail: vkmuliya@yahoo.com.

Introduction

Ayurveda is said to be a world medicine and is the most holistic or comprehensive medical system (Tirth, 1998). Before civilization, ayurveda was in practice only in the applied form. In due course of time various changes like elaboration, refinement and system organization of the subject had taken place. Although ayurveda is a practical science yet it requires thorough textual knowledge (Gaur, 2006). According to Vogel (1970), Indians have perpetuated an empirical science of herbology in relation to health which has been essentially ignored during these days of great advances in biomedicine. In the international peer reviewed journals ayurveda is always ignored and workers in this field are concentrating more on herbs of Indian medicine rather than formulations or preparations of ayurveda and that could be the reason that many times the desired result is not found in clinical trials. The plant species mentioned in the ancient texts of these Ayurveda and other Indian systems of medicines may be explored with the modern scientific approaches for better leads in the health care (Mukherjee and Wahile, 2006). Moreover, old literature available on this subject deals with the local name of the plant in particular language at the same time people following/speaking that particular language are not that much familiar with local name or creates confusion because of same name more than one plant. According to Patwardhan *et al* (2003) we must increase and improve the publications related to quality, safety and efficacy of Ayurvedic medicines in international peer-reviewed journals and this is a matter of serious introspection and debate for ayurvedic, pharmaceutical and medical scientists (Baghel, 2006).

"Aryabhishak athva Hindustan no Vaidhraj" is a one of the such old book written in Marathi by Late Ayurved-martand Shastri Shankar Daji Pade in 1894 and is translated in Gujarati language by Shri Harikrishna Bhagvanlal Vyas. This book contains detailed account of uses of medicinal plant, salts and animal product in ayurveda and its first part "Subodh Vaidak-Purvardh" is deals with the preparations and utilization of ayurvedic formulations of medicinal plants.

Ancient text described uses of whole plant or many plant in single formulation and claiming synergistic effect. There are some experimental evidences for synergy and buffering in certain whole plant preparations (Vicker and Zolman, 1999). The use of folk beliefs and knowledge of traditional healer is a short cut to the discovery and isolation of pharmacologically active compound (Holland, 1996). In the following paper discussion has been made about relationship of formulation mentioned with modern dosage forms used in modern medicine system.

Plant Powder Mixed with Boiled Rice Water: Remedy for Colon Diseases

1. Ankol (*Alangium lamarckii*) root bark is triturated with honey and mixed with boiled rice water for antidiarrheal activity.
2. In case of bleeding hemorrhoid, seed of *aghedo* or *andhi jhara* (*Achyranthus aspara*) is crushed with boiled rice water.

Boiled rice water is used as antidiarrheal in modern medicines (Ricetral, a product of FDC) and this plant may be used as antimicrobials or to cure other elements which are causing colon disease.

Plant Powder Given with Ghee or Butter: Concept of Enteric Coating

1. In case excess *vatta* condition in colon or gastritis, (*Apium graveolens*) along with *Piper longum*, *Tinospora cordifolia*, Ginger, *Tylophora asthmatica*, *Withania somnifera* and *Asparagus* is given in ghee.
2. *Caesalpinia bonducella* powder is given with ghee for anthelmintic property.
3. *Tinospora cordifolia* is given with butter for excessive *vatta* condition.

When powder is given with ghee or butter, they will coat the powder and not allow to get digested in stomach so that powder will start disintegration in colon which is almost related to principle of enteric coating.

Plant Powder in Oil for External Use: As an Ointment

1. Fine powder of *Withania somnifera* is mixed with oil and applied on skin for various skin diseases.
2. Powdered roots of castor are mixed with ghee and applied on wounds for healing.
3. Leaves of *Aristolochia indica* mixed with castor oil is used for fungal infection on skin.

Here when powder is mixed with oil, fat soluble component will be extracted not others and action will be slow as it is there in ointments.

Nasal Preparation

1. In case of cold and fever, drops of leaf extract of *Agathio* (*Sesbania grandiflora* (L.) Pers) are applied in nose.

This preparation is directly indicating itself as nasal drops of modern medicine system.

Plant Powders with Honey: Expectorant Effect

1. In case of cold and cough, aghedo (*A. aspara)* and black pepper powder is mixed with honey and orally taken (without water or other liquid).
2. *Aconitum heterophyllum* or *Echinops echinatus* powder is also recommonded with honey for cough.
3. *Barleria prionitis* extract is mixed with honey as remedy for cough.
4. Decoction of *Tinospora cordifolia* is given with honey for cough.

Here mixing plants powder with honey gives soothing effect and act locally as expectorant.

Plant Powder with Hot Water: Carminative Effect

1. In case of spasm and dyspepsia, carum (*Trachyspermum ammi* (L.) Sprague) or ajmoda (*Apium graveolens*) is taken orally and then warm water should be taken on it.
2. *Piper longum,* rock salt, *Terminalia belerica* fruit, zingiber powder is given with warm water for dyspepsia.

Here warm water should be given for liberation of volatile component of carum to give carminative and antispasmodic effect.

Plant Preparation Applied on Skin for Internal Medicine: Topical Root for Administration

1. *Tinospora cordifolia* and guggul (*Cinnamomum camphora*) is mixed with castor leaf, crushed and applied on abdomen for anthelmintic effect.
2. In case of migraine extract of *Blumea lacera* is applied on head.
3. Sunflower oil is applied on abdomen and vertebra for purgative effect.

In this case active ingredient is absorbed through the skin and giving systematic effect which is related to modern root of topical administration.

Plant Decoction for Gargling: Gargle

1. Fruit skin of *Cordia rothii* is crushed in water and used as gargle for toothache.
2. Stem bark of *Anthocephalus cadamba* is used for gargle in case of stomatitis.

Gargle or mouthwash is commonly prescribed in modern medicine and plant decoction is also used for same purpose.

Plant Extract with Honey for Local Action in Mouth: As Gum Paint

1. *Barleria prionitis* extract is mixed with honey and applied in mouth to prevent bleeding form the gums.

This formulation is like gum paints of modern medicine system.

Plant Decoction for Internal Use: Mode of Sustain or Controlled Release

1. Coriander and zingiber decoction is given directly for dyspepsia
2. Neem leaf decoction is directly given in case of hyperacidity

In case of decoction, fibers, tannins etc are present along with active ingredients. Presence of tannins will slow down the absorption from gastrointestinal tract giving controlled or sustained release of active ingredient.

Challenges

There are several such formulations in ayurveda where plant decoction or powder is given with sugar or jaggery (gur) or honey. Why these types of formulations were prepared? Either it was giving some pharmacological action or giving synergistic effect or it was for antagonistic effect for some harmful component other than active ingredient. There may be a probability of binding of additives to those receptor where action is not needed. Many times same plant is given with salts rather than sugars. Was it for instant release of active ingredient? There is an urgent need to study the pharmacokinetics and pharmcodynamics of ayurvedic formulations rather than herbal medicines. Bioavailability of herbal medicine is another area of considerable importance (Pal and Shukla, 2003) but ancient formulations are known for their effects indicate bioavailability of active ingredient in sufficient concentration. Dahanukar *et al* (2000) has reviewed the pharmacology of medicinal plants but there is very less study of formulations based on ayurveda. Clinical assessment of ayurvedic medicine should be done by its own theoretical framework as well as with conventional medicine and then there should be comparisons of results for efficacy for different systems as well as traditional practices (Baghel, 2006).

Conclusion

In ayurveda medicines are given mainly in a formulation rather than an individual plant. It shows concept of individual medicine. Modern experiments are design to study for herbal medicine and are mainly dealing with single ingredient rather than entire formulation. Thus, there is an urgent need to correlate traditional composition or preparation of dosages with the parameters of modern medicine system and to develop new parameters to study ayurvedic formulations.

References

Baghel, M.S., 2006. Ayurvedic assessment criteria for clinical researchers. In: *Souvenir of 5th International Seminar on Ayurveda*, Gujarat Ayurved University, Jamnagar, pp 41–43.

Dahanukar, S.A., Kulkarni, R.A. and Rege, N.N., 2000. Pharmacology of medicinal plants and natural products. *Indian Journal of Pharmacology*, 32: S81–S118.

Gaur, B.L., 2006. Literary research in ayurveda: Need of hour. In: *souvenir of 5th International Seminar on Ayurveda*, Gujarat Ayurved University, Jamnagar, pp 41–43.

Holand, B.K., 1994. Prospecting of drugs in ancient text. *Nature*, 369: 702.

Mukherjee, P.K. and Wahile, A., 2006. Integrated approaches towards drug development from Ayurveda and other Indian system of medicines. *Journal of Ethnopharmacology*, 103: 25–35.

Pade, S.D., 2005. *Aryabhishak*. Sastu Sahitya Vardhak Karyalay, Mumbai (In Gujarati), pp. 38–41.

Pal, S. and Shukla, Y., 2003: Herbal medicine: Current status and the future. *Asian Pacific Journal of Cancer Prevention*, 4: 281–288.

Patvardhan, B., Chopra, A. and Vaidya, A.D.B., 2003. Herbal remedies and the bias against Ayurveda. *Current Science*, 84(9): 1165–1166.

Tirtha, S.S.S., 1998. *The Ayurveda Encyclopedia: Natural Secrets to Healing, Prevention and Longevity*. Sri Satguru Publications, New Delhi, pp. 3

Viscker, A. and Zollman, C., 1999. ABC of complementary medicine: Herbal medicine. *British Medical Journal*, 319: 1050–1053.

Medicinal Plants: Conservation, Cultivation and Utilization (2007) *Pages 199–205*
Editors: **A.K. Chopra, D.R. Khanna, G. Prasad, D.S. Malik and R. Bhutiani**
Published by: **DAYA PUBLISHING HOUSE**

Chapter 27

Development of a Database for Identification of Powdered Crude Drugs

S.P. Bhatnagar[1] and V. Kaushik[2]
[1]Department of Pharmaceutical Sciences,
Birla Institute of Technology, Ranchi – 835 215
[2]Department of Pharmaceutical Sciences,
S.B.S.PG.I of Biomedical Sciences and Research, Balawala, Dehradun – 248 161 (UA)

ABSTRACT

In the present era, information storage and retrieval, is a science in itself, and manual searches of literature being an impossible long procedure, that is why it is necessary to rely on computer both for information retrieval and for current literature scanning. Herbal drugs are gaining importance currently in health care system as well as research for drug discovery and development, so it is necessary that there should be a computerized authentication and standardization of herbal drugs.

In the present communication microscopical characteristics of powdered crude drugs has been reported with the aid of digital microscope and image processing softwares by making database using oracle 8i as back end and visual basic as front end. The information regarding the microscopical characteristics of powdered crude drugs has been collected from textbooks, Pharmacopoeias, journals and lab work. This database provides detailed diagnostic powder drug characteristics on searching the botanical name or diagnostic powder drug characters.

This database has enormous applications as, it can be used by scientists, authors and pharmacognosists for extensive study of herbal drugs, standardization of different powdered crude drugs available in the local areas, detection of adulteration and establishment of identity of powdered crude drugs.

Introduction

India is blessed with a vast treasure of flora and fauna. Due to vast potential in its botanical resources, India has the advantage of traditionally rich knowledge of the medicinal plants. An increase in the awareness of the people towards the various traditional systems of medicine like Ayurveda, Siddha, Unani, Chinese, Tibetan etc., since last four decades, has lead to an increase in the demand of herbal medicines. For meeting these healthcare demands of the world community the herbal formulations need to be formulated at a large scale. The demand for herbal drugs has also created an increase in awareness of their quality. This quality control procedure requires the assessment of the various parameters of which, microscopical identification and evaluation is an important parameter and plays a significant role. All this requires a systematic and scientific study of medicinal plants. Manual search of literature of medicinal plants is a tedious and time-consuming job. In current times, information storage and retrieval is a science in itself and manual searches of literature is being replaced by computer-based searches. Computerized storage, authentication and standardization of herbal drugs and medicinal plants are essential for quick reference and easy accessibility.

However, this will require collection of detail information about microscopical characteristics of different powdered crude drugs and preparation of an extensive database, which shall store all relevant information comprehensively.

Methodology

The information regarding the microscopical characteristics of powdered crude drugs has been collected from textbooks of pharmacognosy, Pharmacopoeias, journals and lab work. Compound microscope, Leica microscope with digital camera and a computer (IBM Corp.) with Pentium IV processor and image processing softwares were used for the microscopy of powdered crude drugs. Oracle 8i and visual basic 6 were the softwares used for the preparation of database.

Experimental

Microscopical Studies for Powdered Crude Drugs

Following Microscopical Structures were found to be Present in Powdered Crude Drugs

Leaf Drugs

Epidermis with stomata, and not very abundant small sized vascular elements. Frequently trichomes, palisade cells and crystals of calcium oxalate are also present.

Bark Drugs

Cork cells, fibers, calcium oxalate, stone cells, medullary rays, and starch grains.

Root and Rhizome Drugs

Cork cells, vascular tissue in varying amount, abundant parenchyma, which often contains starch grains in large amount, occasionally stone cells and calcium oxalate crystals are also found.

Fruit Drugs

Stone cells, calcium oxalate, more highly developed vascular tissue, starch grains and occasionally trichomes.

Computer Programming in the Database-using Oracle 8i as Back-end and Visual Basic 6 as Front-end is Divided into Two Parts for the Assessment of Crude Drugs

GRAPHICAL INTERFACES IN VISUAL BASIC 6

Login Form

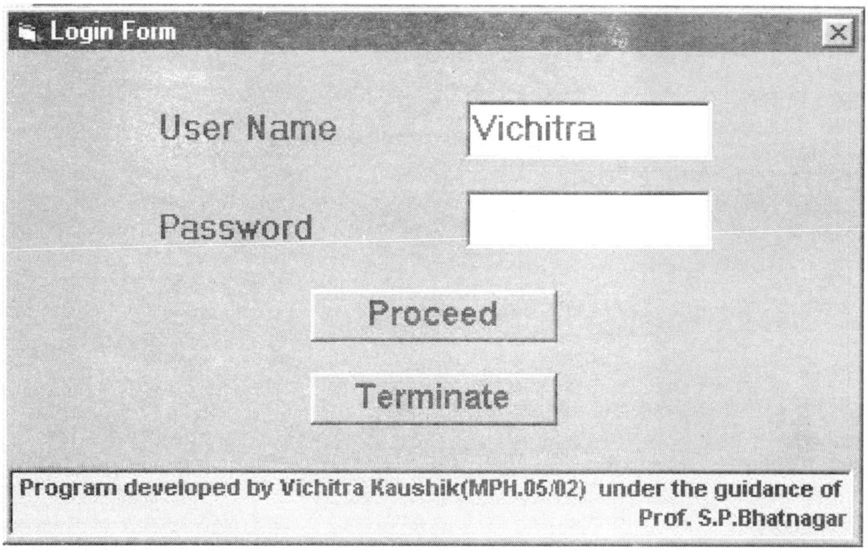

Main Form

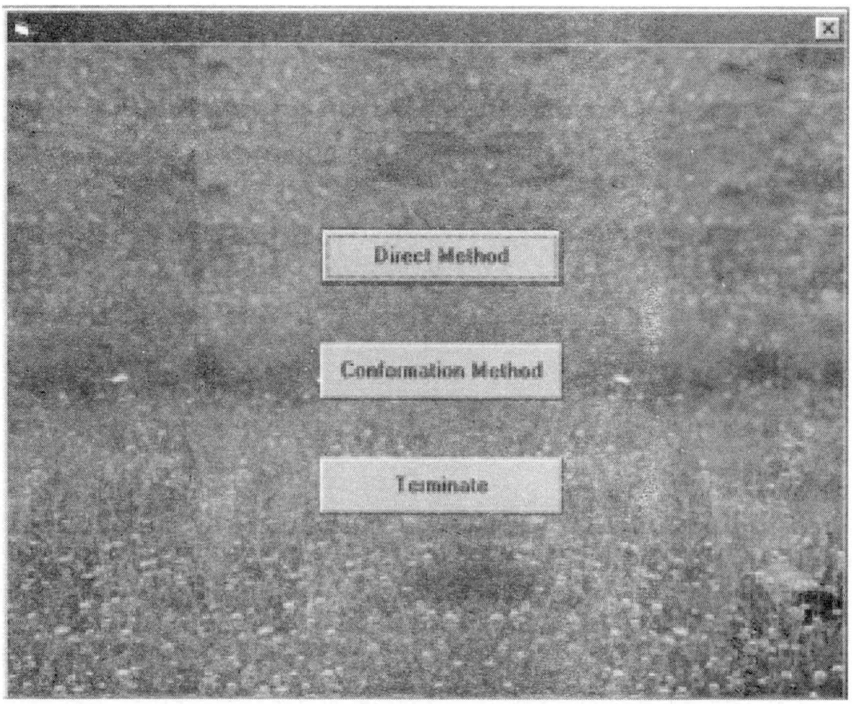

Form for the Selection of Crude Drug

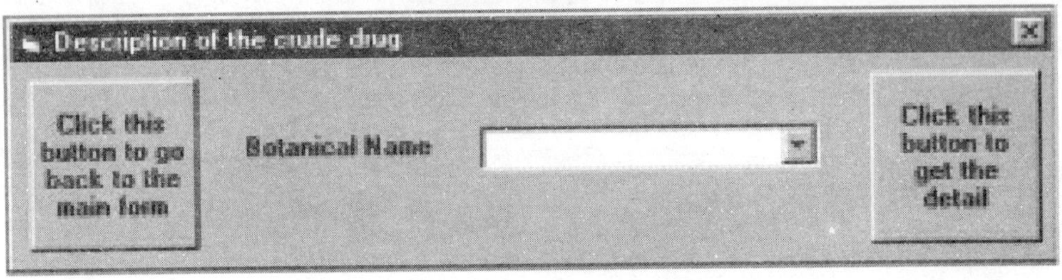

Form for the Description of Crude Drug

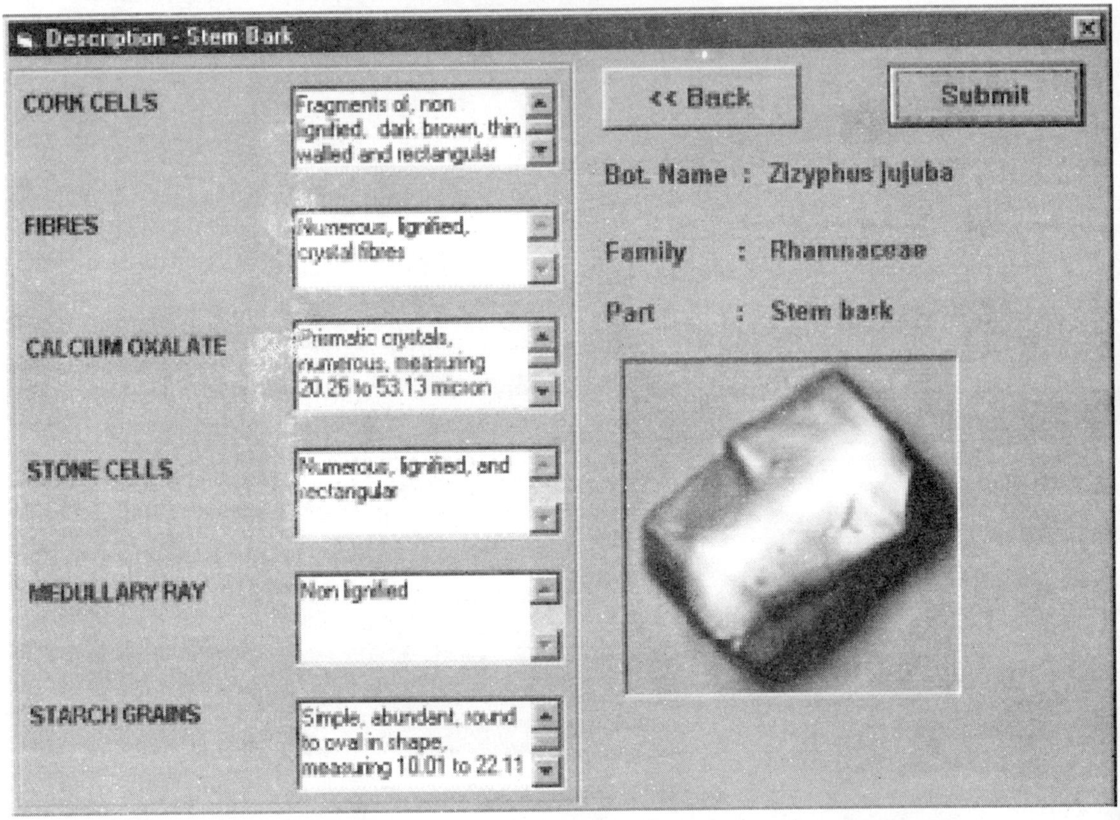

Direct Method

In this method Microscopical characteristics of powdered crude drugs can be assessed directly through their botanical name.

Conformation Method

Preliminary Conformation

It involves assessment of eight diagnostic characteristics *i.e.*, stomata, trichomes, calcium oxalate stone cells, fibers, starch grains, cork cells, and xylem vessels. On the basis of the conclusion drawn by

Preliminary Confirmation Form

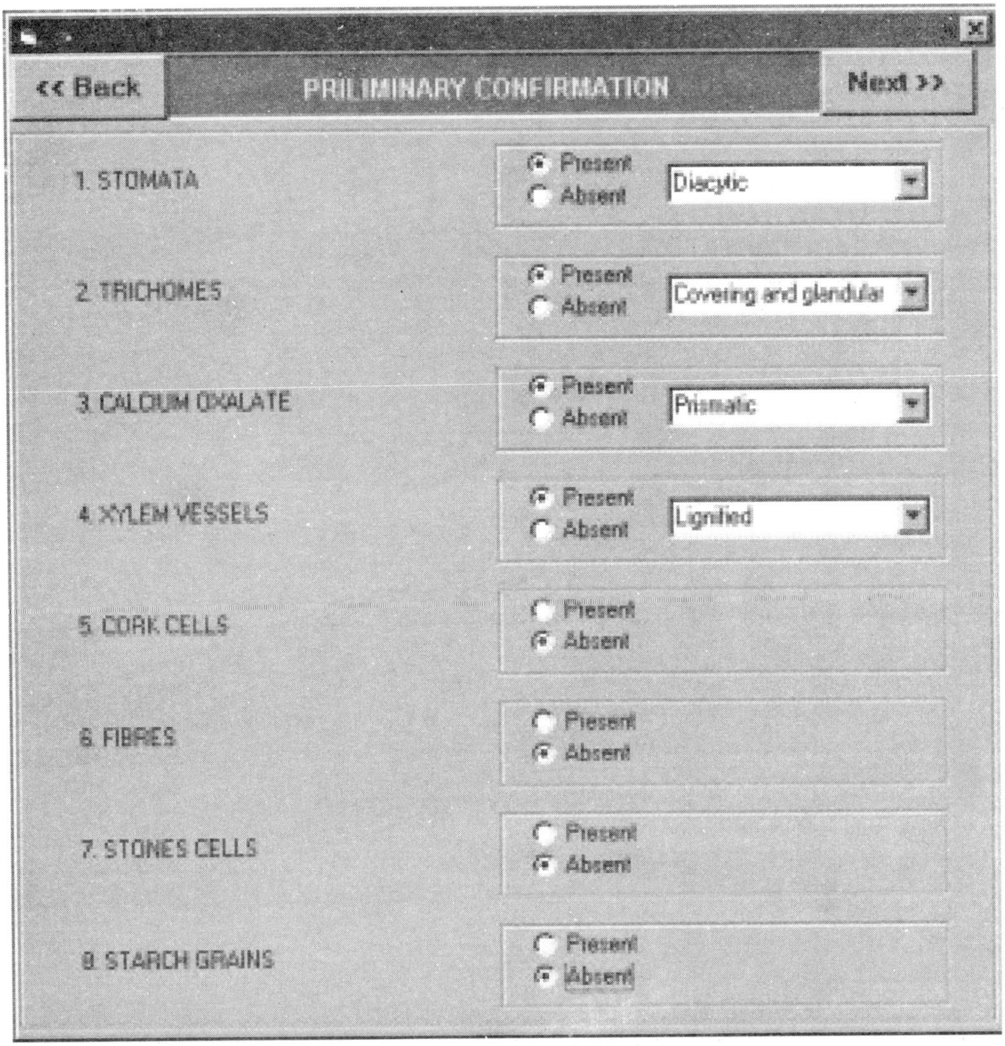

Form for the Conclusion of Preliminary Confirmation

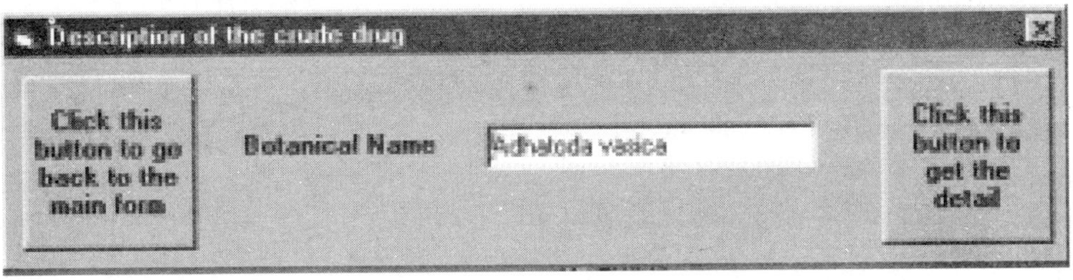

Form for the Final Confirmation of Leaf Drugs

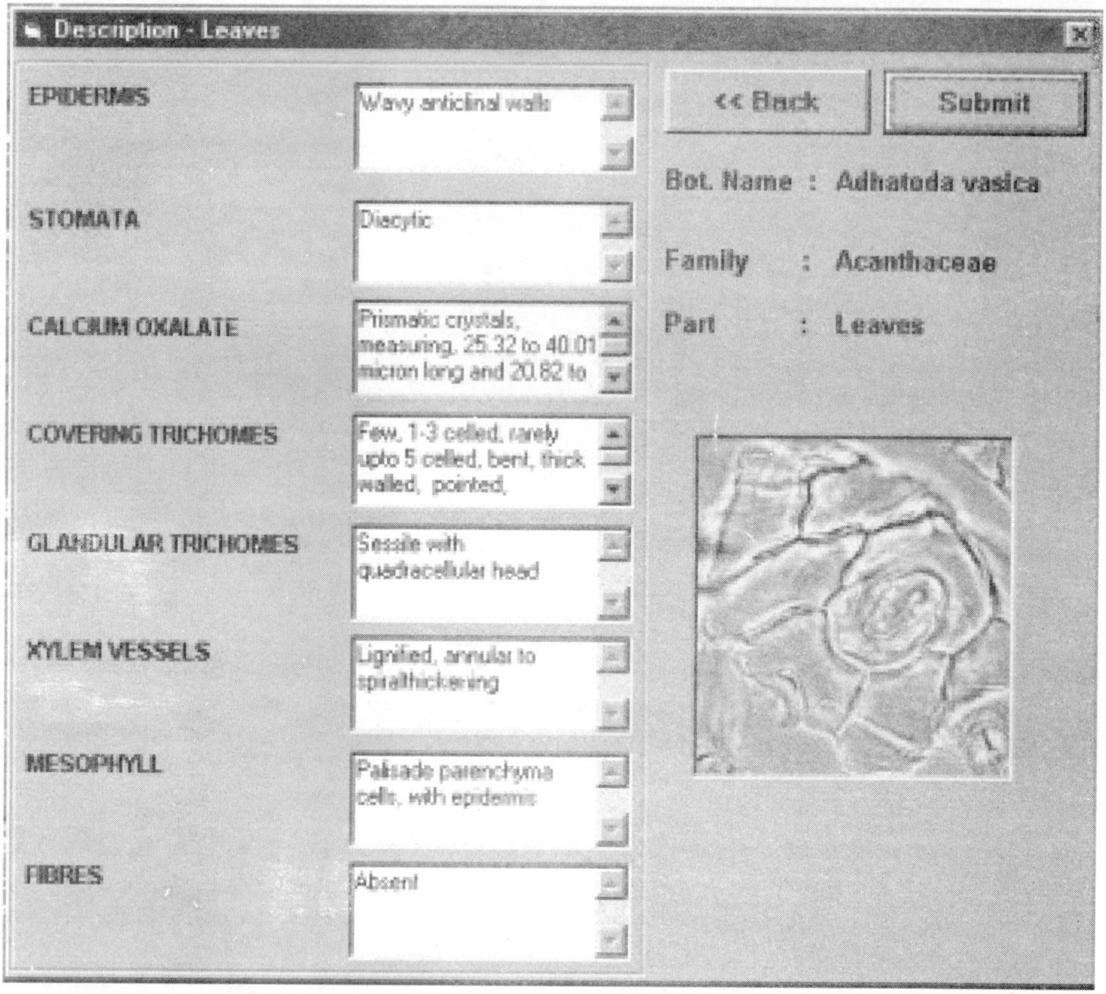

the presence and type of above diagnostic characteristics the software will provide preliminary confirmation of the particular crude drug.

Final Conformation

It includes the description of the specific diagnostic characteristics present in powdered crude drugs along with their corresponding images.

Conclusion

Few unions would appear to have dimer prospects of success than the one, between the rigorous and highly mathematical applications of computers and descriptive, empirical and often intuitive approach of the microscopist. Nevertheless, the computer has certain features, which permit it to assist in identification problems. It can have an extremely large, permanent and reliable memory. It calculates quickly and the information in its memory can be accessed when required. The computer is not influenced by recent experience and personnel bias. It can be updated easily.

With the help of Information Technology, the enormous large list of herbal drugs can be transformed into a database, by which, an individual can get quick information about the herbal drugs and their authenticity.

This database can be a good tool for the rapid identification of the crude drugs and can also be a better option for the analyst involved in the analysis.

With the help of this database one can include microscopical characteristics of powdered crude drugs with their images, since microscopic examination is not only essential for the study of adulterants but also is indispensable in correct identification of crude drugs.

Acknowledgement

The authors thankfully acknowledge the financial help provided by A.I.C.T.E., New Delhi, India during the course of study.

References

Bayross, I., 2002. *SQL, PL/SQL: The Programming Language of Oracle*, 2nd edn. BPB Publications, New Delhi.

Bronson, G., 2001. *Introduction to Programming Using Visual Basic 6*, 2nd edn. Scott Jones Publishers, Caliphornia, USA.

Date, C.J., 1981. *An Introduction to Database System*, 3rd edn. Narosa PublishingHouse, New Delhi.

Datta, S.C. and Mukerji, B., 1949. *Pharmacognosy of Indian Root and Rhizome Drugs*. Govt. of India Press, Calcutta.

Evans, W.C., 1996. *Trease and Evans, Pharmacognosy*, 14th edn. Harcourt Brace and Co. Asia Pvt. Ltd.

Indian Herbal Pharmacopoeia, 1998. Vol.-2, Regional Research Laboratory, Jammu Tawi, and Indian Drug Manufacturers Association, Mumbai.

Iyenger, M.A., 1980. *Pharmacognosy of Powdered Crude Drugs*, 2nd edn., Manipal.

Jerke, N., 1999. *Visual Basic 6: The Complete Reference*. Tata McGraw Hill, New Delhi.

Kokate, C.K., 1996. *Practical Pharmacognosy*, 3rd edn. Nirali Prakashan, Pune.

Kokate, C.K., Purohit, A.P. and Gokhale, G.B., 1997. *A Textbook of Pharmacognosy*, 7th edn. Nirali Prakashan, Pune.

Lalla, J.K. and Mamania, H.M., 2001. Triphala churna: From raw materials to finished products. *Indian Drugs*.

Loney, K. and Koch, G., 2000. *Oracle 8i: The Complete Reference*, 10th edn. Tata McGraw Hill, New Delhi.

Muller, R.J., 1997. Oracle *Developer 2000 Handbook*, 2nd edn. Tata McGraw-Hill, New Delhi.

Wallis, T.E., 1997. *TextBook of Pharmacognosy*, 5th edn. J and A Churchill Limited, London.

Medicinal Plants: Conservation, Cultivation and Utilization (2007) *Pages 207–211*
Editors: A.K. Chopra, D.R. Khanna, G. Prasad, D.S. Malik and R. Bhutiani
Published by: DAYA PUBLISHING HOUSE

Chapter 28

Ethnomedicinal Flora of West Nimar (Khargone) District, M.P., India

S.K. Pathak[1] and Sunita Pathak[2]
[1]Department of Zoology, [2]Department of Economics
Government P.G. College, Mhow

ABSTRACT

Among the plant wealth the ethnomedicinal flora have a key position. The rural population including tribal population of West Nimar is still dependent on the ethnomedicinal flora of their vicinity for curing disease. The medicine men have developed their own way of treatment by collecting the knowledge from their ancestors. The present investigation gives an account of the medicinal plants used by rural population of West Nimar (Khargone) district of M.P. The information of 30 plants along with vernacular names and its medicinal application in the treatment of disease and ailment like fever, cough, common cold, back ache, swelling, skin disease, eczema, vomiting, abdominal and cholic pain, dysentery, diarrhea, jaundice, arthritis, bronchitis, asthma, migraine, tumor, urinary disorder, menstrual disorder, abortion, sexual impotency, venereal disease, tumor etc.

Introduction

The life of human civilization influenced by plants. The people are using various plants and their products for their benefits especially for cloth, food, shelter and medicinal purpose (Kaushik and Dhiman, 2000). About 80 per cent of world population used plant based traditional medicines system for the treatment of various diseases and refer as indigenous health care system. In Asian countries including India this system occupies an important part/role in national healthcare programme because billions of people depend upon traditional because billions of people depend upon traditional health system. Today 90 per cent of Indian rural population depends on Local Village Health Practitioners (LVHP) for curing the various disease (Yadav and Patil, 2001). Rural population including tribals believed on local 'Vaid'and 'Bhagat' which use local plants for curing human ailments.

In Indian literature Rigveda, Atharveda, Sushruta Samhita also indicate medicinal use of plants. In India, ethnomedicinal use of regional plants reported by Chopra *et al.* (1956), Girach *et al.* (1994), Bhattacharjee (1998), Maikhuri *et al.* (1998), Tewari (1999), Dhiman and Khanna(2001), Yadav and Patil(2001) Patil *et al.* (2003), Patil (2004).

Ethnomedicinal studies of West Nimar district especially in Sirwel hills were pioneered by S.K.Mahajan (1990). A preliminary survey on anthelmintic plant used by tribes of West Nimar done by Mahajan *et al.* (2003).

The West Nimar (Khargone) district lies between 21° 22' to 22° 35' latitude and 75° 19' to 76° 14' longitude. It is situated 309 M above the mean sea level. It occupies an area of 6541.870 Sq. kilometers and has a population 1529954 with 7 towns and 1170 villages.

Methodology

The present article includes a survey of tribal area of West Nimar district. About 40 plants were collected from remote areas of each blockhead quarters of the district. However, this paper includes only 30 important medicinally used plants. The study involved fieldwork, interviews with local practitioners and Bhagat, and collection of ethnomedicinal plants specimens. The ethnomedicinal information and vernaculars of the plants was first gathered from local medicinal practitioners and peasants, and then confirmed through standard literature.

Results

The rural and tribal population strongly believed in Vaidji and Bhagat for curing various diseases. Table 28.1 shows the results of a study carried out in West Nimar (Khargone) district.

Discussion

Many local practitioners were found to have knowledge and competence for treatment of common as well as serious ailments. The medicinal flora are capable of curing various disease such as fever, cough, common colds, backache, swelling, skin diseases, eczema, vomiting, abdominal and colic pain, dysentery, diarrhea, jaundice, arthritis, bronchitis, asthma, migraine, tumor, urinary disorder, menstrual disorder, abortion, sexual impotency, venereal disease, tumor etc.

After detailed consultations with the local practitioners of plant medicines, their prescriptions for various ailments were carefully studied. It was noticed that plants are used either rows, or powdered form or juices an extracted form or decoction of various parts as per requirement. In some cases combinations of plant extracts are used to treat patients. These remedies have been successfully administered for many centuries and the local tribals and villagers have been benefiting from them. So much so, it tuned out that more than 65 per cent of population in west nimar depends solely on the ethnoremedies for curing even some of the serious ailments.

The common tribal and villagers have reported the beneficial effects of their ethnomedicinal formula and believe in preparations made by practicing persons. The maximum population of tribal area used ethnoremedies for treatment of any disorder of body and even in emergencies. More than 65 per cent of population of West Nimar (Khargone) district recognized ethnoremedies.

Table 28.1: List of Vernacular Names, Botanical Names of the Plants, their Parts Used, and Diseases

Sl.No.	*Vernacular Name*	*Botanical Name*	*Parts Used*	*Diseases*
1.	Neem	*Azadirachta indica*	Leaves, Stem, Bark	Fever, Antihelminthatic, Jaundice, Skin infection, Swelling of gum, Snake bite
2.	Palas	*Butea monosperma*	Leaves, Seeds, Flower, Gum	Wormicide, Pimples, Impotency, Seminal strength
3.	Amaltas	*Cassia fistula*	Leaves, Stem, Bark	Pustules Suppuration
4.	Dhatura	*Datura stramonium*	Leaves, Seeds	Cough, Backache, Swelling on feet and hand, Child birth, Dysentery
5.	Gular	*Ficus glomerata*	Leaves, Stem, Root, Bark, Fruit, Seeds	Piles, Vomiting, Skin disease, Rhinitis, Diabetes, Mumps, Backache
6.	Jamun	*Eugenia jambolana*	Leaves, Stem, Bark, Fruit, Seeds	Eczema, Menstrual disorder, Dysentery, Urinary disorder, Diabetes, Liver tonic
7.	Arandi	*Rincinus communis*	Leaves, Seeds, Roots, Seed oil	Rheumaticfever, Joints pain, Renal, Colic, Constipation
8.	Kaner	*Nerium odorum*	Leaves, Roots	Ring worm, Leprosy, Ulcer on genitals
9.	Giloe	*Tinospora cordifolia*	Leaves, Seeds	Fever, Jaundice, Urinary trouble, Diabetes
10.	Satyanashi	*Argemone maxicana*	Leaves	Skin disease
11.	Gvarpatha	*Aloe vera*	Whole plant pulp	Jaundice, Common cold, Easy lactation
12.	Bel	*Aegle marmelos*	Roots, Bark, Ripe fruit	Fever, Digestive stimulation, Piles, Constipation, Heart palpitation
13.	Mathi	*Trigonella foenumgraecum*	Leaves, Seeds, Flowers	Migrain, Bronchitis, Asthma, Tumour, Dysentry, Diarrhea, Rheumatism
14.	Aak	*Calotropis*	Stem, Leaf, Bark	Asthmatic cough, Insect bite, Ulcers, Applied in swelling and painful joints
15.	Makoi	*Solanum nigrum*	Leaves, Fruit, Roots	Fever, Skin disease, Liver tonic, toothache
16.	Hadjode	*Ceasus quadrangularis*	Stems	Arthritis, Bone related ailments
17.	Safed musli	*Chlorophytum borivilianum*	Roots	Physical weakness, Lactation increase, Diabetes, Diseases after delivery
18.	Kali musli	*Curculigo orchioides*	Roots	Sexual impotency, Urinary disease, Venereal disease, Health tonic, Asthma, Jaundice, Piles, Stomach ache, Diarrhoea
19.	Kaunch	*Mucuna pruriens*	Leaves, Roots, Bark, Fruit, Seeds	Antihelmenthatic, Liver and Bile Disorder, Diuretic
20.	Nager motha	*Cyprus scariosus*	Roots	Pain keelar, Fever, Piles, Epilepsy, Venereal disease, Lactation increase
21.	Adusa	*Justicia adatoda*	Leaves, Flowers, Fruit, Roots	Caugh, Dehydration, Jaundice, Heartdisease, Bronchitis, Asthma, Abortion
22.	Ashva gandha	*Withania somnifera*	Roots	Children growth, Retard aging, Haematin tonic, Aphrodigiac

Contd...

Table 28.1–Contd...

Sl.No.	Vernacular Name	Botanical Name	Parts Used	Diseases
23.	Gudmar	*Gymnema sylvestre*	Leaves, Roots	Fever, cough, Liver tonic, Dysentery, Diabetes, Abdominal Pain, Abdominal disease, Heart Disease, Leprosy
24.	Sataver	*Asparagus racemosus*	Roots	Diarrhoea, Dysentery, Sexual Weakness, Health tonic, Epilepsy, Stimulation of lactation
25.	Bathua	*Chenopodium album*	Leaves, Flowers, Seeds	Blood purifier, Skin disease, Anthelmintic, Hepatic disease, Spleen enlargment, Intestinal Ulcers, Abortion
26.	Dudhi	*Euphorbia hirta*	Leaves, Stems, Seeds, Latex	Dysentery, Colic, Bronchitis, Asthma, Leucorrhoea, actation Increase, Urino-genital disease
27.	Sadabahar	*Catheranthus roseus*	Leaves, Roots	High blood pressure, Cancer
28.	Bavchi	*Psoralea corylifolia*	Seeds, Seed oil	Skin disease, Leucoderma, Antimicrobial and Antifungal
29.	Lajvanti	*Mimosa pudica*	Leaves, Roots	Hydrocoel, Glandular swelling, Piles, Fistula, Sores
30.	Jangli bhindi	*Abelmoschus ficulneus*	Fruit, Roots	Urine stone, Control of early Ejaculation of semen

Much more attention is required in the field of medicinal research for testing authenticity of these ethnoremedies. The following necessary steps requires for popular of this pathy:-

1. Indigenous medicinal plants are of great help to us since they provide much more simple, convenient and inexpensive remedies for a variety of ailments.
2. It is essential that an authentic documentation of indigenous ethnomedicinal plants and their respective use in the treatment of various diseases is made known to the coming generations.
3. It is also necessary that all relevant scientific information regarding to the locally available medicinal flora is made known to far and wide as a part of the progressive educational programme.
4. It is also to make people in general and cultivators in particular better in forms about the local medicinal plants, it is admissible that nurseries of medicinal plants are set up in every block quarters of the district through out the country.
5. Freshly extracted juices from medicinal plants provide a much quicker remedy to the patients.
6. An organized and widespread cultivation of medicinal flora will certainly provide much needed employment opportunities in the country.
7. Cultivation, pharmaceutical production, marketing and finally clinical use of ethnomedicinal

9. The Govt. also gives technical support or assistance to farmer to get more yields of ethno medicinal plants.
10. They also help to conserve the endangered ethnomedicinal plants.

References

Bhattacharjee, S.K., 1998. *Handbook of Medicinal Plants*. Pointer Publishers, Jaipur, India.

Chopra, R.N., Nayar, S.L. and Chopra, I.C., 1956. *Glossary of Indian Medicinal Plants*. National Institute of Science Communication. Dr. K.S. Krishnan marg, New Delhi, India.

Dhiman, A.K. and Khanna, D.R., 2001. Notes on medicinal flora of Guru Nanak Dev University campus Amritsar. *Environ. Conserv. J.*, 2(1): 45–57.

Mahajan, S.K., 1990. A Preliminary ethnobotanical survey in the Sirvel hills of western M.P. *Natl. Seminar on Ethnobotany of Tribes of M.P.* Abst. No. 14.

Mahajan, S.K., Patel Puspa, Singh, P.P. and Sapru, T., 2003. Preliminary survey of the anthelmintic plants used by the tribes of west Nimar, M.P. In: *Natl. Seminar Organised at Goa University on Plant Diversity, Human Welfare and Conservation, Proceeding*, p. 289–292.

Maikhuri, R.K., Nautiyal, S., Rao, K.S. and Saxena, K.G., 1998. Role of medicinal plants in the traditional health care system:A case study from Nanda Devi biosphere reserve. *Curr. Sci.*, 75(2): 152–157.

Patil, U.S., Manik, S.R. and Pachkhede, A.U., 2003. Morphotaxonomic authentication of ethnomedicinal plants from Amravati district, M.S. *J. Comp. Toxicol. Physiol.*, 1(2): 118–126.

Patil, U.S., 2004. Some less known ethnomedicinal plantsused by tribals of Amravati district, Maharashtra. *J.Comp. Toxicol. Physiol.*, 1(3 and 4): 277–283.

Tewari, D.N., 1999. Medicinal plants for health care. *Yojana June*, 99: 8–11.

Yadav, S.S. and Patil, N.S., 2001. Traditional medicines and health care system of tribals of satpuda region, Maharashtra state. *Plant Archives*, 1(1 and 2): 111–118.

Medicinal Plants: Conservation, Cultivation and Utilization (2007)
Editors: A.K. Chopra, D.R. Khanna, G. Prasad, D.S. Malik and R. Bhutiani
Published by: DAYA PUBLISHING HOUSE

Chapter 29

Makoi (*Solaum nigrum*) and Punarnava (*Boerhavia diffusa*): Effective Herbal Drug in Liver and Kidney Disorders

D.R. Khanna, Pradeep Sharma and Pramod Kumar
Department of Zoology and Environmental Science
Gurukul Kangri Vishwavidyalaya, Haridwar – 249 404, U.A.

ABSTRACT

Plant products and extracts are being used in India since time of immemoriable. In Vedas, Upnishads, Puranas and other ancient books plants have been considered like God. Medicinal uses of plants have been discussed in Rigveda and Ayurveda etc. Maharishi Charaka and Sushruta told about medicinal properties of plants and their uses for human beings. This paper include the study of use of Makoi(*Solanum nigrum*) and Punarnava(*Boerhavia diffusa*) for the treatment of liver and kidney disorders. Swelling in body due to these disorders have been treated by the use of extracts of Panchang of Makoi and Punarnava.

Introduction

Makoi (*Solanum nigrum*) is the member of family solanaceae (Potato Family) while Punarnava is the member of family Nycto-ginaceae. Both of these plants are being utilized for medicinal purposes since time immemoriable. Medicinal values of these plants have been discussed in Charak Samita, Ayurveda etc. the medicinal value of Punarnava is discussed in "Bhavaprakash" followingly.

पुनर्नवा भवेदुष्णा तिस्तारूक्षा कफायहा।
संशोधपाण्डु हृद्रोकासोर चमत बमदज क्षतशुलनत।।

(भावप्रकाश)

The literal meaning of this shloka is "Punarnava is antipyretic, Analgesic, Cardiostimulator, Calmand Diuretic. So it is used for the treatment of fever cardiac disorders, urinary disorders and Jaundice (Liver disorders).

काकमाची (मकोय) ध्वाङ्क्षमाची काकाह्वा चैव वायसी।
काकमाची त्रिदोशह्नी स्निग्धोश्णा स्वरशुक्रदा।। 246
तिक्ता रसायनी शोथकुष्ठार्शोज्वरमेहापित चमत बमदज ।
कटुर्नेत्रहिता हिक्काच्छर्दिह्द्रोगनाशनी।। 247

(भावप्रकाश)

It means Makoi is hot in potency and Pungent bitter in taste. It cures dropsy, Piles, Leucoderma and Leprosy.

Medicinal values of these plants have been studied by oliver (1980), *Rawat et al.* (1994), Chude *et al.* (2001), Khanna and Dhiman (2001, 2002), Dhiman (2004 and 2005).

Makoi is commonly known as black night shrub. It is found in cultivated grounds, waste areas and damp shady spots it is an brital stemmed need that grows up to a meter tall. It has ovate leaves tiny white star shaped flowers and small round black berries that are green when unripe. Panchang *i.e* Leaf, stem, root, flower and fruit is used for the treatment of various disorders.

Phytochemistry

The Panchang of Makoi specially green berries and leaves contain glycol-alkaloid-Solanine or Solasodine. It is Diaphoretic, Purgative, Narcotic, Sudorific and Anti inflammatory hence used for Hepato-Renal disorders, Leaves are used for the treatment of Ulcers or skin infections, Green berries are recommended for Herpes.

Punarnava

It is a perennial herb flowernig in Jan-Dec. It is found in dry Sandy soil, flowers are hermaphrodite. Panchang this plant is used for the treatment of various disorders.

Phytochemistry

Main medicinal part of Punarnava alkaloid known as Punarnavine. It is 0.04 per cent in roots, other alkaloids are 6.5 per cent. Its roots have sterones which are unable to dissolve in water. β-cytosterol and α-2 Cytosterol are main sterones. Beside these it also has organic acids and salts per cent Amongst acids steavic acid and Palmitic acid and amongst salts KNO_3, Na_2SO_4 and Nacl are main components. All of these constituents are combindly responsible for following effects of Punarnava.

1. Diaphoretic and Diuretic
2. Emetic and Expectorant
3. Laxative and Rejuvenative
4. Stomachic, Antihelminthic and Purgative

Chude *et al.* (2001) studied Hypoglycemic effect of the aqueous extract of Punarnava and proved that it is helpful for lowering blood glucose level.

Methodology

To Study the Hepato-Renal effects of Makoi and Punarnava we have made an experiment. In which combination of panchang of Makoi and punarnava was given to the patients suffering from various liver and kidney disorders. The extract of panchang of these two plants was mixed and it was given to patients. We know that swelling take place in body due to kidney and Liver disorders. It our experiment combination if extract was given 10-20 gm 2/3 time daily to patients of different age groups and the effects are shown in following table.

Observation

Effect of combination of extracts of Makoi *(Solanum nigrum)* and Punarnava (Boerhavia diffusa) upon Hepate–Renal disorders are shown in Table 29.1

Table 29.1

Sl.No.	Age Group of Patients	No. of Patients	Recovery					Total Days of Treatment
			0 Days	3 Days	5 Days	7 Days	14 Days	
1.	10–20	4	–	20	40	50	75	20 Days
2.	21–30	5	–	20	35	50	70	25 Days
3.	31–40	5	–	15	30	45	65	25 Days
4.	41–50	8	–	15	30	45	60	30 Days
5.	51–60	10	–	10	20	40	50	40 Days

Results and Discussion

On the basis of Table 29.1, it is clear that combination of extracts of Makoi and Punarnava is highly effective for Hepato Renal disorders.

In age group 10-20 yrs, the swelling was completely recovered in 20 days. In age groups, 21-30 and 31-40 yrs. 25 days are required for this recovery. While in age group 41-50, 30 days and in age group, 51-60 yrs. 40 days are required for complete appoximately recovery from swelling. This difference is due to reduced power of immunity caused by the process of ageing with advancing age.

Makoi (*Solanum nigrum*) and Punarnava (*Boerhavia diffusa*) are being used for medicinal purposes since time of Charaka and Sushruta studies of various research workers prove that both of them are still effective for the treatment of above mentioned various disorders. Various types of commercial medicines have been made from them. Extracts, Kwath, Punarnava Mandur, Punarnava kshar, Punarnava ashtak, Punarnva asav, Punarnava churna, Powder of seeds, Panchang etc are main commercial preparations (Dhiman, 2004).

On the basis of all these facts we can say that both of them should be used for the treatment of various disorders and their cultivation, extraction and use as a medicine should be promoted for better health of people.

References

Chopra, R.N. Nayar, S.L. and Chopra, I.C., 1986. *Glossary of Indian Medicinal Plants (including the supplement)*. C.S.I.T., New Delhi.

Chude, M.A., Orisakwe, O.E., Afonne, O.J., Gamaniel, K.S., Vongtau, O.H. and Obi, E., 2001. *Indian Journal of Phamacology*, 33: 215–216.

Dhiman, A.K. and Khanna, D.R., 2001. Notes on medicinal Flora of Guru Nanak Dev University Campus, Amritsar. *Environment Conservation Journal*, 2(1): 45–57.

Dhiman, A.K., 2004. *Common Drug Plants and Ayurvedic Remedies*. References Press, New Delhi.

Dhiman, A.K., 2004. *Medicinal Plants of U.A. State*. Chowkhamba Sanskrit Series Office, Varanasi.

Dhiman, A.K., 2005. *Wild Medicinal Plants of India*. Bishan Singh Mahendra Pal Singh, Dehradun.

Jain, S.P. and Singh, S.C., 1994. Ethnomedical botanical survey of Ambikapur District, M.P. Ethnobiology in human Welfare. *Abstracts of the 4th International congress of Ethnobiology Lucknow, Uttar Pradesh, India*. 17th –21st November, pp. 293.

A.K., Oliver, B., 1980. Oral hypoglycemic plants in west Africa. *J. Ethnopharm.*

Khanna, D.R. and Dhiman, A.K., 2002. A floristic survey of the vegetation of university campus of Guru Nanak University, Amritsar. *Flora and Fauna*, 7(1): 214.

Singh, M.K., Usha, S. Singh, S.C. and Singh, U., 1994. Phytosergical investigations of *Boerhavia diffusa* Linn. of Darbhanga district, Bihar. *Neo-Botanical*, 2: 61–64.

WHO, 1980. Expert committee on diabeties mellitus. *Technical Report Service* No. 646.

Medicinal Plants: Conservation, Cultivation and Utilization (2007) *Pages 217–220*
Editors: A.K. Chopra, D.R. Khanna, G. Prasad, D.S. Malik and R. Bhutiani
Published by: DAYA PUBLISHING HOUSE

Chapter 30

Isolation of New Isoflavonoids from *Bowdichia virgiliodes*

C.P. Singh, Ashuthosh Sharma, C. Shekhar and Alok Gupta
Research Division, Chemistry Department, Sahu Jain College, Najibabad (U.P)

ABSTRACT

Two new isoflavonoids 7,8,4′-trimethoxyisoflavone and 7,8,4′-trimethoxyisoflavanone and calycosin (7,3′-hydroxy-4′-methoxyisoflavone) were isolated from the wood of the leguminous tree *Bowdichica virgilioides* by usual chromatographic procedures. Besides these compounds were also obtained the pterocarpane(-)-maackianin, isoliquiritigenin (4,2′,4′-trihydroxychalcone), and the hydrobenzylfuran derivative bowdenol. The structures of these new compounds were determinated by MS and 1D and 2D NMR spectral analysis.

Keywords: *Bowdichia virgilioides, Leguminosae, Isoflavones, Isoflavanone.*

Introduction

Bowdichia virgilioides Kunt. (Leguminosae, subfamily Papilionoideae, tribe Sophoreae) is a tree native to tropical South America ranging from Venezuela to Eastern Brazil (Polhill, 1981). In Brazil it is popularly know as "sucupira" and "sucupira-acu" (Correia, 1984). The plant is used as medicine, its barks being employed for arthritis, diabetes, as anti-rheumatic and for diarrhoea (Correia, 1984). Previous phytochemical investigations with the barks and roots of this species revealed the presence of piperidine alkaloids (Torrenegra *et al.*, 1989; Marinho *et al.*, 1994), triterpenes (Arriaga *et al.*, 2000; Velozo *et al.*, 1999; Torrenegra *et al.*, 1985), dihydrobenzofurane derivative (Melo *et al.*, 2001) and flavonoids, specially isoflavonoids (Velozo *et al.*, 1999; Torrenegra *et al.*, 1985). This work describes the isolation and spectrometric characterization of two new isoflavonoids, the 7,8,4′-trimethoxyisoflavone (1) and the 7,8,4′-trimethoxyisoflavanone (2).

Experimental

General Experimental Procedures

NMR spectra were recorded on Varian Gemini 300 and a Brucker AMX400 spectrometers. El Mass spectra were obtained on HP 5973 mass detector. Optical rotation were recorded on Zeiss polarimeter using MeoH as solvent.

Plant Material

The wood of *B. virgilioides* was collected in the Campus of the Universidade Estadual de Feira de Santana (EA), Brazil in September of 1999. The plant material was identified by comparing with specimens housed the Herbarium of the Department of Biological Sciences of that University (acronym HUEFS). Voucher material (*L.P. de Queiroz* 2877) is stored at the same herbarium under the number 12672.

Extraction and Isolation

The air dried wood of *B. virgilioides* (1.8 Kg) was twice extracted with MeOH for 2 days. The crude extract was concentrated and partitioned with hexane and $CHCl_3$. The $CHCl_3$ phase (12.3 g) was fractionated on C.C. on silica gel 60 eluting with different mixtures of $CHCl_3$: AcOEt and collected 30 fractions of 50 ml. From the fractions eluted with a 7 : 3 mixture of $CHCl_3$: AcOEt it was obtained the mixture of flavonoids that were separated by CCDP developed with $CHCl_3$: MeOH (96 : 4). This procedure allowed to isolated (-) maackianin (142.7 mg) (Agrawal and Bansal, 1989) as well as the compound 1 (8.0 mg) and the 2 (4.9 mg). The fraction (562 mg) of main CC eluted with $CHCl_3$: AcOEt (3 : 2) was subjected to a CC on silica gel 60 and eluted with $CHCl_3$: MeOH (95 : 5). Subfractions were submitted to a CCDP $CHCl_3$: MeOH (92 : 8) and this procedure afforded isoliquiritigenin (11.8 mg) (Yenesew *et al.*, 1998), calycosin (6.0 mg) (Ma, *et al.*, 2003) and bowdenol (78.8 mg) (Melo *et al.*, 2001).

7,8,4′-Trimethoxyisoflavone (1)

EIMS *m/z* (rel. int.): 312 [$M^{+\bullet}$ (Arriaga *et al.*, 2000)], 283 (100), 132 (70), 123 (45). ^{1}HNMR (Aceton-d_6, 400 MHz): δ 8.26 (*s*, H-2),7.82 (*d*, J = 8.8 Hz, H-5), 7.05 (*d*, J = 8.8 Hz, H-6), 7.57 (*d*, 2H, 1 = 8.9 Hz, H-2′ and H-6′), 6.99 (*d*, 2H, J = 8.9 Hz, H-3′ and H-5′), 3.84 (*s*, 6H, 4′ and 7 OCH_3), 3.97 (*s*, 3H, 8-OCH_3).

^{13}CNMR (Aceton-d_6, 100 MHz)

δ 153.22 (C-2), 124.75 (C-3), 175.72 (C-4), 122.04 (C-5), 110.56 (C-6), 155.30 (C- 7), 135.81 (C-8), 151.83 (C-9), 119.39 (C-10), 125.41 (C-1′), 131.04 (C-2′), 114.40 (C-3′), 131.04 (C-6′), 61.71 (8-OCH_3), 56.25 (7-OCH_3), 55.55 (4′-OCH_3).

7,8,4′-Trimethoxyisoflavanone (2)

EIMS *m/z* (rel. int.) 314 [$M^{+\bullet}$ (Torrenegra *et al.*, 1989)], 296 (100), 355 (10), 132 (10). ^{1}HNMR (Aceton-d_6, 400 MHz): δ 4.18 (*m*, 2H, H-2), 4.65 (br*d*. J = 3 Hz, H-3), 7.82 (*d*, J = 8.8 Hz, H-5), 7.05 (*d*, J = 8.8 Hz, H-6), 7.57 (*d*, 2H, J = 8.7 Hz, H-2′ and H-6t), 6.99 (*d*, 2H, J = 8.7 Hz, H-3′ and H-5′), 4.05-4.18 (*m*, 2H), 4.65 (*d*, indt.), 3.83 (*s*, 3H, 4′-OCH_3), 3.84 (*s*, 3H, 7-OCH_3), 3.97 (*s*, 3H, 8-OCH_3). ^{13}CNMR (Aceton-d_6, 75 MHz): O 72.19 (C-2), 54.07 (C-3), 187.68 (C-4), 122.04 (C-5), 110.50 (C-6), 155.30 (C-7), 135.81 (C-8), 151.83 (C-9), 119.39 (C- 10), 125.41 (C-1′), 131.04 (C-2′ and C-6′), 114.40 (C-3′ and C-5′), 160.48 (C-4′), 160.48 (C-4′), 61.71 (8-OCH_3), 56.25 (7-OCH3), 55.55 (4′-OCH_3).

Results and Discussion

The ion molecular (*m/z* 312) recorded in the mass spectra of 1 and data of NMR (^{1}H, ^{13}C and DEPT experiments) were in agreement with the molecular formulae $C_{18}H_{16}O_5$. The ^{13}C NMR spectra of this compound showed 15 C*sp*^{2}, and the CH signal at δ 153.22 besides the singlet at δ 8.26 observed in the ^{1}HNMR spectra permitted assigned the isoflavone skeleta for 1. The NMR spectra data and the isoflavonoid moety was proposed by presence of two *orto* dublets (0 7.82 and 7.05). However this proposal was confirmed by bidimensional espectral analysis (HMQC and HMBC), especially multiple bond ^{1}H and ^{13}C correlations. The two most important correlations observed was between H-5 (δ 7.05) with carbonyl (δ 175.72) and C-7, and the correlactions of H-6 (07.05) and the signals at 119.39 (C-10) and 135.81 (C-8) (Figure 30.1). These data permitted to unequivocally assign all the NMR data and identify 1 as being 7,8,4'-trimethoxyisoflavone.

The mass spectra of compound 2 showed molecular ion at *m/z* 314 ($C_{18}H_{18}O_5$). The NMR data were similar to 1. This compound was identified as being isoflavanone by presence of signals at ^{13}CNMR spectrum of carbonyl at δ 187.68 and an oxymethylene (δ 72.19) and benzylic (δ 54.07) carbons which are characteristic of this skeletal (Jain and Prasad, 1988). In order to confirm the proposed structure HMQC and HMBC spectra were recorded and the latter permitted to identify this, compound as being 7,8,4'-trimethoxyisoflavanone.

Recent phylogenetic surveys in the Leguminosae using DNA markers had, demonstrated that the tribe Sophoreae is not monophyletic and that *Bowdichia* is related with *Acosmium*, another South-American genus, basally nested within a group also including the Genisteae (Pennington *et al.*, 2003). This finding was also strongly supported by data from quinolizidine alkaloids (vanWick, 2003). On

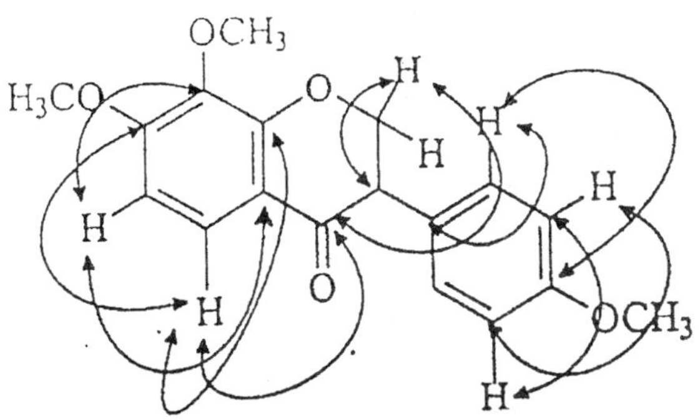

(1)

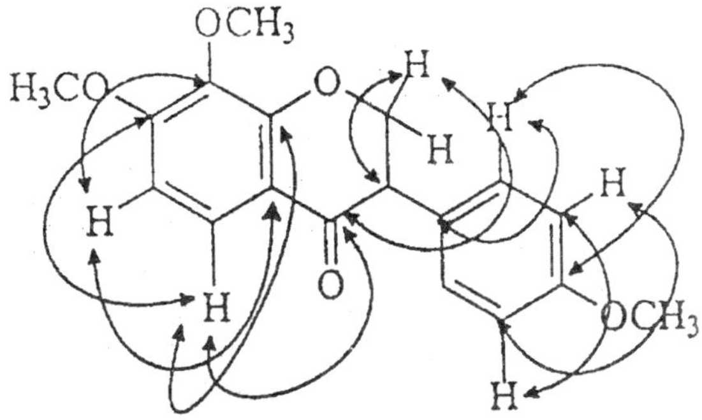

(2)

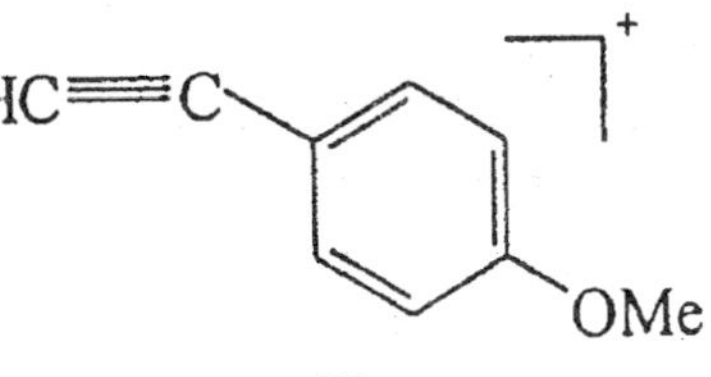

(3)

Figure 30.1: Long Range Correlations Observed in the HMBC Spectra of 1 and 2

the other hand, isoflavonoid data show a erratic evolutionary pattern difficult to interpret in a taxonomic framework (vanWick, 2003) but the representatives of the Sophoreae producing isoflavonoids were found to form a basal group inside a Genistoid group (Wink and Mohamed, 2003). To there is no report of isoflavonoid occurence in *Acosmium*. However it was also isolated from *A. qijugum* pterocarpanes (Silva *et al.*, 2001). So, similar studies in *Acosmium*, a putative related–genera, could bring light the chemical evolution in Genistoid legumes and allies.

Acknowledgements

We are greatly indebted to Dr. Dioneia C. Rodrigues (USP-Rib. Preto, Brazil) for the bidimensional spectra and we also thank to CNPq and FAPESB by the scholarships and grants.

References

Agrawal, P.K. and M.C. Bansal, 1989. Isoflavonoids. In: *Carbon-13 NMR of Flavonoids*, (Ed.) P.K. Agrawal. Elsevier, Amsterdam, p. 218.

Arriaga, A.M.C., G.A. Gomes and R. Braz-Filho, 2000. *Fitoterapia*, 71: 211–212.

B.-E. van Wick, 2003. *Biochemical Systematics and Ecology*, 31: 875–884.

Correia, M.P., 1984. *Diciondrio das Plantas Uteis do Brasil.* V. VI, Imprensa Nacional, Rio de Janeiro, p. 149.

Jain, A.C. and A.K. Prasad, 1988. *Indian Journal of Chemistry*, 26B: 622–624.

Ma, X., P. Tu, Y. Chen, T. Zhang, Y. Wei and Y. Ito, 2003. *Journal of Chromatography* A, 992: 193–197.

Marinho, L.C., C.M.T.M. da Cunha, G. Thomas and J.M. Barbosa-Filho, 1994. *Fitoterapia*, 65: 475.

Melo, F.N., V.R. Navarro, M.S. da Silva, E.V.L. Da-Cunha, J.M. Barbosa-Filho, R. Braz-Filho, 2001. *Natural Product Letters*, 15,261-266.

Pennington, R.T., M. Lavin, H. Ireland, B. Klitgaard, J. Preston and J.-M. Hu., 2003. *Systematic Botany*, 26: 537–556.

Polhill, R.M., 1981. Papilionoideae. In: *Advances in Legume Systematics Part I*, (Eds.) R.M. Polhill and P.H. Raven. Royal Botanic Gardens, Kew, p. 191–208.

Silva, V.N.T., F.M. de Oliveira and L.M. Conserva, 2001. *Biochemical Systematics and Ecology*, 29: 1189–1192.

Torrenegra, R., P. Bauereiss and H. Achenbach, 1989. *Phytochemistry*, 28: 2219–2221.

Torrenegra, R., S. Escarria, P. Bauereiss and H. Achenbach, 1985. *Planta Medica*, p. 276–277.

Velozo, L.S.M., B.P. da Silva, R.R. Bernardo and J.P. Parente, 1999. *Phytochemistry*, 52: 1473–1477.

Wink, M. and G.I.A. Mohamed, 2003. *Biochemical Systematics and Ecology*, 31: 897–917.

Yenesew, A., J.O. Midiwo and P.G. Waterman, 1998. *Phytochemistry*, 47: 295–300.

Medicinal Plants: Conservation, Cultivation and Utilization (2007) *Pages 221–230*
Editors: A.K. Chopra, D.R. Khanna, G. Prasad, D.S. Malik and R. Bhutiani
Published by: DAYA PUBLISHING HOUSE

Chapter 31

Ayurvedic Quick Remedies

Arun Chugh*
Navoday Ayurved and Panchkarm, A-29, Sri Ram Nagar Colony, Opposite Railway Station, Jwalapur – 249 407, Haridwar, U.A.

Ayurved means (*Ayur,* 'life' and *Veda,* 'knowledge'), the traditional medical system of India. It is derived in part from *Vedas,* and from later text of the fifth and second centuries BC. It is promoting physical health, Ayurvedic medicine, encompasses moral, religious, and social education. The ayurvedic system spread to the north, where it influenced Chinese medical thoughts, and to the west, where it influenced early Greek medicine.

The Ayurvedic system aims for a balance of the influence of the five elements (air, water, earth, fire, ether) on the five senses of the body.

During old period the Herbal system was accepted globally. After independence the government policies degraded it by encouraging the Alleopathy.

It was and is always stated that Ayurvedic system dose not have remedies which can effect immediately on the illness. But this is not true. Comparative to the European drugs the herbal system is very economical.

I am briefing here the *"Ayurvedic Quick Remedies"*, which will help you during emergency and general problems of minor nature, as coughs, colds, sore throat, sore eyes, indigestion, breathing problem, acne, shock, sinusitis, constipation, headache, acidity etc. Most of the ingredients are homely used. At our Navoday Ayurved and Panchkarm, opposite Railway Station, Jwalapur (Haridwar), we are using these quick remedies frequently with excellent efficiency.

* Member of Asthma and Bronchitis Association of India; Panchkarm Expert; Phone: 9219838164.

Acne

1. Mix half teaspoon turmeric, sandalwood, rose petals, milk and glycerin. Make paste and apply.
2. Add five teaspoon of aloe vera in wheat floor. Make *roti* of it and eat daily till Acne vanishes.
3. Drink hair cup of gulab-Jal daily.

Asthma

1. Add ginger juice (5 teaspoon), tulsi leaf juice (2 teaspoon), turmeric (1/4 teaspoon), kala namak (1/4 teaspoon) in a cup of hot water and drink.
2. Drink two teaspoon of vinegar with eight spoon of onion juice.
3. Apply warm sesame oil with a pint of salt over the chest and back region.
4. Mix 5 grains of alum in ½ ounce of rose water and drink.
5. Make pill of camphor and asfoedita in equal quantity and swallow with water.
6. Arusha leaves (dried) 2 ounce and make cigarettes and smoke.
7. Dalchini 60 grains, saunf 60 grains, mulathi 60 grains munaka 180 grains, sweet, almond 120 grains, sugar 60 grains. Powder all the drugs well and make into a pill mass. 5 grains three times a day.

Acute Muscular Pain

1. Do vasti karma with calamus oil and castor oil.
2. Apply castor oil mixed with a pint of Hing and camphor.
3. Hot fomentation.
4. Cover the area with crape bandage.

Abortion

1. Boil ashoka bark 100 grams, milk 4 ounce, water 1 pint to 1/4th strain and drink.
2. Tankan 30 grains, cinnamon powder 10 grains. Take it with conjee.

Acidity

1. Add slaked lime ½ ounce in 2 pint of water. Shake well and allow to deposit for 12 hours. Mix with equal parts of milk. Take 3–4 teaspoon of it after meal.

Amenorrhoea

1. Make pill of Asafoetida 1 grain and aloes 1 grain. Take it with water.

Anaemia

1. Take kasis 20 grains, kala mirch 20 grains, honey q.s. Make 10 pills of it. Take one pill twice a day with water.
2. Aloes 12 grain, kasis 12 grains, ilachi 30 grains, honey q.s. Make 12 pills of it. Take one pill twice a day with water.

Antispasmodics

1. Rock salt, hing and harr choti in equal parts. Make fine powder and take ½ teaspoon with water.
2. Hot fomentation with dhatura leaves boiled in water.
3. Make pills of hing and camphor in equal quantity. Swallow with warm water.
4. Ajwain 1 dram, ilachi 1 dram, kala mirch 30 grains sonth 30 grains. Make powder and take twice a day with warm water.

Aphthae

1. Apply sohaga 1 dram in honey 1 ounce with honey.

Backache

1. Apply lemon juice, ginger juice and eucalyptus oil over the effected area.
2. Hot fomentation.

Bleeding

1. Spray alum powder over the bleeding site.
2. Apply ice.
3. Apply burned powder of old wool.

Bleeding Gums

1. Apply mustard oil mixed with a pinch of salt.
2. Add 2–3 pinch of alum powder in warm water and gargle.
3. Massage gums with majuphal powder and lemon juice.

Burning Eyes

1. Apply ice cube over the eyes.
2. Instill 3–4 drops of rose water.
3. Move on green grass early morning naked feet daily.

Boils

1. Apply poultice made of jaggry, wheat floor and mustard oil.
2. Make paste of turmeric, gandhak powder and water. Apply to the effected area.

Burns

1. Apply ice cube over the burn area.
2. Camphor with coconut oil can also be used.
3. Make paste of til oil 2 ounce and limewater 2 ounce and apply.

Bed Sores

1. Make fine powder of sohaga, zinc oxide and starch of equal quantity. Dust over the effected area.

2. Sohaga 1 dram, paraffin 1 ounce–mix it and apply.
3. Piney resin 4 ounces, Wax 2 ounces, and Lard 8 ounces. Heat gently and stir while cooling. Apply it.

Blister

1. Apply on a cloth piece Root bark (Lal chita) 2 drams mixed in wheat or rice water for 20 minutes.
2. Apply camphor and multani mitti paste over it.

Bronchits

1. Make infusion of ginger 5 grains, black pepper 5 grains, sugar 10 grains, adhatoda 10 grains. Drink 1 ounce three times a day.
2. Anantamul 5 grains, syrup of liquorice 1 dram and water 1 ounce. Make infusion and drink 1 ounce three times a day.
3. Make pills of liquorice root 1 grain, black pepper 1 grain, gum babul 1 grain, common salt 1 grain. Suck 2-3 pills three times a day.
4. Make infusion of nausader 1 part, liquorice syrup 2 ounces and water 4 ounce. Drink 1 ounce three times a day.
5. Make pills of liquorice root, ginger, nausader, long pipul, sugar in equal quantity. Suck 2–3 pills three times a day.
6. Take morning and evening kakra singhi 5 grains and triphla 5 grains.

Cough and Cold

1. Gargle with Luke warm water mixed with a pinch of salt, turmeric and eucalyptus oil.
2. Burn little sugar over the charcoal and inhale.
3. Drink a cup of lemon mixed tea.

Constipation

1. Take gulkand 2 teaspoon, black resin 5 and anjeer 2 with hot milk at bedtime.
2. Take senna leaves half teaspoon, flax seeds one teaspoon with warm water at night.
3. Drink 3–4 glass of water early morning everyday.

Carminative

1. Camphor 1 dram, water 1 pint. Drink 1 ounce of it three times a day.
2. Sonth 3 grains, kala mirch 3 grains, sonf 5 grains kala namak 10 grains. Powder it and take after meal.

Conjunctivitis

1. Alum 5 grains, water 1 ounce. Drop for eyes twice a day.
2. Instill gulab jal in eyes 2–3 times a day.

Convulsions

1. Suhaga 1.0 grains, ualchini 10 grains. Powder and take three times a day.
2. Nausader 10 grains, water 1 ounce. Give during convulsions.

Cystitis

1. Isaphgul seeds 2 grain, water 1 pint. Boil for 10 minutes, strain and give 2 ounce thee times a day.

Diarrhoea

1. Drink a cup of tea with two spoon of curd added to it.
2. Mix two drops of mentha oil to two spoon of fresh ginger juice in half cup of warm water and drink.
3. Drink boiled rice water with a pinch of salt added to it.
4. Boil bruised majuphal 1 ounce in 1 pint of hot water for 10 minutes and drink
5. Powder har choti, pipul and sendha namak in equal quantity. Take ½ teaspoon full after each meal.
6. Chalk 2 dram, gum acacia 2 dram and infusion cinnamon 8 ounce. 1 ounce three times a day.

Diarrhoea of Children

1. Tutiya (copper sulphate) 2 grains, arak-of-ajawain 2 ounce. Give 1 teaspoonfuls three times a day.

Diarrhoea with Blood

1. Macerate for two hours katha 3 drams dalchini 1 dram, boiling water 8 ounces and strain. Give 2 teaspoonfuls three times a day.
2. Make powder of alum 4 grains, katha 5 grains and bael 20 grains. Take three times a day with curd.

Diarrhoea with Dysentry

1. Boil Pomegranate rind of fruit (bruised) 2 ounce, cloves 2 dram, and water 1 pint for 15 minutes strain and drink.
2. Powder katha 10 grains, dalchini 10 grains. Take three times a day.
3. Palas gond 15 grains dalchini 5 grains, powder and take three times a day.

Digestive Powder

1. Haldi 10 grains, papal 10 grains, sonth 5 grains, ilachi 10 grains, kali mirch 5 grains. Powder and take three times a day.
2. Har, anwala, ajawain, sonf, sonth, send ha namak, jira, namak. Powder equal parts of each and take 1–2 teaspoonful after meal.
3. Triphla (har, bahera, anwala) sugar, pipul, black salt in equal quantity. 30 grain after meal.

Debility after Fever

1. Kiryet stem ½ ounce, bach 1 dram, soya 1 dram, boiling water ½ pint. Infuse for an hour and strain. Take 1 ounce three times a day.

Delerium

1. Mix kapur 3 grains, kasturi 3 grains honey 1 teaspoonful. Place it on the tongue.
2. Take kasturi, jaiphal, jai patri, pipul, kali mirch in equal quantity and make pills of 5 grain. One tablet in a day.
3. Kapur, hing 3 grain each. 1 pill at bedtime.

Diaphoretic

1. Ajowain 8 grains, madar bark 1 grain, shora 8 grains soda-bi-carb 16 grains. For child 4 grains and for adult 10 grains.

Dropsy

1. Shora 10 grains shajna root infusion 1 ounce. 1 ounce three times a day.
2. Braleria root 1 ounce, water 1 pint. Boil for 10 minutes and strain. Drink during the day.

Earache and Tinitus

1. Instill 3–4 drops of clove and garlic oil in the ear.
2. Hot fomentation.

Exhaustion and General Debility

1. Drink a glass of fruit juice or coconut water.
2. Drink a glass of lemon and sweet water.
3. Drink a glass of milk with 10–15. Black resin.

Eczema

1. Make lotion of alum, borax and water. Apply on cloth to skin.
2. Mix sulphur, borax, kamala, soda-bi-carh in equal quantity. Dust over the effected area.

Erysipelas

1. Kasis 20 grains, alcohol 2 grains. Paint to the effected area.

Fever

1. Atis 15 grains, kala mirch 10 grains kaladana 10 grains. One powder twice a day.

Flatulence

1. Mix ¼ teaspoon of kala namak, ginger juice 2 tea spoon, limejuice 2 teaspoon and soda-bi-carb in a glass of water and drink.
2. Infusion of five gram of ajwain, a pinch of hing and pinch of salt in a cup of water is very effective.
3. Apply hing paste over the naval region.

Flatulency of Children

1. Infuse soya 3 drams in ½ pint of water, strain and drink.
2. Apply paste of hing on the naval region.
3. Make powder of dalchini, sonth and cardamom of equal quantity. Half teaspoonful three times a day.

Gonorrhea

1. Shora 10 grains, decoction of bhindi 2 ounce. One ounce three times a day.
2. Kababchini 30 grains, alum 5 grains. One powder three times a day.

Headache

1. For vataj headache apply sandal powder paste over the frontal and temporal region.
2. For kaphaj headache apply ginger powder paste.
3. For pittaj headache apply sandal powder, camphor paste.
4. Inhale lime mixed nausader.
5. Instill eucalyptus oil mixed with camphor into the nostrils.
6. Apply lotion of camphor, vinegar and water locally.

Hepatitis

1. Give infusion of nausader 20 grains, shajna 1 ounce. One ounce three times a day.
2. Give infusion of 20 grams of punarnava three times a day.
3. 50 cc of radish juice three times a day.

Hysterical Fits

1. Karpor, hing in equal quantity. Make pills of 8 grain one pill two times a day.
2. Make twelve pills of musabar 20 grains, hing 20 grains in honey. 1 pill two times a day.

Indigestion

1. Infusion of kali mirch powder 5–6, jira ½ teaspoon, ginger powder ½ teaspoon is very effective.
2. Take a spoon of honey with 5 drops of garlic and a pinch of salt.
3. Suck jaggry mix ginger lounges.
4. Do langhan.
5. Har, anwala, pippal, sendha namak in equal quantity can be taken after meal.

Influenza

1. Give infusion of dalchini 1 teaspoonful, cloves 5, ginger ½ teaspoonful three times a day.
2. Make linctus of atis 5 grains, pipul 5 grains, kakra sringi 10 grains and honey 10 dram. Give 1 teaspoonful three times a day.

Insects Bite and Poisoning

1. Remove the sting.
2. Give infusion of coriander seeds.
3. Apply calamus oil and camphor over the bite.
4. Apply nausader over the site.

Insomnia

1. Drink infusion of nutmeg, jatamansi and bhrami.
2. Slowly massage the soles of feet and head with warm bhrami oil.
3. Instill 3–4 drops of badam rogan in both ears.
4. Drink milk with 2–3 teaspoon of ghee.
5. Make pills of kapur 3 grains, hing 3 grains. 1 pill twice a day.

Leprosy

1. Chaulmoongra oil 2 ounce, neem oil 2 ounce. Apply to the effected area.
2. Chaulmoongra oil 5 drops, cod liver oil 30 drops. Twice a day after food.

Leucorrhoea

1. Mix shora 10 grains, alum 5 grains in 1 ounce of water. Take this dose three times a day.
2. Boil pomogranate fruit rind 3 ounces, cloves 2 dram in 2 dram water for 15 minutes and add 2 pint of alum to it. Use it as injection for cleaning.

Lice

1. Make ointment of sufed damar 1 dram, oil of tepertine ½ ounce, til oil 1 ounce and apply locally.

Lumbago

1. Camphor 1 ounce sweet oil 8 ounce. Apply locally.
2. Lemon grass 1 ounce, linseed oil 1 ounce. Apply locally.
3. Gandhak 2 ounce neem oil 1 ounce 1 pint. Apply over effected area.
4. Sulphur sublimate 10 grains, soda-bi-carb 10 grains, powder sublimate 1 grain. Take orally twice daily.

Malaria

1. Kaladana 20 grains, black pepper 5 grains and atis 15 grains. Powder it and take it twice a day.

Mouth Ulcer

1. Take tutiya 5 grains and honey 1 ounce. Apply to the ulcer.
2. Borax 5 grain, glycerin ½ ounce. Mix and apply to the ulcer.

Nipples (Cracked)

1. Borax 1 dram, bees wax 1 ounce. Apply 2–3 times a day.

Pharyngitis

1. Apply alum 30 grains; honey 1 ounce, and decoction galls 8 ounces mixture to the pharynx.
2. Pomegranate rind 2 ounce, cloves 1 dram water 1 dram. Boil for 15 minutes and add alum to it. Gargle 2–3 times a day.

Piles

1. Kaladana 15 grains, sulpur 15 grains. One powder every night.
2. Alum 1 dram, water 1 pint. Apply on the cloth form 15 minutes.
3. Har, bahera, aonwla, sonf, sonth all in equal quantity, salsa and kala namak ½ dram each. Powder it and take 1 dram at bedtime with milk.

Scabies

1. Sulphur 1 dram, til oil 1 ounce. Apply to the effected area.
2. Sulphur 2 dram, kamla 4 dram. Dust on the effected area.

Shock

1. Inhale nausader mixed with chuna.
2. Inhale onion or garlic.
3. Sprinkle cold water on the face.
4. Rub hand and feet sole rapidly.

Sinusitis

1. Instill 9–10 drops of cow's ghee mixed with a pinch of salt in nose
2. Introduce 4–5 drops of badam rogan into the nose and ears.
3. Inhale Eucalyptus oil or instill 3–4 drops in the nostrils diluted in sesame oil 4 Apply paste of ginger, tulsi leaves, kali mirch ad ghee over the effected area.

Swelling

1. Hot fomentation with salted water.
2. Drink infusion of punarnava and barley water.
3. Apply paste of turmeric, salt and mustard oil (in equal quantity) to the effected area.

Throat Infection

1. Gargle with alum water.
2. Massage ghee mixed with a pinch of salt externally.

Toothache

1. Massage mustard oil mixed with a pinch of salt to it.
2. Plug clove oil pack to the tooth cavity.

3. Tooth powder–Make fine powder of alum, majupha, kasis, katha sohaga, salt, karpur of equal quantity.

Ulticaria

1. Mix camphor, alcohol and apply.
2. Apply pulp of aloe vera over the effected region.
3. Drink half cup of aloe vera.
4. Drink the infusion of coriander seeds.
5. Keep 2–3 cardamoms in the mouth and suck at regular intervals.

Medicinal Plants: Conservation, Cultivation and Utilization (2007) *Pages 231–235*
Editors: A.K. Chopra, D.R. Khanna, G. Prasad, D.S. Malik and R. Bhutiani
Published by: DAYA PUBLISHING HOUSE

Chapter 32

Approach to Cure Tamak Shwas (Asthma) by Panchkarma

Arun Chugh*
Navoday Ayurved and Panchkarm, A-29, Sri Ram Nagar Colony, Opposite Railway Station, Jwalapur – 249 407, Haridwar, U.A.

ABSTRACT

In modern medicine, Asthma has no specific medicine to cure, so claimed as incurable disease. Ayurved believes that 'Sum dosh-Sum agni-Sum dhatu' (Primary bio-factors which carry out metabolism of the body) develops strong immune system. Ayurveda treatment consist in restoring of harmony between the Tridosha theory of Kapph, Pitta and Vata *i.e.* Growth factor of life, Consuming factor of life and Motive factor of life. A study over 120 cases of Tamak Shwas was conducted at Navoday Ayurved and Panchkarm Centre. The cure rate was observed by the herbal and panchkarma treatment at different age group.

Introduction

Tamak Shwas or Asthma due to allergy is a chronic disease, characterized by inflammation the airways. The inflammation causes associated increase in the existing airway hyper responsiveness to variety of stimuli, such as allergens, cold air and virus. Exposure of the patient to these stimuli provokes a variety of changes in airways including broncho constriction, wheezing, breathlessness, chest, tightness and coughing experience by the patients with Asthma, particularly at night and in early morning, is usually associated with airflow obstruction.

* Member of Asthma and Bronchitis Association of India; Panchkarm Expert; Phone: 9219838164.

Maharishi Charak illustrates the symptoms of shwas rog as:

प्रतिलोम यदा वायुः स्त्रोतासि प्रतिपद्यते ।
ग्रीवा शिरस्व संग हय श्लष्माणं समुदीय च ।।

(चरक–चि0 स्थान 54–91)

Asthma can occur at any age and individuals with its difference in frequency and degree of symptoms. Some people have only an occasional attack *i.e.* mild in degree and of brief duration and otherwise are entirely free of symptoms. Other have mild coughing and wheezing most of the time, triggered by several attacks following exposure to known allergen, infection or certain stress conditions.

Asthma can go unnoticed in people with the history of any allergic disorder who suffer from recurrent wheezing.

Ayurveda the ancient system of medicine believes in prevention from the disease. It has versatile approach to root out many incurable problems.

In Ayurveda, Asthma is known as Shwas Rog, It is described as:

1. Maha Shwas
2. Urdhva Shwas
3. Chhina Shwas
4. Tamak Shwas
5. Ksudra Shwas

Among these five types of Shwas first three are fatal and not curable. The last two Tamak and Ksudra Shwas are curable. More than 70 per cent of Asthma cases belong to Tamak Shwas and Ksudra Shwas group.

Samprapty of Tamak Shwas

दोष – कफ, पित्त

दूष्य – रस

स्त्रोतस – रसवह, प्राणवह

अग्नि – जठराग्नि एवं रसाग्नि

आम – जठराग्निजन्य एवं रसाग्निजन्य

व्याधि – क्षमत्व, अल्प

Patients and Methods

At Navoday Ayurved and Panchkarma Centre, situated near bank of Ganges, Jwalapur, Haridwar (U.A.). 120 cases of Tamak Shwas, from different part of India and of different age group was included in the study.

1. Age: 10 yrs to 75 year
2. Sex M/F: 72/48
3. Weight: 15 Kg to 92 Kg

4. Duration of illness: 6 months--20 yrs
5. Alcoholic addiction: 12 per cent
6. Tobacoo addiction: 10 per cent

Treatment was started by appointment for panchkarma.

During Acuteness

1. Oleation–Applied luke warm sesam oil with a pint of rock salt over the chest and back region.
2. 1 grain of Asafoetida in water applied on navel region softly.
3. Kept both feets in salted hot water
4. Zinger Powder–1/4th teaspoon
   Black paper–6 in nos. (Powder)
   Black salt–1/4th teaspoon
   Holy basil–5 in 4 number
   Somlata powder–½ teaspoon

The mixture was boiled in 200 ml of water and reduce to 50 ml. Filtered and given to sip.

For Childrens

Zinger juice–1 teaspoon

Basil leaves juice–1 teaspoon

Honey–1 teaspoon

Warm water–½ cup

This mixture was given 2--3 times a day.

During Normal Phase

Internal Oleation–Vasa Ghrit in Khiedi was given in following order.

1st day–25 ml.

2nd day–50 ml.

3rd day–75 ml.

4th day–100 ml.

After fourth day the internal oleation continued to achieve Samyak Snehyan. Lower age group received lower dose.

External Oleation

Sesame oil was applies over the trunk and extremities for external oleation.

Sudation

After Samayak Snehyan and Sarvang Abhyang medicated steam bath (Swedan) was given to widen the channels and eliminate the toxins of the body.

Vaman (Emesis)

Purv Karm

Patients were given sesame oil for three days in increasing order with initial dose of 30ml. The stool become oily. Kaphgenic diet was given to aggrevate, kaph in the system.

A day before Vaman patients were given oil massage and fomentation. Next morning vaman is done with Madan Phal Kalp*.

**Madan Phal Preparation*: Add 10 gm of Madanphal and 10 gm. of pippli to 200 ml of Mulathi Kwath. This decoction is kept throughout the night. Add 10 gms of sendhev and 20 gms of Honey to it in the morning. This mixture is Madan Phal Kalp.

Vamari Procedure: At morning patients were asked to drink milk full stomach and then given Madan Phal kalp. Vomiting was induced and continued till pittant was achieved.

Paschyat Karm

Complete rest and fasting.

Sansarjan Karm: Peya, Velapi, Yush or meat soup is given to the patient.

Virechan: Virechan was done after 15 days. Both external and internal oleation was done regularly for three days. Snehpan was given in this order

1st day–150 ml.

2nd day–100 ml.

3rd day–50 ml.

Virechan Kalp* was used to remove the dosh of bowl till Kaphant was achieved.

***Virechan Kalp Preparation**

Kutki–20 gm.

Nishoth–20 gm.

Choti Harer–20 gm.

Make Kwath of this mixture in 200 ml of water. Add 20 ml of castor oil and give to the patient empty stomach.

After Virechan Sansarjan Karm was done accordingly.

Following Instructions–were given to the patients that they:

1. Should avoid the factors, places, business that causes Asthma.
2. Should avoid common cold, cold drinks and moist places.
3. Must go for daily morning walk, do yoga exercises (Surya Namaskar and Pranayam).
4. Must go to sleep in time at night.
5. Should avoid mental tension.
6. Must brush teeth every morning after every meal and have good hygiene life.
7. Must avoid Tobacoo, wine and smoking habits.
8. Must avoid over eating and take light dinner one hour before going to bed.

9. Should not over load house with furniture and carpets.
10. Should keep room ventilated and use exhaust fan in the kitchen.
11. Should avoid air conditioner, cooler and direct air of fan.
12. Must avoid perfumes, aggarbatti, mosquito repellents that aggrevets attack.
13. Must not over exercise, over do sex, over do work, eat rough food, take excess emesis and laxative and suppress toilet urge.
14. Must drink boiled water in excess.
15. Must avoid those medicines which aggravets asthmatic symptoms.
16. Patients of Asthma children were advised to inform the schools teacher to keep their ward out of aggravating activities.

Advise Given for

What to Eat?

Hot soup of Bengal gram, Gram flour mixed with wheat flour, Garlic, Black pepper, Asafoetida, Clove, Basil leaves, Long pepper, Mint leaves, Papaya, Carrot, Carrot juice, Radish, Apple, Black resin, fig, Dates, Almond, Barley flour, Honey, Spinach, Rock salt, Cumin seeds, Lemon Grass Tea.

What Not to Eat?

Beans, Pea, Excess pulses, Cheese, Banana, Oranges, Water melon, Curd, Rice, Oily food, Bread, Jam, Pickels.

Medicines Used

Shwas kas Chintamani Ras, Shwas Kutar Ras, Sitopladi Churn, Talisadi Churn, Vasavakha, Chawanprash.

Krimi Mudgar Ras was given as antihelminthic.

Results

The results show remarkable changes in all the patients. The panchkarma reestablished the immunity of the bio-system. Hence, the change in the clinical picture were outstanding. The absolute eosinophyl count was elevated in 90 per cent of cases. After panchkarma and treatment 75 per cent showed normal. The Hb was shown below the normal level in 35 per cent cases. Most of them were children and females. A course of Antihelmint was given to intestinal infestation cases prior to panchkarm. The medication was given for three month. There was no relapse of wheezing after three month in 82 cases, 12 cases had wheezing once or twice during the course 10 cases did not respond well and six cases discontinued:

Total cases of Tamak Shwas–120

Cured–Excellent–92

Cured–Good–12

Poor–10

Discontinued–No result–6

Medicinal Plants: Conservation, Cultivation and Utilization (2007) *Pages 237–257*
Editors: A.K. Chopra, D.R. Khanna, G. Prasad, D.S. Malik and R. Bhutiani
Published by: DAYA PUBLISHING HOUSE

Chapter 33

Status of Medicinal Plants Found in a Montane Forest of Garhwal Himalaya

Asha Dobhal[1], Pramod Kumar[2], G.S. Rajwar[3] and Manisha Dobhal[4]
[1]Department of Botany Govt. P.G. College, New Tehri, Tehri Garhwal – 249 001
[2]Department of Botany HNB Garhwal University Campus, B. Thaul, Tehri Garhwal – 249 199
[3]Department of Botany, Govt. P.G. College, Rishikesh, Dehradun – 249 201
[4]Department of Chemistry, HNB Garhwal University Campus, B. Thaul, Tehri Garhwal – 249 001

ABSTRACT

Status of medicinal plants of an oak forest in Arakot-Khadikhal area of Chamba block of Tehri district were analysed on the basis of the quantitative data collected (during August 2000 to July 2002) from different slope sites. The study area is belonging to mid-montane forest of Garhwal Himalaya rich with a number of medicinal plants. 155 species of medicinal importance were observed as common, 110 rare, 30 frequent, 17 escape from cultivation and 6 endangered. Most of the rare and endangered plant species of the present investigation have been recorded as rare or endangered in the flora of District Garhwal. Over-exploited species of medicinal importance was 18. Endangered or rare medicinal plants must be conserved with the help of *in-situ* and *ex-situ* conservation methods.

Introduction

India is one of the main centre of the ancient human civilization in the world, where plants have been used for medicinal purposes. Out of about 17,500 flowering plant species that occur in India, about more than 3000 are recognized with their medicinal uses and in which over 1600 are used in traditional medicinal system. The Indian pharmaceutical industry is using over 500 plant species in their different formulations which have been collected from the natural habitat, and most of these medicinal plants grow in marginal mountain areas of India, such as the Himalaya.

A large number of medicinal plants of the Himalaya received significant attention in the ancient treatise such as Rigveda, Ayurveda, Charak Samhita, Agni Puran, Nighantus, Meghadoota, Shustra, Brikshaveda etc., which sung the glory of Himalayan herbs and drugs. The plants which are highly medicinal and already in use in the indigenous Ayurvedic system and herbal industries grown in different parts of the Garhwal Himalaya, are facing the problem due to over-exploitation and collections by tribal and migratory communities of the region such as Bhotiyas, Gujjars, Marchiyas (shepherds) etc. They collect the medicinal plants from the wild habitat when livestock graze in forests and pastures. Most of the collected medicinal species comes in the queue of rare and endangered flora of that region. As per current estimates more than 10 per cent of the plants fall in the threatened category and due to absence of any serious exploratory work (Gaur,1999).

On a global basis, the International Union for Conservation of Nature and Natural Resources (IUCN) has estimated that about 10 per cent of world's vascular plant species totaling to about 20,000-25,000 species are under varying degrees of threat. Simultaneously, to include information on threatened biological species, the IUCN has started publication of Red Data Book (Nayar and Sastry, 1987-1990). In India, out of an estimated 15000-16000 species of flowering plants about 1500 (10 per cent) have already come under various categories of threatened plants (Rao, 1994). According to Nayar and Sastry (1987-90) Extinct (Ex) category is only used for species which are no longer known to exist in the wild after repeated searches of the type localities and other known or likely places, Endangered (E) includes the taxa whose numbers have been reduced to a critical level or whose habitats have been so drastically reduced that they are deemed to be in immediate danger of extinction, Vulnerable (V) category includes the taxa of which most or all the populations are decreasing because of over-exploitation, extensive destruction of habitat or other environmental disturbance; taxa with population that have been seriously depleted and whose unlimited security is not yet assumed; and taxa with populations that are still abundant but are under threat from serious adverse factors throughout their range, while Rare (R) are the taxa with small world population that are not at present endangered or vulnerable. Taxa known to be extinct, endangered, vulnerable or rare but where there is not enough information to say which of the four categories comes in Intermediate (I) category. Whereas, taxa formerly included in one of the categories, but which are now considered relatively secure because effective conservation measures have been taken or previous threat to their survival has been removed are included in Out of Danger Category (O), and taxa that are suspected but not definitely known to belong to any category because of the lack of information are counted in Insufficiently known (K).

According to a cumulative estimate, the Garhwal Himalaya has more than 3500 species of flowering plants most of which are in forests or alpine meadows. Increasing pressure on the plant resources due to anthropogenic activities like grazing beyond the carrying capacities, increasing human population, increasing demands of fire-wood and cultivation land, increase in demand of timber and other construction wood, forest fires, exploitation of medicinal plants in addition to the invasion by ubiquitous weeds and other natural causes have tremendously affected the plant diversity of the Garhwal Himalaya (Rawat *et al.*, 2001). Ever increasing human and domestic animal population pressure in the arable land, natural resources and lack of well defined land management strategy are further leading to deforestation with serious environmental, social, economic and biological consequences (Khoshoo, 1992). It has also been noticed that though economic plants receive prime concern on account of their over exploitation, the other species facing difficulties in perpetuation due to ecological and phenological events are usually ignored when the rare or threatened taxa are listed, often leading to the un-noticed loss of taxa of the area (Gaur *et al.*, 1993).

The present study attempts to describe the vegetation study area with a view to status of medicinal plant that exist at Arakot-Khadikhal area of Tehri district of the Garhwal Himalaya where no such studies were attempted earlier. The work may be helpful to the explorers, ethnobotanists, scholars, naturalists and planners working for various aspects of the vegetation and landscape study and for planning and management purposes.

Study Area

The study area includes an oak forest at Arakot-Khadikhal in Chamba block of district Tehri Garhwal lying between geo-coordinates 30° 20′ N latitude and 78° 26′ E longitude, at an elevation ranging from 1550 to 2100 m. The northern part of the study area is highly disturbed due to interference by Gujjars and local shepherds who cross it with their cattle during early summer and late rainy season. The unscientific road construction has also affected the vegetation of the study area. The chief constituents of the forest were *Quercus leucotrichophora, Myrica esculenta, Rhododendron arboreum, Benthamidia capitata* and *Lyonia ovalifolia.*

Maximum precipitation was observed from May to September in both the years, whereas January and February of year 2002 also showed maximum rainfall. Mean monthly temperature ranged from 11.8 to 24.9°C and 9.9 to 27.1°C and the minimum from 2.1 to 16.4°C and 1.6 to 17.0°C for the first and second years respectively. Relative humidity ranged from 52.2 (April) to 94.6 per cent (August) for 2000-2001, and from 24.5 (June) to 96.5 per cent (August) for 2001-2002. The wind velocity was found higher during winter season due to dry and cline environmental condition. In comparison to other months of both years, the highest value of wind speed was found during August to December.

Methods

The data on phytosociology of medicinal plants belonging to tree, shrub and herb layers of the vegetation were used to measure their population size in terms of density. There are no hard and fast rules for classifying the plants into various categories because reproductive capacity of different species shows variations in different site conditions, habitat locations and pressure gradients and for plants of various layers (trees, shrubs, herbs). In the present study, the density and frequency data were used for categorizing medicinal species into four categories given below. The data were used for the study area only and was also compared with their status given in the floras of the adjacent Himalayan region and the Red Data Book.

Frequent (F)

These species had highest values of the density and frequency and were found in nearly all the sites consistently. Such species can also be called much common.

Common (C)

These species were present in most of the sites of the study area and had a relatively higher value of density and frequency.

Rare (R)

These species had a low density and were present in few stands of the study area.

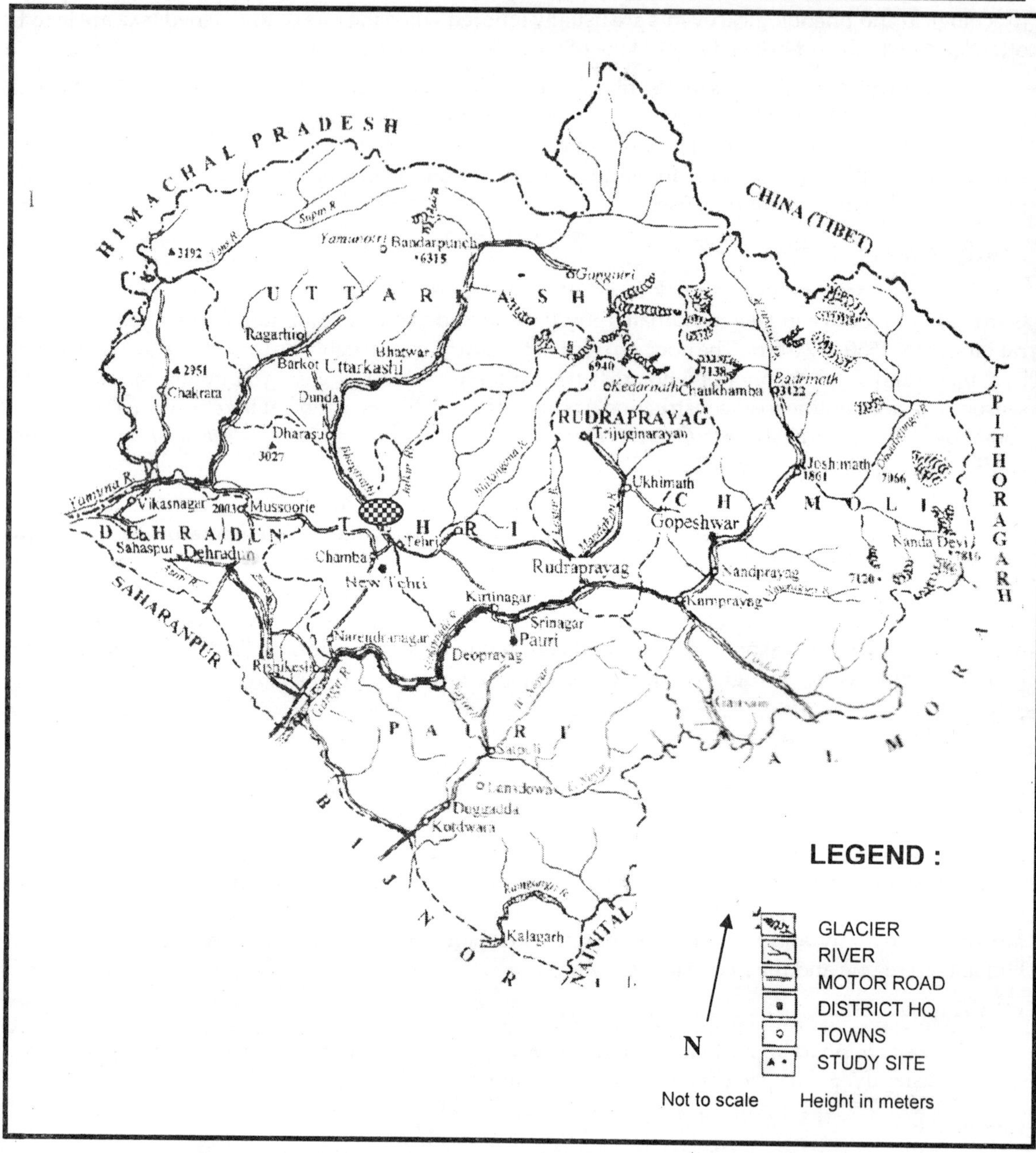

Figure 33.1: Location of the Study Site and Map of the Garhwal Himalaya

Endangered (E)

The species with a very low density and frequency values and whose survival in the area is in danger were classified as endangered species.

Escape from Cultivation (EC)

These includes cultivated species that were of medicinal importance and were found in the study area as an escape from the cultivated condition. These plants represented low frequency values.

Results

Total number of 318 species with 219 genera were recorded as medicinal plants from the study area, out of which 39 species and 30 genera of trees, 63 species with 44 genera, and 6 species with 2 genera of dicots and monocots respectively of shrubs, and 179 species belonging to 118 genera of dicotyledons, and 24 species with 20 genera of monocotyledons of herbs and only 7 species with 5 genera belonging to pteridophytes (Table 33.1).

Table 33.1: Vegetational Status of Medicinal Plants of the Study Area

Habit	*Genera*	*Species*
Trees	30	39
Shrubs		
Dicots	44	63
Monocots	2	6
Herbs		
Dicots	118	179
Monocots	20	24
Ferns	5	7
Total	**219**	**318**

Results on status of medicinal plants were based on density and frequency values and field observation. Out of 318 species of medicinal importance in the study area, 6 were endangered, 110 rare, 155 common, 30 frequent and 17 escape from cultivation (Table 33.2). Most of the rare and endangered species of the study area have been observed as rare or endangered in the flora of District Garhwal. Among endangered species of the study area, only *Acer oblongum* (which was noted as non-medicinal tree species) has been listed as endangered in the red data book. Out of 6 endangered species of medicinal importance, 2 belonged to tree category and 4 to herb category. Among 110 rare species which were recorded in the study area, the maximum species were herbs (73) followed by shrubs (27), trees (8) and ferns (2). Most of the medicinal plants were observed as common in the area of present investigation, out of which the highest number belonged to herbaceous layer (107) followed by shrubs (36), trees (8) and ferns (4) (Table 33.3). Frequent species of medicinal importance were found in almost all the stands of the study sites. The number of species of this category of plants enumerated as 16, 8, 5 and 1 belonged to herbs, trees, shrubs and fern respectively. A total of 17 species of medicinal plants were recorded as escape from cultivation category and most of which belonged to trees (13) followed by herb (3) and shrub (1) layers. Table 33.5 indicates that the common category of medicinal plants had highest value of percentage (48.74 per cent) in the study area followed by rare (34.59 per cent), frequent (9.43 per cent), escape from cultivation (5.35 per cent) and endangered (1.89 per cent) (Table 33.3).

Table 33.2: Status of Medicinal Plants in the Study Area Showing their Frequency (per cent) and Density (ha^{-1}) Values and Comparison with Red Data Book (Nayar and Sastry 1987–1990) and in District Garhwal Flora (Gaur 1999)

Name of Species	*Habit*	*NW*		*NE*		*N*		*S*		*SE*		*SW*		*Status*
		D	*F*	*D*	*F*	*D*	*F*	*D*	*F*	*D*	*F*	*D*	*F*	
Achyranthus aspera L.	H	–	–	–	–	1000	10	2500	15	3500	25	2000	10	C
Achyranthus bidentata Blume	H	2000	20	6000	20	1000	10	3000	30	–	–	–	–	C
Adiantum edgeworthii Hook.	TF	–	–	–	–	–	–	3000	20	–	–	3000	10	R
Adiantum incisum Forrsk	H		–		10		–		20		–		10	C
Adiantum venustum D.Don	TF	–	–	6000	20	–	–	–	–	–	–	–	–	R
Agrimonia aitchisonii Seh.-Temery	H		–		–		10		–		–		10	C
Agrimonia pilosa Ledebour	H	–	–	2000	20	1000	10	–	–	–	–	–	–	R
Ainsliaea aptera DC.	H	–	–	17000	100	1000	10	–	–	–	–	–	–	C
Ainsliaea latifolia (D.Don) Schultz-Bipontinus	H	30500	75	6000	30	17700	100	3000	80	9000	70	32000	90	F
Ajuga bracteosa Wallich ex Benth.	H	3500	30	8000	40	6500	45	11000	50	5500	35	4000	35	F
Ajuga parviflora Benth	H	–	–	–	–	–	–	2000	10	2000	20	7000	40	C
Albizia julibrissin Durazzini	T	–	–	–	–	–	–	10	10	–	–	–	–	R
Alnus nepalensis D.Don	T	10	10	20	20	10	10	–	–	–	–	10	10	C
Amaranthus tricolor L.	H		–		–		–		10		–		–	EC
Ampelocissus rugosa (Wallich) Planchon	Cl.S		–		40		10		10		30		–	C
Anagallis arvensis L.	H		–		–		10		10		–		10	C
Anagallis pumila Swartz	H		–		–		–		10		10		10	C
Anaphalis adnata Wallich ex DC.	H		–		10		–		10		–		10	C
Anaphalis busua (Buch.-Ham. ex D.Don) DC.	H	12000	70	5000	40	4000	30	3000	30	2500	20	6000	35	F
Anaphalis margaritacea (L.) Benth.	H	–	–	2000	20	–	–	–	–	–	–	–	–	R
Anaphalis triplinervis (Sims) C.B. Clarke	H		10		10		20		–		10		–	C
Anemone rivularis Buch.-Ham. ex DC.	H		10		–		10		–		–		–	C
Anemone tetrasepata Royle	H		–		10		–		–		–		–	C
Anemone vitifolia Buch.-Ham. ex DC.	H	–	–	3000	30	1000	10	4000	40	2000	20	2000	20	C
Arabis amplexicaulis Edgew.	H		–		10		–		10		–		–	C
Argemone mexicana L.	H		–		–		–		–		–		10	R
Arisaema concinnum Schott	H		–		–		–		10		–		–	R
Arisaema flavum (Forsk.) Schott	H		–		–		10		–		–		–	R
Arisaema jacquemontii Blume.	H	–	–	–	–	–	–	–	–	1000	10	–	–	R
Artemisia capillaris Thunb.	H		–		–		–		–		10		–	R

Contd...

Table 33.2–Contd...

Name of Species	Habit	NW		NE		N		S		SE		SW		Status
		D	F	D	F	D	F	D	F	D	F	D	F	
Artemisia japonica Thunb.	H		–		–		–		–		10		20	C
Artemisia nilagirica (C.B. Clarke) Pamp.	H	–	–	–	–	4000	30	–	–	–	–	–	–	R
Artemisia roxburghiana Wallich ex Besser	H	2000	15	3000	25	1000	10	1000	10	3500	20	7000	40	F
Asparagus adscendens Buch.-Ham. ex Roxb.	S	120	20	40	10	80	10	–	–	80	10	–	–	C
Asparagus curillus Buch.-Ham. apud Roxb.	S	–	–	40	10	–	–	–	–	–	–	280	30	R
Asparagus filicinus Buch.-Ham. apud Roxb.	S	40	10	–	–	–	–	80	20	–	–	40	10	R
Asplenium dalhousiae Hook.	TF	2000	15	1500	10	–	–	–	–	2000	10	3000	10	C
Aster peduncularis Wallich ex Nees	H	–	–	–	–	–	–	3000	20	–	–	–	–	R
Barleria cristata L.	H		–		10		–		40		–		20	C
Begonia picta Smith	H	–	–	2000	20	–	–	–	–	–	–	–	–	R
Benthamidia capitata (Wallich ex Roxb) Hara	T	2300	90	90	60	140	90	40	20	10	10	30	30	F
Berberis aristata DC.	S	960	60	240	40	560	60	280	40	360	40	–	–	C
Berberis asiatica Roxb. *ex* DC.	S	–	–	–	–	120	20	680	80	680	60	760	70	C
Berberis chitria Edward	S	720	50	1840	90	1080	90	–	–	120	20	800	80	C
** *Berberis lycium* Royle	S	600	50	440	60	–	–	1120	80	480	70	440	40	C
Bergenia ciliata (Haworth) Sternberg	H	3500	25	4000	25	2500	20	5000	20	2000	10	5000	40	F
Bergenia ligulata (Wallich) Engl.	H		–		10		–		–		–		–	R
Boehmeria macrophylla D.Don	S	–	–	–	–	–	–	–	–	–	–	80	10	R
Boehmeria rugulosa Wedd.	T	–	–	–	–	–	–	–	–	60	10	10	10	R
Boenninghausenia albiflora (Hook.) Reichb. ex Meisn.	H	31000	60	15700	60	61000	65	23500	45	7000	30	21500	50	F
Boerhavia diffusa L.	H		–		–		–		–		10		–	R
Bupleurum hamiltonii Balakrishnan	H	–	–	–	–	–	–	1000	10	1000	10	2000	20	R
Cardamine impatiens L.	H	2000	20	–	–	–	–	–	–	–	–	–	–	R
Carpesium nepalense Lessing	H	1000	10	–	–	–	–	–	–	–	–	–	–	R
Caryopteris foetida (D.Don) Thellung	S	280	30	800	80	1120	60	200	40	680	60	1040	90	F
Cassia pumila Lam.	H		10		–		–		10		–		–	C
Cedrus deodara (Roxb.exD.Don) G.Don	T		–		–		10		–		–		–	R
Centella asiatica (L.) Urban	H		10		–		30		–		–		10	C
Chaerophyllum reflexum Lindley	H		–		–		–		10		–		–	R
Chenopodium album L.	H	–	–	–	–	1000	10	–	–	–	–	–	–	EC

Contd...

Table 33.2–Contd...

Name of Species	*Habit*	*NW*		*NE*		*N*		*S*		*SE*		*SW*		*Status*
		D	*F*	*D*	*F*	*D*	*F*	*D*	*F*	*D*	*F*	*D*	*F*	
Cirsium wallichii DC.	H		10		10		20		–		–		10	C
Cissampelos pareira L.	Cl.S		20		–		–		10		10		–	C
** *Clematis acuminata* DC.	Cl.S		–		–		–		10		–		–	R
Clematis buchananiana DC.	Cl.S		10		–		–		–		–		–	R
Clematis connata DC.	Cl.S		–		–		10		–		–		–	R
Clematis grata Wallich	Cl.S		–		–		–		20		–		10	C
Clinopodium umbrosum (M.Bieb.) C.Koch	H	3000	30	–	–	–	–	6000	20	5000	30	5500	25	C
Clinopodium vulgare L.	H	–	–	–	–	4000	30	–	–	–	–	–	–	R
Colebrookia oppositifolia J.E. Smith	S		–		–		–		10		20		10	C
Conyza canadensis (L.) Cronquist	H	2000	10	–	–	11000	30	3000	25	4500	35	10500	45	C
Conyza stricta Willd.	H		–		–		10		–		10		–	C
Coriaria nepalensis Wallich	S		–		10		–		–		–		–	R
Cosmos bibinnatus Cav.	H		–		–		–		10		–		–	R
Cotinus coggygria Scopoli	S		10		–		30		–		10		40	C
Cotoneaster bacillaris Wallich	S	–	–	–	–	8000	50	–	–	–	–	–	–	R
Cotoneaster microphyllus Wallich ex Lindley	S	120	30	960	60	40	10	–	–	1000	50	160	30	C
Crotalaria alata Buch.-Ham. ex D.Don	H		–		–		10		–		10		–	R
Crotolaria albida Heyne ex Roth.	H		10		40		–		40		–		10	C
Cupressus torulosa D.Don	PT		–		–		–		10		–		10	EC
Cuscuta europaea L.	PClH		–		–		–		–		60		10	C
Cyathula capitata Maq.	H		–		–		10		–		–		–	R
Cynodon dactylon (L.) Persoon	H		–		10		–		20		10		40	C
Cynoglossum glochldiatum Wallich ex Benth.	H	–	–	–	–	4000	20	4000	20	1000	10	–	–	C
Cynoglossum lanceolatum Forsk.	H	–	–	–	–	2000	20	–	–	–	–	–	–	R
Cynotis cristata (L.) D.Don	H	5500	35	2000	20	6000	30	4000	30	–	–	3000	20	C
Cyperus rotundus L.	H	–	–	–	–	–	–	–	–	25000	80	13000	40	C
Daphne papyracea Wallich ex Steudel	S	400	60	200	40	–	–	–	–	400	40	240	30	C
Datura stramonium L.	H		–		–		–		–		10		–	R
Delphinium roylei Munz.	H		–		10		–		–		–		–	E
Desmodium elegans DC.	S		–		–		20		–		10		–	C
Deutzia staminea R.Br. ex Wallich	T	–	–	–	–	–	–	20	20	–	–	–	–	R
Dicliptera bupleuroides Nees	H	–	–	6000	10	–	–	4500	25	11000	45	5000	25	C

Contd...

Table 33.2–Contd...

Name of Species	*Habit*	*NW*		*NE*		*N*		*S*		*SE*		*SW*		*Status*
		D	*F*	*D*	*F*	*D*	*F*	*D*	*F*	*D*	*F*	*D*	*F*	
Dipsacus inermis Wallich	H	2000	20	–	–	–	–	–	–	–	–	3000	10	R
Drosera peltata J.E. Smith ex Willd.	H	–	–	–	–	–	–	–	–	5000	10	4000	10	R
Duchesnea indica (Andrews) Focke	H	4000	20	–	–	16000	30	5000	20	–	–	–	–	C
Echinops niveus Wallich ex Royle	H	–	–	–	–	–	–	–	–	–	–	1000	10	E
Elshoitzia ciliata (Thunb.) Hylander	H		–		–		–		40		–		20	C
Emilia sonchifolia (L.) DC.	H		10		–		10		–		10		–	C
Engelhardtia spicata Lesch. ex Blume	T	–	–	–	–	–	–	20	20	–	–	–	–	R
Epilobium brevifolium D.Don	H		10		30		–		10		–		10	F
Epilobium tetragonum L	H		10		–		–		–		10		–	C
Epipactis helleborine (L.) Crantz	H	–	–	3000	30	–	–	–	–	–	–	–	–	R
Erigeron annuvs Pers.	H		–		–		–		10		10		10	C
Erigeron multiradiatus (Lindley ex DC.) C.B. Clarke	H		–		10		10		–		–		–	C
Euonymus tingens Wallich	T		–		10		–		–		–		–	R
Eupatorium glandulosum H.B.K.	H	15300	40	12000	45	11700	55	20300	45	17000	40	21000	55	F
Eùphorbia hirta L.	H	–	–	–	–	–	–	–	–	–	–	2000	20	R
Euphorbia pilosa L.	H	–	–	–	–	2000	10	–	–	1000	10	–	–	R
Ficus palmata Forsk.	T		–		–		–		–		–		10	EC
Flacourtia indica (Burm.f.) Merrill	T		30		10		10		20		10		–	C
Flemingia fruticulosa Wallich ex Benth.	S		–		10		–		–		–		10	C
Flemingia procumbens Roxb.	H	–	–	–	–	–	–	–	–	6000	40	–	–	R
Fragaria nubicola Lindley ex Lacaita	H		10		30		10		–		40		10	F
Fumaria indica (Haus.) Pugsley	H		–		–		–		10		30		–	C
Galinsoga parviflora Cav.	H	–	–	–	–	2000	20	–	–	1000	10	2000	20	C
** *Galium acutum* Edgew.	H		–		–		10		–		–		–	R
Galium aparine L.	H	14000	60	–	–	–	–	4000	20	6500	25	6000	30	C
Galium asperifolium Wallich	H	11000	35	6000	20	17000	50	14000	55	–	–	10700	35	C
Galium asperuloides Edgew.	H	14000	40	–	–	–	–	–	–	–	–	–	–	R
Galium elegans Wallich	H	12000	60	–	–	–	–	19000	50	9000	50	10500	45	C
Galium vestitum D.Don	H	–	–	10000	50	–	–	9000	50	6000	40	–	–	C
Gamphogyne sp.	H		–		–		10		–		–		–	R
Gentiana aprica Decne.	H		10		–		30		10		–		10	C
Gentiana pedicellata (D.Don) Wallich	H		–		–		–		10		20		30	C
Geranium nepalense Sweet	H	7500	35	9000	40	6000	30	4000	30	4000	20	6500	45	F

Contd...

Table 33.2–Contd...

Name of Species	*Habit*	*NW*		*NE*		*N*		*S*		*SE*		*SW*		*Status*
		D	*F*	*D*	*F*	*D*	*F*	*D*	*F*	*D*	*F*	*D*	*F*	
Geranium ocellatum Cambess	H	–	–	–	–	9000	60	–	–	–	–	–	–	C
Geranium wallichianum D.Don ex Sweet	H	–	–	2000	20	5000	25	3000	20	–	–	–	–	C
Gerbera gossypina (Royle) G. Beauv.	H	10500	45	–	–	5500	30	6000	40	23700	65	10700	50	C
Gerbera maxima (D.Don) G. Beauv.	H	–	–	1000	10	1000	10	–	–	2500	20	1000	10	C
Geum elatum Wallich ex G.Don.	H	–	–	–	–	1000	10	–	–	–	–	–	–	R
Goodyera repens (L.) R.Br.	H		–		10		–		–		–		–	R
Grewia optiva J.R. Drummon ex Burret	PT		–		–		–		–		10		–	EC
Habenaria intermedia D.Don	H	9000	50	4000	20	–	–	–	–	–	–	–	–	C
Habenaria latilabris (Lindley) Hook.f.	H	2000	10	1000	10	3000	20	–	–	–	–	–	–	C
Hartmannia rosea G.Don	H		–		30		–		10		–		10	C
Hedera nepalensis K. Koch.	Cl.H		10		–		40		–		10		–	C
Hedychium spicatum Buch.-Ham. ex J.E. Smith	H	–	–	1000	10	–	–	–	–	–	–	–	–	E
Herminium lanceum (Thunb. ex Swartz) Vuijk	H	4000	30	–	–	–	–	–	–	–	–	–	–	C
Himalrandia tetrasperma (Roxb.) Yamazaki	S	600	60	280	30	360	50	560	60	240	40	560	50	F
Hoya lanceolata Wallich ex D.Don	Cl.S		–		–		10		–		–		–	R
Hypericum choisianum Wallich ex N.	S		–		–		10		–		–		–	R
Hypericum oblongifloium Choisy	S	–	–	40	10	–	–	–	–	–	–	–	–	R
Hypericum perforatum L.	H	–	–	–	–	1000	10	–	–	–	–	2000	10	R
***Hypericum podocarpoides* N. Robson	S	840	80	80	10	–	–	–	–	320	50	–	–	C
Hypericum uralum Buch.-Ham. ex D.Don.	S	120	20	–	–	120	20	–	–	–	–	160	30	C
Hypoxis aurea Lour.	H		–		10		–		–		–		–	R
Impatiens bicolor Royle	H		–		–		20		10		–		–	C
Impatiens scabrida DC.	H		10		–		10		–		–		–	C
Imperata cylindrica (L.) P.Beauv.	H		–		60		–		10		10		–	C
Indigofera cassioides Rottler ex DC.	S	–	–	–	–	160	20	–	–	40	10	–	–	R
Indigofera dosua Buch.-Ham. ex D.Don	H		–		–		–		–		10		10	C
Indigofera heterantha Wallich ex Brandis	S	40	10	40	10	–	–	–	–	–	–	40	10	C
Inula cappa (Buch.-Ham. ex D.Don) DC.	S	–	–	–	–	–	–	440	40	–	–	–	–	R

Contd...

Table 33.2–Contd...

Name of Species	*Habit*	*NW*		*NE*		*N*		*S*		*SE*		*SW*		*Status*
		D	*F*	*D*	*F*	*D*	*F*	*D*	*F*	*D*	*F*	*D*	*F*	
Inula cuspidata (DC.) C.B. Clarke	S	–	–	–	–	–	–	120	20	360	20	400	50	C
Ipomea nil (L.) Roth.	H	–	–	2000	10	12000	40	–	–	–	–	1000	10	C
Jasminum humile L.	S	720	40	520	50	400	50	–	–	600	50	600	50	C
Jasminum officinale L.	S	–	–	320	30	–	–	–	–	–	–	–	–	R
Julgans regia L.	T	–	–	–	–	10	10	–	–	–	–	–	–	EC
Lantana camara L.	S		–		–		–		–		–		10	R
Leea asiatica (L.) Ridsdale	S	–	–	–	–	–	–	80	10	80	20	–	–	R
Lepidium virginicum L.	H		10		–		20		10		–		30	C
Leptodermis lanceolata Wallich	S	360	50	120	20	760	40	–	–	–	–	–	–	C
Lespedeza gerardiana Graham ex Maxim	H	–	–	–	–	–	–	–	–	6000	30	–	–	R
Lespedeza juncea (L.f.) Persoon	H	–	–	–	–	4000	20	3000	20	–	–	2000	20	C
Leucas lanata Benth.	H	–	–	–	–	–	–	3500	25	5000	25	6000	20	C
Lindenbergia indica (L.) Vatke	H	–	–	–	–	5000	40	–	–	–	–	–	–	R
Liparis nervosa (Thunb.) Lindley	EpH		10		–		–		–		–		–	R
Lonicera quinquelocularis Hardwicke	S	–	–	240	30	240	30	40	10	360	20	–	–	C
Lyonia ovalifolia (Wallich) Drude	T	30	20	80	70	70	60	70	60	30	30	40	40	F
Malaxis acuminata D.Don	H	–	–	–	–	2000	20	–	–	–	–	–	–	R
Malva verticillata L.	H		–		–		–		–		10		40	C
Malvastrum coromandelianum (L.) Gurcke	H		–		–		–		10		–		10	C
Marsdenia lucida Edgew. ex Madden	Cl.S		–		10		–		–		–		–	R
Mazus pumilus (Burm.f.) van Steenis	H	4000	30	2000	20	5000	30	1000	10	–	–	–	–	C
Melia azedarach L.	T		–		–		–		–		10		–	EC
Micromeria biflora (Buch.-Ham. ex D.Don) Benth.	H	–	-	–	-	–	-	22000	30	48300	65	10300	10	C
Morus alba L.	T		–		–		–		–		10		–	EC
Murraya koenigii (L.) Sprengel	S	–	–	–	–	–	–	240	20	–	–	–	–	R
Murraya paniculata (L.) Jack	S	–	–	–	–	40	10	40	10	–	–	40	10	R
Myriactis nepalensis Lessing	H		–		–		10		–		–		–	R
Myrica esculenta Buch-Ham ex D.Don	T	110	70	140	90	120	70	110	70	50	50	70	60	F
Myrsine africana L.	S	37120	100	16160	100	16000	100	10480	100	8000	100	7800	90	F
Nasturtium officinale R. Br.	H		–		–		10		–		–		–	R
Nicandra physalodes (L.) Gaertner	H		–		–		–		–		10		10	C

Contd...

Table 33.2–Contd...

Name of Species	Habit	NW		NE		N		S		SE		SW		Status
		D	F	D	F	D	F	D	F	D	F	D	F	
Ophiopogon intermedius D.Don	H	–	–	–	–	4000	30	7000	60	–	–	–	–	C
Origanum vulgare L.	H	–	–	–	–	–	–	1000	10	7000	30	–	–	R
Osbeckia stellata Buch.-Ham. ex D.Don		S		–		–		10		–		–		–R
Oxalis acetosella L.	H		40		10		20		30		10		10	F
Oxalis corniculata L.	H	6000	30	7000	25	8000	25	6700	20	7000	15	5700	40	F
Oxalis dehradunensis Raizada	H		–		20		10		–		–		–	C
Parnassia nubicola Wallich ex Royle	H		–		–		10		–		–		–	R
Parnassia ovata Ledeh.	H		–		–		–		10		–		–	R
Pedicularis bifida (Buch.-Ham. ex D.Don) Pennell	H		–		–		–		10		40		20	C
Pedicularis gracilis Wallich ex Benth.	H		–		–		10		–		–		–	R
Perilla frutescens (L.) Britton	H		–		10		–		30		–		10	C
Persicaria chinensis (L.) H.Gross	S		–		–		–		–		–		10	R
Phyllanthus parvifolius Buch.-Ham. ex D.Don	S		–		–		–		10		30		10	C
Pimpinella acuminata (Edgew.) C.B. Clarke	H	4000	30	–	–	2000	10	–	–	–	–	–	–	R
Pimpinella diversifolia DC.	H	3000	20	–	–	2000	20	4000	30	–	–	–	–	C
Pinus roxburghii Sorgent	T	20	20	10	10	–	–	60	40	50	40	30	20	C
Pinus wallichiana A.B.Jackson	T	–	–	–	–	20	20	–	–	10	10	–	–	R
Plantago depressa Willd.	H		–		–		10		–		–		–	R
Plantago lanceolata L.	H		–		20		–		10		–		10	C
Polygala arvensis Willd.	H		40		–		–		30		10		20	C
Polygala crotalaroides Buch.-Ham. ex DC.	H		–		10		–		–		30		20	C
**Polygonatum cirrhifolium* (Wallich) Royle	H		–		10		–		–		–		–	R
Polygonum plebeium R. Br.	H		–		–		–		10		–		–	EC
Polygonum recumbens Royle ex Babcock	H		–		–		10		10		–		20	C
Polypodium microrhizoma Clarke	H		–		–		10		10		–		40	C
Polystichum squarrosum (D.Don) Fee	TF	7300	25	6300	20	8000	20	7000	20	3500	10	6000	10	F
Potentilla argyrophylla Wallich ex Lehm.	H		–		–		–		10		–		–	R
Potentilla fulgens Wallich ex Hook.	H	10000	40	–	–	5000	25	–	–	2000	20	–	–	C

Contd...

Table 33.2–Contd...

Name of Species	Habit	NW		NE		N		S		SE		SW		Status
		D	F	D	F	D	F	D	F	D	F	D	F	
Potentilla gerardiana Lindley ex Lehmann	H	–	–	3000	10	6000	30	11000	20	7500	35	6500	30	F
Potentilla leschenaultiana Sev.	H	–	–	4000	30	4000	10	–	–	–	–	7000	20	C
Potentilla nepalensis Hook.f.	H	–	–	10000	40	5000	40	–	–	–	–	–	–	C
Primula denticulata Smith	H		–		10		–		–		–		–	R
Primula floribunda Wallich	H	–	–	–	–	1000	10	–	–	–	–	–	–	R
Primula microphylla D.Don	H		–		–		10		–		–		–	R
Prinsepia utilis Royle	S	–	–	–	–	–	–	–	–	–	–	80	10	R
Prunus armeniaca L.	T		–		–		–		10		–		–	EC
Prunus cerasifera Ehrhart	T		–		10		–		–		–		–	EC
Prunus cerasoides D.Don	T	20	20	30	30	30	20	60	50	40	40	30	20	F
Prunus cornuta (Wallich ex Royle) Steudel	T		–		10		10		–		–		–	EC
Prunus persica (L.) Batsch	T		–		–		–		–		–		10	EC
Pteracanthus alatus (Clarke) Bre.	S		–		–		10		–		60		–	C
Pteracanthus angustifrons (Clarke) Bre.	S		–		10		–		10		–		40	C
Punica granatum L.	T	–	–	–	–	–	–	–	–	–	–	10	10	EC
Pyracantha crenulata (D.Don) M. Roemer	S	280	20	–	–	120	10	–	–	–	–	120	20	C
Pyrus malus L.	PT		–		–		10		–		–		–	EC
Pyrus pashia Buch.-Ham. ex D.Don	T	10	10	20	20	20	20	140	80	80	50	60	50	F
Quercus leucotrichophora A. Camus	T	1190	100	1310	100	1190	100	1300	100	1210	100	1090	100	F
Rabdosia lophanthoides (Buch.-Ham.ex D.Don) Hara	H	3000	30	–	–	5000	30	5000	40	1000	10	3000	20	C
Ranunculus hirtellus Royle	H	2000	20	–	–	1000	10	–	–	–	–	–	–	R
Ranunculus laetus Wallich ex D.Don	H		10		–		10		–		–		–	C
Reinwardtia indica Dumortier	H	4500	25	2500	15	2500	20	11300	50	–	–	4000	30	C
Remusatia vivipara (Roxb.) Schott.	H	–	–	–	–	–	–	1000	10	1000	10	–	–	R
Rhamnus purpureus Edgew	S		–		–		–		10		–		10	C
Rhamnus triqueter (Wallich) Lawson	T	–	–	–	–	–	–	–	–	10	10	–	–	R
Rhododendron arboreum Smith	T	160	80	180	90	120	80	70	60	10	20	40	40	F
Rhus javanica L.	T	20	20	10	10	30	20	–	–	20	10	10	10	C
Rhus parviflora Roxb.	S	–	–	–	–	–	–	160	30	160	20	160	30	C
**Rhus punjabensis* J.L. Stewart	T	–	–	–	–	–	–	–	–	10	10	–	–	E

Contd...

Table 33.2–Contd...

Name of Species	Habit	NW		NE		N		S		SE		SW		Status
		D	F	D	F	D	F	D	F	D	F	D	F	
Ricinus communis L.	S		–		–		–		–		–		10	EC
Rosa brunonii Lindley	S	80	10	440	50	360	50	–	–	–	–	–	–	C
Rosa macrophylla Lindley	S	–	–	40	10	200	30	–	–	–	–	–	–	R
**Roscoea alpina* Royle	H	8000	50	16000	80	15000	70	4000	30	–	–	3000	20	C
Roscoea purpurea J.E. Smith	H		10		20		–		10		–		–	C
Rotala densiflora (Rolt.) Koehre	H		–		–		–		–		10		–	R
***Rubia manjith* Roxb. ex Fleming	H	3000	30	5000	30	2000	20	4000	35	2000	20	4000	20	F
Rubus ellipticus Smith	S	560	70	760	70	640	70	1600	80	1720	80	840	80	F
Rubus foliolosus D.Don	Cl.S		–		–		–		10		–		–	R
Rubus niveus Thunb.	S	760	60	440	50	720	70	360	40	280	50	800	60	F
Rubus paniculatus Smith	S	–	–	920	70	560	50	120	20	–	–	120	20	C
Rumex hastatus D.Don	H		–		10		–		20		–		40	C
Rumex nepalensis Sprengel	H		–		–		50		–		10		–	C
Saccharum spontaneum L.	H		–		–		–		–		40		10	C
Saliva nubicola Wallich ex Sweet	H		–		–		–		40		10		20	C
Salvia lanata Roxb.	H	–	–	–	–	–	–	–	–	3000	20	–	–	R
Sanicula elata Buch.-Ham. ex D.Don	H	–	–	5000	20	–	–	–	–	–	–	–	–	R
Satyrium nepalense D.Don	H	–	–	–	–	–	–	–	–	–	–	1000	10	R
Saussurea heteromalla (D.Don) Hand.-Mazz.	H		–		–		–		10		40		–	C
Scurrula elata (Edgew.) Danser	PS		20		10		–		10		–		–	C
Scutellaria scandens Buch.-Ham. ex D.Don	H	117000	60	–	–	–	–	–	–	–	–	–	–	C
Sedum multicaule Wallich ex Lindley	H	–	–	27500	30	25000	70	1000	10	2500	10	4000	15	C
Senecio rufinervis DC.	H		–		10		–		–		–		–	R
Sida cordata (Burm.f.) Berss.	H		10		–		–		40		–		20	C
Siegesbeckia orientalis L.	H	3000	30	–	–	4000	30	–	–	–	–	–	–	C
Smilax aspera L.	S	200	30	–	–	160	20	–	–	160	40	–	–	C
Smilax glaucophylla Klotzsch	S	1440	80	1080	60	280	30	–	–	–	–	–	–	C
Smilax menispermoidea A.DC.	S	–	–	80	10	80	10	120	10	–	–	–	–	C
Solanum nigrum L.	H	–	–	–	–	1000	10	–	–	–	–	–	–	R
Solena amplexicaulis (Lam.) Gandhi	H	2000	20	–	–	–	–	–	–	–	–	–	–	R
Sonchus oleraceus L.	H		–		–		–		10		–		10	C
Spermadictyon sauveolens Roxb.	S	–	–	–	–	–	–	120	20	–	–	–	–	R
Spiraea vacciniifolia D.Don	S		–		10		–		–		40		–	C

Contd...

Table 33.2–Contd...

Name of Species	Habit	NW		NE		N		S		SE		SW		Status
		D	F	D	F	D	F	D	F	D	F	D	F	
Sporobolus diander (Retz.) P. Beauv	H		–		–		–		60		–		10	C
Stellaria media (L.) Villars	H	–	–	18000	50	15000	20	–	–	5000	10	2000	10	C
Stephania elegans Hook. f. and Thomson	Cl.H		–		–		–		20		–		–	R
Swertia alata (Royle ex D.Don) C.B. Clarke	H	–	–	5000	30	–	–	2000	10	1000	10	–	–	C
Swertia angustifolia Buch.-Ham. ex D.Don	H		–		–		10		40		40		–	C
Swertia chirayita (Roxb. ex Fleming) Karsten	H	1000	10	–	–	–	–	–	–	–	–	–	–	E
Swertia ciliata (D.Don ex G.Don) Burtt.	H	–	–	–	–	–	–	–	–	–	–	2000	20	R
Swertia cordata (G.Don) C.B. Clarke	H		–		–		–		10		–		–	R
Swida macrophylla (Wallich) Sojak	T		10		–		10		10		–		30	F
Swida oblonga (Wallich) Sojak	T	–	–	–	–	–	–	20	10			–	–	C
Tagetes minula L.	H		–		–		–		–		10		–	R
Taraxacum officinale Weber	H	–	–	–	–	–	–	–	–	15000	10	–	–	R
Tectaria coadunata (Wallich.ex Hook. et. Grev.) C.Chr.	TF	–	–	–	–	11000	20	–	–	–	–	–	–	C
Teucrium quadriforium Buch.-Ham. ex D.Don	H	7000	30	–	–	–	–	3000	20	2000	15	–	–	C
Thalictrum foliolosum DC.	H	–	–	1000	10	–	–	–	–	–	–	–	–	R
Thalictrum javanicum Blume	H	2500	10	2000	20	3500	30	3000	20	–	–	2000	10	C
Thalictrum saniculaeforme DC.	H	3000	20	–	–	–	–	–	–	–	–	–	–	R
Thuja orientalis L.	PT		–		–		–		–		–		10	EC
Tillaea pharnacesides Fischet	H	–	–	–	–	–	–	–	–	2000	10	–	–	R
Toona serrata (Royle) M. Roemer	T	–	–	20	20	–	–	10	10	–	–	10	10	C
Trifolium pratense L.	H		–		10		–		–		–		–	R
Trifolium repens L.	H		10		–		30		–		10		–	C
Urtica ardens Link	H		–		–		–		–		–		10	R
Urtica dioica L.	H		–		–		10		–		20		30	C
Valeriana hardwickii Wallich	H	15000	70	7000	40	23000	70	–	–	–	–	–	–	C
Valeriana jatamansii Jones	H	–	–	–	–	6000	30	5000	40	1000	10	10000	50	C
Valeriana roylei Kdotz and Greeke	H	7000	40	2000	20	5000	30	–	–	–	–	–	–	C
Valeriana stracheji C.B. Clarke	H	1000	10	18000	60	1000	10	–	–	–	–	–	–	C
Verbascum thapsus L.	H	–	–	–	–	–	–	–	–	1000	10	–	–	R

Contd...

Table 33.2–Contd...

Name of Species	Habit	NW		NE		N		S		SE		SW		Status
		D	F	D	F	D	F	D	F	D	F	D	F	
Vernonia cinerea (L.) Lessing.	H	–	–	17000	70	–	–	1500	10	2000	10	2000	10	C
Veronica persica Poiret	H		10		–		–		–		–		–	R
Viburnum continifolium D.Don	T	40	40	30	20	30	30	–	–	–	–	–	–	C
Viburnum cylindricum Buch.-Ham. ex D.Don	T		10		10		–		10		–		–	C
Viburnum mullaha Buch.-Ham. ex D.Don	T	10	10	30	30	20	20	–	–	–	–	–	–	C
Vigna vexillata (L.) A. Richard	H		–		–		–		10		–		20	C
Viola betonicifolia J. Smith	H	3000	20	36000	90	12000	40	–	–	–	–	14000	50	C
Viola biflora L.	H	–	–	4000	10	8000	40	–	–	11000	40	–	–	C
Viola canescens Wallich	H	15000	70	17000	40	6600	55	9500	50	14000	60	5000	30	F
Viola pilosa Blume	H	8000	30	4700	25	25000	50	9000	65	11300	50	12000	60	F
Viscum nepalense Spreng.	PS		–		10		–		–		20		–	C
Vitex negundo L.	S		–		–		10		–		–		–	R
Woodfordia fruticosa (L.) Kurz.	S	–	–	–	–	–	–	–	–	–	–	120	20	R
Zanthoxylum armatum DC.	S	200	30	160	30	160	30	160	30	–	–	–	–	C

*: Categorised as Endangered in District Garhwal; **: Categorised as Rare in District Garhwal.

Status: E: Endangered; R: Rare; C: Common; F: Frequent EC: Escape from Cultivation.

Life forms: H:Herbs; S: Shrubs; T: Trees; CIH: Climbric Herbs; CIS: Climbric Shrubs; TF: Terrestrial Ferns; PCIH:Parasitic Climbric Herb.

Table 33.3: Number of Medicinal Plants in Various Categories in the Study Area

Category	Trees	Shrubs	Herbs	Ferns	Total
Frequent	8	5	16	1	30
Common	8	36	107	4	155
Rare	8	27	73	2	110
Endangered	2	–	4	–	6
Escape from cultivation	13	1	3	–	17

The number of over-exploited species was 18 in the study area, in which 11 were herbs and 7 shrubs (Table 33.4). These species had been exploited maximum for the collection of medicinal plants in large quantities in the recent years. Notable among these species were all four species of *Berberis* followed by *Asparagus, Valeriana, Swertia* and *Viola* (each with two species) found in the study area.

Discussion

As a result of active field study, 318 medicinal plants were recorded from the study area which were categorized in 5 categories on the basis of frequency and density *viz.* frequent (F), common (C), rare (R), endangered (E) and escape from cultivation (EC). The frequent species had maximum values of density and frequency and occurred in most of the study sites while, common species had relatively higher values of population density and frequency in comparison to rare, endangered and escape from cultivation categories of medicinal plants. Out of 6 endangered species, 4 belonged to herbs and 2 to trees. Among rare texa which were recorded from the area of present investigation, the highest percentage number belonged to herbs (66.36 per cent) followed by shrubs (24.55 per cent), trees (7.27 per cent) and ferns (1.82 per cent).

Table 33.4: Percentage Distribution of Medicinal Plants in Various Categories in the Study Area

Sl.No.	*Categories of Medicinal Plants*	*Percentage in the Study Area*
1.	Frequent	9.43
2.	Common	48.74
3.	Rare	34.59
4.	Endangered	1.89
5.	Escape from cultivation	5.35

Table 33.5: List of Over-exploited Medicinal Species of the Study Area

Botanical Name	*Common Name*	*Family*
Ajuga bracteosa Wallich ex Benth.	Neelkanthi	Lamiaceae
Asparagus curillus Buch.Ham. apud Roxb.	Karu	Liliaceae
Asparagus filicinus Buch.Ham. apud Roxb.	Kaunta	Liliaceae
Berberis aristata DC.	Kingor	Berberidaceae
Berberis asiatica Roxb. *ex* DC.	Kingor	Berberidaceae
Berberis chitria Edward	Kingor, Totar	Berberidaceae
Berberis lycium Royle	Kingor	Berberidaceae
Bergenia ciliata (Haworth) Sternberg	Silparu	Saxifragaceae
Habenaria intermedia D.Don	Rhidi-Bidhi	Orchidaceae
Rubia manjith Roxb. ex Fleming	Manjeth	Rubiaceae
Swertia chirayita (Roxb. ex Fleming) Karsten	Chirayte	Gentianaceae
Swertia ciliata (D.Don ex G.Don) Burtt	Chiraita	Gentianaceae
Thalictrum foliolosum DC.	Kirmuli	Ranunculaceae
Valeriana hardwickii Wallich	Shammia	Valerianaceae
Valeriana jatamansii Jones	Sumaya	Valerianaceae
Viola biflora L.	Vanfsa, Dundi-Birali	Violaceae
Viola canescens Wallich	Vanfsa	Violaceae
Zanthoxylum armatum DC.	Timru	Rutaceae

A total of 427 species of flowering plants has been listed under various categories in Indian Red Data Book (Nayar and Sastry, 1987-1990), of which 30 species have been found distributed in the Garhwal Himalaya (Table 33.6), but only *Acer oblongum* was found as endangered species from the present study area which is non-medicinal tree in nature. Any rare species of medicinal importance was also not included in the present study which had been listed as rare in the Red Data Book.

According to new IUCN Red List Criteria in conservation and management assessment plant (AMP) meeting held in Lucknow (U.P.), *Berberis aristata* is an endangered plant of medicinal importance which was common in present study area but reported as endangered by Kala (1998) from the buffer zone of Valley of Flowers National Park, Garhwal Himalaya and as rare by Sharma (1998) from the Western Himalaya. *Hedychium spicatum* which was recorded as endangered in the study area was reported as rare by Sharma (1998) from Western Himalaya.

Table 33.6: Species which are Present in Garhwal Himalaya According to Red Data Book (Nayar and Sastry, 1987-1990)

Name	*Family*	*RDB Status*	*Altitudinal Range (a msl)*	*Distribution in Himalaya*
Acer caesium Wall. ex Brandis	Aceraceae	Vulnerable	1500-2700	J&K, HP, G, K
* *A. oblongum* Wall. ex DC.	Aceraceae	Endangered	1500-1800	G
A. osmastonii Gamble	Aceraceae	Endangered	800-2400	EH, G
Aconitum falconeri Stapf	Ranunculacsae	Vulnerable	3600-4000	HP, G, B
Allium stracheyi Baker	Liliaceae	Vulnerable	2500-3000	J&K, HP, G, K, N
Aphyllorchis gollani Duthie	Orchidaceae	Endangered or Extinct	2400-3000	G
A. parviflora King and Patling	Orchidaceae	Rare	3400-3600	G, N, S
Archineottia microglottis (Duthie) Chen.	Orchidaceae	Rare	2000-2400	G
Arenaria curvifolia Majumdar	Caryophyllaceae	Endangered	3550-3650	G
Berberis osmastonii Dunn	Berberidaceae	Rare	1700	G
Calanthe mannii Hook. f.	Orchidaceae	Rare	1300-2200	G, K, N, S, B Khasi Hills
C. pachystalix Reichb. f. ex Hook. f.	Orchidaceae	Endangered	2000	HP, G, N
Catamixis baccharoides Thorns.	Asteraceae	Vulnerable	300-800	G, N
Cyananthus integer Wall. ex Benth.	Campanulaceae	Rare	2800-3800	K, G
Cypripedium cordigerum D. Don	Orchidaceae	Rare	2500-3500	J&K, HP, G, K, N, S, B
C. elegans Reichb. f.	Orchidaceae	Rare	2500-4000	G, K, S, N, B
C. himalaicum Rolfe	Orchidaceae	Rare	3100-4000	G, K, S, N, B
Didicea cunninghamii King et Prain ex King et Patling	Orchiclaceae	Rare	2000-2500	G, S
Dioscorea deltoidea Wall. ex. Griseb.	Dioscoreaceae	Vulnerable	2000-2500	J&K, HP, G, K, N, S, EH
Eria occidentalis Seidenf.	Orchidaceae	Rare	1200-1500	G, K
Eulophia machinnonii Duthie	Orchidaceae	Rare	300-800	G
Hedysarum microcalyx Baker	Fabaceae	Vulnerable	3000-4500	J&K, HP, G
Microschoenus duthiei Clarke	Cyperaceae	Indeterminate	4572-4876	G
Nardostachys grandiflora DC.	Valerianaceae	Vulnerable	3200-4600	HP, G, K, N, S, B
Picrorhiza kuffooa Royle ex Benth.	Scrophulariaceae	Vulnerable	3000-4500	HP, K, G
Pittosporum eriocarpum Royle	Pittosporaceae	Indeterminate	1200-2400	G, K
Saussurea bracteata Decne.	Asteraceae	Rare	3500-5000	J&K, HP, G, K
S. costus (Falc.) Lipschitz	Asteraceae	Endangered	2500-3500	J&K, HP, G, K
Silene kumaonensis Williams	Caryophyllaceae	Rare	2500-4000	J&K, HP, G, K

B: Bhutan; G: Garhwal; K: Kumaon; J&K: Jammu and Kashmir; HP: Himachal Pradesh; N: Nepal; S: Sikkim; EH: Eastern Himalaya; RDB: Red Data Book.

* Found in the present study area.

Among the rare species observed in the study area *Climatis acuminata* and *Galium acutum* were medicinal plants also categorised as rare, while *Rhus punjabensis* was classified as endangered in the flora of District Garhwal (Gaur, 1999). Most of the rare or endangered species of medicinal importance recorded in the study area were also reported by Pandey *et al.* (1993) under similar categories for medicinal plants of Kumaon Himalaya. Some species such as *Rubus manjith, Berberis lycium, Hypericum intermedia, Potentilla fulgens, Swertia alata* and species of *Valeriana* and *Viola* categorised as common or frequent in present study area were reported as threatened species from the different parts of the Himalaya (Shah and Kapoor, 1978; Rajwar, 1982, 1984; Goel and Bhattacharya, 1983; Biswas, 1991; Gaur, 1993; Pandey *et al.*, 1993; Sharma, 1998; Kala, 1998; Gaur, 1999 and Nautiyal *et al.*, 2001). The most dominant category of medicinal plants was common (48.72 per cent) in the study area, of which 69.03 per cent belonged to herbs, 23.23 per cent to shrubs, 5.16 per cent to trees and 2.58 per cent to ferns. Most of the species recorded as common in the study area have also been classified in the same category in the flora of District Garhwal. Gaur (1999) reported more than 10 per cent of the plants fall in the threatened category from the District Garhwal (47 species endangered and 164 species as rare out of 2035 species) and concluded that the original vegetation of Himalaya is more prone to the disturbances as compared to any other phyto-geographical region, the actual number of threatened category of plant is much larger. According to Lucas and Synge (1978), a plant is considered vulnerable when it is believed likely to move into endangered category in the near future if the causal factors continue operating, including the taxa of the population which are decreasing because of over exploitation, extensive destruction of habitat or other environmental disturbances.

Most common medicinal plants which were collected legally by the Government authorized co-operative agencies and unauthorized by some local people and contractors from the study area were *Ajuga bracteosa, Asparagus curillus, Asparagus filicinus, Berberis aristata, B. asiatica, B. chitria, B. lycium, Bergenia ciliata, Habenaria intermedia, Rubia manjith, Swertia chirayita, Swertia ciliata, Thalictrum foilosum, Valeriana hardwickii, Valeriana jatamansii, Viola biflora, Viola canescens* and *Zanthoxylum armatum*. Among these *Berberis asiatica* and *Valeriana hardwickii* were reported as over-exploited plants from Garhwal Himalaya by Rajwar (1989), and Rao and Datt (1993), *Berberis aristata, Bergenia ciliata* and *Valeriana hardwickii* from Chamoli district of the Garhwal Himalaya by Sharma and Khali (1998). Similar data of over-exploited medicinal plants of the Himalaya have been recorded by Sinha (1982), Uniyal and Malhotra (1982), Shah (1983), Silas and Gaur (1986), Singh (1993), Gaur *et al.* (1993, 1994), Gaur and Raiwani (1995), Dangwal *et al.* (1995), Sharma (1998) and Rawat *et al.* (2001). The over-exploitation of endangered or vulnerable species is an alarming situation in this area because this condition may further reduce their population to negligible number or they may deplete from this area. These species have been exploited to such an extent that their very existence was threatened generally due to over-exploitation besides loss of natural habitat and other biotic pressure such as over-grazing by domestic animals, forest fire, road construction and tourism.

For the conservation of medicinal plants, they should be planted in nurseries, botanical gardens, and in natural habitats, or germplasm of endangered and other medicinal plants must be conserved with the help of *in-situ* and *ex-situ* methods. A national policy on medicinal plant conservation and their development can be a mile-stone against the preservation of endangered or threatened plant species. Sharma and Khali (1998) suggested that NGOs can play a very vital role as they work in close co-operation with the local population in such a way that sustainable exploitation of these species could be organised besides activating the communities in protection/checking of the ruthless and unauthorized extraction of these vital resources by the outside agencies.

References

Biswas, Sas, 1991. Rare and endangered flora of Eastern Himalaya and the measures for its conservation. In: *Advances in Himalayan Ecology*, (Ed.) G.S. Rajwar. Today and Tomorrow's Printers and Pub., New Delhi, p. 267–273.

Dangwal, L.R., Rawat, D.S. and R.D. Gaur, 1995. Some rare and interesting plants of Fabaceae from Garhwal Himalaya. *Ind. J. For.*, 18: 225–257.

Gaur, R.D., 1999. *Flora of the District Garhwal North-West Himalaya (with Ethnobotanical notes)*. TransMedia, Srinagar (Garhwal).

Gaur, R.D. and Sukriti Raiwani, 1995. A preliminary report on the threatened arborescent taxa of Garhwal Himalaya. *J. Indian Bot. Soc.*, 74: 283–292.

Gaur, R.D., Dangwal, L.R. and D.S. Rawat, 1994. Some rare plants of Fabaceae from Garhwal Himalaya. *Ind. J. For.*, 17(1): 80–83.

Gaur, R.D., Rawat, D.S. and L.R. Dangwal, 1993. Status of some vulnerable plant species from Garhwal Himalaya. In: *Himalayan Biodiversity: Conservation Strategies*, (Ed.) U. Dhar. G.B. Pant Institute of Himalayan Envir. and Dev., Kosi, Almora.

Goel, A.K. and U.C. Bhattacharya, 1983. Rare flowering plants of Garhwal Himalaya. In: *An Assessment of Threatened Plants of India*, (Eds.) S.K. Jain and R.R. Rao. B.S.I., Howrah, p. 13–17.

Kala, C.P., 1998. *Ethnobotanical Survey and Propogation of Rare Medicinal Herbs from Farmers in the Buffer Zone of Valley of Flowers National Parks, Garhwal Himalaya.* Report Submitted to International Centre for Integrated Mountain Development (ICIMOD), Kathmandu and Wildlife Institute of India, Dehradun.

Khoshoo, T.N., 1992. *Plant Diversity in the Himalaya: Conservation and Utilization.* G.B. Pant Inst. of Himalayan Environment and Development, Kosi, Almora.

Lucas, G.Li and S. Synge, 1978. *IUCN Plant Red Data Book*. Gland, Switzerland.

Nautiyal, S., Maikhuri, R.K., Rao, K.S. and K.G. Saxena, 2001. Medicinal plant resources in Nanda Devi biosphere reserve in the Central Himalayas. *J. Herbs, Spices and Medicinal Plants*, 8(4): 47–64.

Nayar, M.P. and A.R.K. Sastry, 1987–90. *Red Data Book of Indian Plants.* Vols. I–III. B.S.I., Calcutta.

Pandey, N.K., Tewari, K.C., Tewari, R.N., Joshi, G.C., Pande, V.N. and G. Pandey, 1993. Medicinal plants of Kumaun Himalaya and strategies for conservation. In: *Himalayan Biodiversity: Conservation Strategies*, (Ed.) U.Dhar. G.B. Pant Institute of Himalayan Env. and Dev., Kosi, Almora.

Rajwar, G.S., 1982. Endangered or rare plants of Garhwal and Kumaun Himalaya. *Himal. J. Sci.*, 2: 38–40.

Rajwar, G.S., 1984. Exploitation of medicinal plants of Garhwal Himalaya. *Sci. and Environ.*, 6: 37–41.

Rajwar, G.S., 1989. Human impact on the forests of Garhwal Himalayas. In: *Advances in Forestry Research in India*, (Ed.) Ram Prakash. International Book Distributors, Dehradun, p. 229–241.

Rao, R.R., 1994. *Biodiversity in India: Floristic Aspects.* Bishen Singh Mahendra Pal Singh, Dehradun.

Rao, R.R. and B. Datt, 1993. Distribution and diversity of the family Berberidaceae in the Himalaya. In: *Himalayan Biodiversity: Conservation Strategies*, (Ed.) U. Dhar. G.B. Pant Institute of Himalayan Envir. and Dev., Kosi, Almora, p. 267–278.

Rawat, D.S., Bhandari, B.S. and R.D. Gaur, 2001. Vegetational wealth. In: *Garhwal Himalaya: Nature, Culture and Society,* (Eds.) O.P. Kandari and O.P. Gusain. TransMedia, Srinagar (Garhwal), p. 125–148.

Shah, N.C., 1983. Endangered medicinal and aromatic taxa of Uttar Pradesh Himalaya. In: *An Assessment of Threatened Plants of India,* (Eds.) S.K. Jain and R.R. Rao. B.S.I., Howrah, p. 40–49.

Shah, N.C. and L.D. Kapoor, 1978. Depletive medicinal plants of Kumaon Himalayas. *Jour. Res. Ind. Med. Yoga and Homoeo.,* 13(3): 38–43.

Sharma, A., 1998. Biodiversity of medicinal and aromatic plants of Western Himalaya, their utilization and strategies for conservation. In: *Himalayan Natural Resourses: Eco-threats and Restoration Study,* (Eds.) B.D. Sharma and Tej Kumar. Indus Publishing Company, New Delhi, p. 121–159.

Sharma, A.K. and R.P. Khali, 1998. Diversity of medicinal flora of Chamoli district of Garhwal Himalaya. In: *Himalayan Natural Resourses: Eco-threats and Restoration Study,* (Eds.) B.D. Sharma and Tej Kumar. Indus Publishing Company, New Delhi, p. 353–376.

Silas, R.A. and R.D. Gaur, 1986. Notes on distribution of rare and little known *Carex ligulata* Nees from North-west Himalaya. *J. Bomb. Nat. Hist. Soc.,* 82: 467–468.

Singh, V.K., 1993. Exploitation and threat to some medicinal plants and folk drugs of Garhwal and Kumaon regions of Uttar Pradesh, India. In: *Himalayan Biodiversity: Conservation Strategies,* (Ed.) U. Dhar. G.B. Pant Institute of Himalayan Envir. and Dev., Kosi, Almora.

Sinha, R.L., 1982. Industrial potential and planned exploitation of Indian medicinal plants in relation of hill eco-types in U.P. In: *The Vegetation Wealth of the Himalayas,* (Ed.) G.S. Paliwal. Puja Publishers, Delhi, p. 241–245.

Uniyal, B.P. and C.L. Malhotra, 1982. Economic exploitation of rare North-western Himalayan plants. In: *The Vegetation Wealth of the Himalayas,* (Ed.) G.S. Paliwal. Puja Publishers, Delhi, p. 221–267.

Medicinal Plants: Conservation, Cultivation and Utilization (2007) *Pages 259–267*
Editors: A.K. Chopra, D.R. Khanna, G. Prasad, D.S. Malik and R. Bhutiani
Published by: DAYA PUBLISHING HOUSE

Chapter 34

Biodiversity of Cultivated Fruits Plants in Jaunpur Development Block of District Tehri Garhwal, Uttaranchal

Pramod Kumar[1], Suman Bisht[1] and Asha Dobhal[2]
[1]Department of Botany, HNB Garhwal University Campus, Tehri Garhwal
[2]Department of Botany, Government Post Graduate College, New Tehri, Tehri Garhwal

Introduction

Uttaranchal is characterized by the great diversity in agro climatic conditions such as sub-montane, montane and alpine. There are 13 district in Uttaranchal. Out of which 11 belonging to Himalayas and this characterized by the highest peeks, mid hills and valleys. The highest living species of plant and animal life found in these areas. The most highly diversified and sharply contrasted ecosystem which fall into ecological region that cover specially a global range of climatic belt from the tropical to the Tundra in brief vertical span of 4 to 5 miles. These are only some of the characteristic features of their range that make the Himalaya unique.

Tehri District of Uttaranchal comprises of three major altitudinal zones *i.e.* submontane, montane and alpine. Presence of these zones makes diversity in cultivated fruit plants. The altitudinal zones extend from 1000 to 9000 ft.

Biodiversity defines present all living organism and ecosystem where they live together *i.e.* plants, Zoo-virus, bacteria, fungus, microbes, arcums under this, it has different forms and many changes.

Types of Biodiversity (Sharma and Shrivastava, 2004)

1. Agro Biodiversity

2. Acclimatized Biodiversity (gramyet)
3. Localized Biodiversity
4. Re-established Biodiversity
5. Microbiological Biodiversity
6. Genetic Biodiversity.

Food is an essential requirement of mankind and plant alone provide upto 95 per cent of the world foods supply directly or indirectly. It is difficult to imagine the existence of human being the availability of plants. Increase in crop production by means of fertilizers, pesticides, irrigation, and better management and in respect of genetic improvement are greatly acknowledged.

According to I.C.M.R., New Delhi, the requirement of fruits for one person is 85 gm, but the availability is only 62 to 65 gm. Biodiversity of cultivated fruit plants reflex variety introduction of a particular area, variability in climate and genetically changes in the genes.

However in district Tehri Garhwal various fruit plants are cultivated in a area of about 3520.88 ha with annual production of 9577.19 quental (Department of Horticulture, Tehri). But it is very necessary to have information on the Biodiversity in fruit plants for detail discussion in a particular area of Tehri district.

Study Area

The study area is situated in the South-East of Chamba town at the distance about 42 km of Tehri district of Uttaranchal at the elevations of ranging from about 350-2500m and geo-coordinates 32'N latitude and 72'longitude. A number of villager which belong to Thathur, Bhavaan, Chamba and Tehri town area replaced or shifted near the forest area of Jaunpur Block and makes new house-building and, so, degradation of soil and forest and weathering of rocks has been highly affected the vegetation of the study area.

Soil

The soil with high organic matter 5-15 per cent formed in temperate and cool humid region and low (1-2 per cent) in soil arid and semi-arid regions. Carbon, nitrogen, calcium, magnesium, potassium are most common minerals present in soil.

Climate

The various climatic elements such as temperature, annual rain fall in different months and humidity reflects a certain types of climatic condition of particular area.

Temperature

It is a continuous element *i.e.* it has always same value and is always an important ingredient of weather and climate. It depends on the balance between incoming and outgoing heat of a place at a given time. The normal temperature recorded for the study area between 21-28 degree centigrade but during winter it may be below to zero degree centigrade.

Rainfall

The average rainfall in a year is between 100-150 cm. The number of rain days is 45-60 days. The rainfall and temperature influences Biodiversity in the fruit plants distribution up to some extent.

Methodology

Study of Biodiversity in fruit plants in a particular area depends on altitude and climatic conditions suitable for their cultivation. Fruit plants are grown in specific climatic conditions and survive for its living. Many fruit plants varieties are specific to temperature, climatic conditions and altitude.

The methodology of Biodiversity comprises introduction of new variety for a particular area and variability in climatic conditions for a particular variety distribution of different types of fruit plants in a particular area.

Biodiversity has been studied as under:

1. Variability of fruit plants in a particular area.
2. Distribution of different varieties in fruit plants.

Results and Discussion

Biodiversity in different fruit plants are reported by scientist. A number of cultivator species shows variability in fruit size, colour, weight, maturity period, quality parameters etc. Variability in different fruit plants are discussed as under.

Apple

Srivastava (1975) classified the cultivers in apple and reported that apple is produced in all the continents of the world. However, 80 per cent of early Sunbarry, Binnani, Cartland, Golden, Relicious, Mcmtosh, Red Delicious, Buckingham, Rymen varities are grown. In the Jaunpur development Block and other places of Tehri District, Early Shunbarry, Fanny, Golden Delicious, Red Delicious, Rymer Green Sweet are grown which gives a high yields of apple and good marketing values. These varieties shows variability in maturity, colour, size and weight. Gautam and Chauhan (1986) also reported such types of observations. Now a day spurvarieties are to be planted in this area like Orange Spur, Red Chief Golden Spur. Anna varieties are also planted in low chilling areas upto 2000 ft.

Bearing parameters of CVs. Co-oper and fellow Spur trees. h.d.p. and m.d.p. from the fourth to sixth years (Table 34.1).

Pear

All the pear cultivars belong to the genus *Pyrus* which is a member of subfamily from oidac in India, Pear occupies about 1400 hectares areas of FAO hodiction years book (Anon, 1987) but the present area has increase many folds, morphological characteristics of *Pyrus* species (Table 34.2).

In Tehri district Gola, Victoria, Baggogosa, Natch varieties are grown and shend variability in fruit long diametical plant height, weight and colour.

Peaches

The important cultivers of Peach being grown in the world for various purposes. Childers, 1975 reported about peaches cultivers:

Table Cultivers

Elberta, J.H. Hale, Babcock, Cardinal, Dixigem, Redtop, Rdhanen, Riooso Gem, Candor, Red Glob, Bafeng.

Table 34.1

Vareity Planting System and Spacing Area	Cropping Zone (tree height in cm)	Fruit/Spurs/Tree					Fruits/Tree					Fruit Set (1)					Fruit Cluster No.		
		Variation No. (yr4=100)					Variation No. (yr4=100)												
		yr4	yr5		Yr6	yr4	yr5			yr6	Yr4		yr. 5		yr6		Yr6		
(A) COOPER 4/M.26																			
HDP	<120	133	–99.	7	–3.	8	23	–95	7	110.	8	2	8	(2)		6	2	1	02
(1.4 m²)	120–240	363	–99–38	87	–1–8	2	71	–95	8	106	3	3	2	–		6	8	1	03
Total and mean		496	–99	6	–1	9	94	–95	8	107	4	3	1	–		6	7	1	02
MDP	<120	45	102	2	–6	7	36	–44	4	43	0	13	3	3	6	6	20	2	1
		132	–38	7	–8	4	82	–30	5	38	4	10	3	1111	77	15	7	1	32
Total and mean		177	–5	1	–8	0	118	–34	8	39	8	11	1	7	6	16	9	1	34
(B)YELLOW SPUR/M.26																			
HDP	<120	188	–71	3	–1	6	39	–2	6	102	5	3	4	11	7	7	1	1	21
(1.4 M²)	120–240	182	78	6	–1	7	57	–57	9	100	0	5	2	10	2	10	6	1	15
Total and mean		370	–74	9	–1	7	96	–36	5	101	.0	4	3	10	9	8	8	1	18
MDP	<120	91	25	2	–57	2	62	45	7	–46	8	11	3	13	1	14	1	1	23
(6.0 M²)	120–240	101	18	8	–57	5	73	42	5	–47	9	12	0	14	4	14	7	1	35
Total and mean		192	21	8	–57	3	135	43	7	–47	4	11	7	13	8	14	4	1	29

Table 34.2

Species	Tree Size (height in m)	Adult Leaf Margins	Juvenile Leaves	Leaf Length (cm)	Fruit			
					Skin	Calyx Type	Fruit Dia (cm)	Carpel No.
P.caucassica	5-6	Crenate	Simple	4.81	Smooth	Persistent	4.70	5
P.communis	5-6	Crenate	Simple	4.95	Smooth	Persistent	3.80	5
P.cordata	2-3	Crenate	Simple	7.87	Russet	Deciduous	1.50	2-3
P.nivalis	3-4	Crenate	Simple	4.87	Smooth	Persistent	5.60	5
P.amygdali formis	1-2	Entire or slight crenate	1-lobed	6.52	Smooth	Persistent	2.60	5
P.elaeagrifolia	3-4	Entire or slight crenate	Simple	5.70	Smooth	Persistent	2.40	5
P.gharbiana		Crenate	Simple	5.15	–			
P.longipes	3-4	Crenate	Simple	3.77	Russet	Deciduous	1.70	3-4
P.mamorensis		Crenate	Simple	4.58		Persistent		
P. synaca	1-2	Crenate	Simple	4.78		Persistent		5
P. pashia	3-4	Crenate	Simple	7.99	Russet	Deciduous	2.39	4-5
P. regelii	1-2	Crenate	Simple	5.80	Smooth	Persistent	2-3.0	5
Pirus salicifolia	1-2	Entire	2-lobed	5.10	Smooth	Persistent	1.90	5
P.bendifolia	5-6	Coarse Serrate	Lacinate	5.74	Russet	Deciduous	0.88	2(3)
P.calleryana	3-5	Crenate	Simple	6.60	Russet	Deciduous	1.06	2
P.dimorphophylla	3-4	Crenate Serrate	1-lobed	7.16	Russet	Deciduous	1.24	2
P. fauriei	1-2	Crenate .	Simple	4.35	Russet	Deciduous	1.34	2
P.hondoensis	3-4	Fine serrate Setose	2-lobed	7.57	Smooth	Persistent	2.80	5
P.psuedopashia	3-4	Crenate	1-lobed	6.42	Smooth	Persistent	4.26	5
P.kawakamii	1-3	Crenate	3-lobed	6.14	Russet	Deciduous	1.04	4(3)
P.pyrifolia	3-5	Fine serrate, Setose	Simple	10.65	Russet	Deciduous	4.10	5
P.ussuriensis	1-3	Coarse serrate, Setose	Simple	8.23	Smooth	Persistent	3.75	5

Canning Cultivers

Cortex, Carolyn, Diocson 1, Halford, Fortuna, Low Chilling Cultivers prefored in India Florda Gold, Flordaking, Flordasun, florda Queen, Sharbati etc.

In Uttaranchal Praredelus of high altitude, Totapure, Prabhat prefers in low chilling of grown in Tehri District (George *et al.*, 1986 and Singh *et al.*, 1984).

Plums

Prunus domestica, Prunus salicina, Prunus einnisitia are grown in world. In Uttaranchal specialy Tehri district Santa Rosa, June Blood, Beaty, Victoria, Golden Drop, Starking Delicious are grown and shows great variability. Growth pattern of different varieties of Pulums in Tehri district is as below:

Table 34.3

Rootstock	*Victoria*			*Marjorie's Seediling*		
	Tree Head Volume (m)	*Yield/Tree (Kg)*	*Fruit Size (g)*	*Tree Head Volume (m³)*	*Yield/Tree (kg)*	*Fruit Size (g)*
St.Julien A	22.0	18.9	40.1	18.1	5.2	51.1
Peshore	26.9	31.1	39.1	24.0	9.1	51.3
Pixy	13.4	16.9	30.4	8.1	3.6	44.1
P. pumila	9.0	8.1	37.0	12.3	5.4	37.8
P.tomentosa	3.1	1.9	20.6	1.2	3.4	49.7

Strawberries

Fragaria cananassa (cultivated) world production of strawberries in 1984 was about 1.9 million tones. In Uttaranchal minor areas are identified and emphasized to its cultivation in Tehri district.

Kiwi Fruits

The Kiwi fruit is native to China and the country of Asian and the center of origin of the genus. Actinidia is in the mountain low ranges of South-West (Ferguson, 1984). In Tehri district the area under this fruit is about 5 hectares and production about 200 quintals/year. The varieties are Bruna, Haywerd, Monty, Alliasen, and Abbott grown and showed great variability in production, size and weight of fruits.

Citrus

Citrus plants are grown in sub-tropical climate of the India. In Uttaranchal the most common varieties cultivated are Malta, Gray fruit, Lemon (Hill Lemon; Galgal; Eureca, Baramasi). Kagzi, Baramasi are grown in the district as large amount. These fruit shows great variability.

Mango

Mangifera indica (family Anacardiaceae) grown upto an altitude of 1200 mt. but fruiting and quantity is poor beyond 600 Mt. The most common varieties which are grown in the areas are Dasheri, Langra, Bombay Green, Amrapali and Safeda.

Litchi

Litchi chinensis also grown in these area. The varieties Dehradun, Calcutta, Rose Scented are inexitence in this district.

Biodiversity in fruit plants in Uttaranchal hills in respect to fruiting time under the conditions prevailing in the apple growing areas of Kumaon and Garhwal hills of Uttaranchal, Srivastava (1975) classified the culitivers as:

Early

Beauty of Bath, Red Astrachan, Early Shanburry, Summar, Golden Pippin, Fanny, Benoni, Devonshire Red, Quarrenden, Green Sweet.

Mid-Season

King of Pippon, Red, Mclntosh, Jonathan Sparthan, Red Delicious, Royal Delicious Cortland.

Late

Golden Delicious, Rymer, Esopus Spitzenberg, Peck's Pleasant, Buckingham.

The cultivars, Tropical Beauty and Parlin's Beauty were judged best in respect of productivity and fruit quality and are recommended for cultivation under mild-hill conditions (Gautam and Chauhan, 1986).

Interrogation and inter-specific hybridization (Bell and Hough, 1986; Layne and Quamme, 1975) specification occurred mainly in Eastern and Central Asia in the Himalayas, Caucasus, Asia minor and Eastern Europe. Vavilov (1951) proposed three centers of origin for the cultivated pears. Hines center, Central Asiatic center and near Eastern center.

Peach is now commercially grown around the world between 25 degree and 45 degree latitudes above and below the equators (Childers, 1975) some of the species *viz. P. jacquimontii, P. undulata, P. salicina* occur commonly in the interior Himalayas (Hooker, 1875-1897).

Watkins (1976) identified five centers of origin for plums. These include Europe for *Prunus domestic* (European plum), Western Asia for *P. insititia* (Damson Plum), Western and Central Asia for *P. cerasifera* (Cherry Plum), China for *P. salicina* (Japanese Plum) and North America for *P. amaricana* (American Plum). European plums require 800 to 1000 hours below 7.2 degree of winter chilling for satisfactory but break in the spring. The cultivate of the Japanese plum require cooperatively less of winter chilling about 700 and 1000 hours below 7.2 degree centigrade.

Most of the cultivated apricots belong to the specific species. *Prunus armeniaca* which is also sometimes called *Armeniaca vulgaris* (Kostina, 1936; Bailey and Hough, 1975).

Strawberries are adapted to different climates *viz.* moderate Mediterranean, subtropical and even at high altitude under tropical climate.

The Kiwifruit is native to China and the center of origin of the genus *Actinidia* is in the mountain ranges of south-Western China (Ferguson, 1984). Lindly (1936) gave the name *Actinidia* to the genus because of the numerous radiating divisions of the style (from the Greek akrits-'ray') and placed in the family Dilleniaceae (Actinidiacae). Liang (1983) has revised the genus recognising over 50 species and 100 distinct taxa.

In 2004 Shailendra Ranjan reported that considerable genetic erosion in mango (*Mangifera indica* L.) is taking place in India, due to urbanization, rapid industrialization and quick spread of commercial cultivators. Although a large number of the cultivers have been conserved in about 20 field gengbands in different parts of the country, still a number of germplasm is to be collected. Central Institute for sub-tropical horticulture, Lucknow has the world's largest collection of mango germplasm numbering nearly 700 accession maintained in field gene bank. Presently, conservation of genetic resources of mango is done in field gene banks only.

Karkara *et al.* (2003) reported that three mango's varieties *viz.* Amrapalim Mallika and Dashehari were planted under high density plantation at Horticultural Regional Research Station at a distance of 3.3 m. (1,1,1 plants/ha) during 1992.

The development Block Jounpur of Tehri district comprise area and production is shown in Table 34.4.

Table 34.4

Sl.No.	*Fruit Crop*	*Area (in ha)*	*Production (in quintal)*
1.	Apple	238.85	7833.70
2.	Pear	8.33	667.00
3.	Peach	18.25	59.15
4.	Plum	16.75	335.85
5.	Walnut	132.78	1850.00
6.	Apricot	32.65	595.30
7.	Mango	95.09	2568.40
8.	Citrus group	42.16	1011.20
9.	Lichi	0.00	0.00
10.	Guava	7.28	673.00
11.	Others	38.87	1073.00
	Total	**631.01**	**16666.60**

Above discussion of review shows great variability in varieties in respect of fruit size, weight of fruit, colour of fruit, bearing behavior. It is also found variability in different fruit plants in respect of climatic conditions where they are grown.

Present study regarding to Biodiversity of cultivated fruit plants in District Tehri Garhwal have great variability in species and varieties in respect of their climatic conditions, where they are grown and variability in fruits, size, shape, weight, colours and bearing behavior. It is also revealed that inter-varietal variation also differs. It is necessary to conserve Biodiversity for better production and ecological development in that particular area. For better living to increase area in different fruit crops.

References

Anon, 1987. FAO Production Year Book, 1986.

Bailey, C.H. and L.F. Hough, 1975. In: *Aowanneas in Fnit Breeding Ceds.*

Bell, R.L and L.F Hough, 1986. *Hort Science*, 21: 62–64.

Childer, N.F., 1975. *Modern Fuit Science.* Hort Pub. Rutgers Uni. Brunshrick, N.J.

Hooker, J.D., 1875–1897. *The Flora of British India*, 7 Vols. L. Reeve and Co., London. Janicle and Moore Purdue University Press, Lafayette, p. 367–383.

Karkara, B.K., Lakhanpal, S.C. and R. Singh, 2004. Performance of mango varieties under high density plantation in Paonta Valley of H.P. Proster paper presented in First Indian Hort. Congress, 6-9 November, pp. 19.

Kostina, K.F., 1936. *Bull. Appl. Bot. Gen. Plant Brdg.*, pp. 3.

Ranjan, S., 2004. Strategies for efficient conservation of genetic diversity in Indian mangoes with minimum repetitiveness. *Poster Paper presented in First Indian Horticulture Congress* 6-9th November, pp. 16.

Sharma, D. and M.N. Srivastava, 2004. Significance of biodiversity in agriculture technology. *Unnat Krisi Patrika*, September–October, pp. 30.

Vavilov, N.I., 1951. *The Origin Variation, Immunity and Breeding of Cultivated Plants*. Ronald Press, New York.

Watkins, R., 1976. In: *Evolution of Crop Plants*, (Eds) N.W. Simmond, Long mans, London, p. 243–246.

Medicinal Plants: Conservation, Cultivation and Utilization (2007) *Pages 269–272*
Editors: A.K. Chopra, D.R. Khanna, G. Prasad, D.S. Malik and R. Bhutiani
Published by: DAYA PUBLISHING HOUSE

Chapter 35

Physico-chemical Screening of *Abutilon indicum* Roots

Shri Krishna[1], Amit Kumar[1] and Navneet[2]
[1]Department of Chemistry, [2]Department of Botany and Microbiology,
Gurukula Kangri University, Hardwar – 249 404, Uttaranchal, India

ABSTRACT

Abutilon indicum Linn. of Malvaceae family is found through out tropical and sub tropical regions. The plant is mentioned in Indian materia medica which is commonly used in the indigenous system of medicine under the name "Atibala" in various ailments. The root is used in Ayurvedic and Unani System of medicine. The physico-chemical studies of the extracts of the root of *Abutilon Indicum* in different solvents *i.e.* petroleum ether, ethyl alcohol and water extracts have been studied. The various compounds present in extract in petroleum ether are steroids and carbohydrates. Ethanolic extract of roots showed steroids, alkaloids, flavinoid, proteins and carbohydrate while the water extract shows the positive test for saponins, proteins and carbohydrate. All the above tests have shown that the root of the plant contains highly medicinal drug properties to cure various ailments. The Physico-chemical properties *i.e.* state, colour, taste, odour, yield, pH, refractive index of extracted material are also given.

Keywords: Abutilon indicum, Root extracts, Medicinal properties.

Introduction

Abutilon indicum Linn. of Malvaceae family is known as Kanghi in Hindi, Atibala in Sanskrit and Country mallow in English is one of the best known drugs of the Indian materia medica (Chopra *et al.*, 1956; Kirtikar and Basu, 1975; Nadkarni and Nadkarni, 1976). This is commonly used in the indigenous system of medicine under the name "Atibala" in various ailments. The plant is under shrub and distributed throughout, tropical and subtropical regions. In India it is cultivated and also occurs naturally as a common weed of roadsides and degraded lands upto 1200 m elevation. The root is used in various Ayurvedic and Unani system of medicine. The decoction of the root is used for chest troubles such as bronchitis and fever. The mucilagenous effect benefits the skin, an infusion of root used for gonorrhoea. The paste made from the powdered root and bark is applied to wounds and used for disorder such as boil and ulcers (CSIR, 1976; Fitotropia, 1985; Sharma *et al.*, 1988). Recent experimental studies on immunological aspects revealed that whole plant has immunostimulating effects. The fixed oils obtained from the petroleum ether extract of roots is reported to contain linolenic, stearic, palmatic, myristic, lauric, capric acid (Sharma *et al.*, 1989; Indrayan *et al.*, 2004), vitamin E., (Arora and Singh, 1999) terpenes, alantolactone, isoalantolactone, gossypetin glucosides, cyanidin 3–rutinoside (British Pharmacopoeia, 1968) have been previously reported.

Materials and Methods

The roots of plant were collected from the local area of Distt. Meerut, and identified by the Botanical Survey of India (BSI), Dehradun, India.

Extraction

The roots of the plant were dried under shade and crushed into small pieces and powdered. The powder of the root was loaded into the soxhlet apparatus and added into it 600 ml petroleum ether, ethyl alcohol and water respectively and subjected to extraction for 48 hours. The extracts were distilled on rotatory evaporator and on water bath, extracts were concentrated to dry residue.

Results and Discussion

The Physico-chemical properties *i.e.* state, colour, taste, odour, yield, pH, refractive index of extracted material are summarized in Table 35.1 and test of natural products are given in Table 35.2. All the three extracts of the root were subjected to qualitative chemical test for the presence of phytoconstituents *i.e.* sterols, saponins, protein, alkaloids, carbohydrates and flavinoids in Table 35.2.

Table 35.1: Physico-chemical Properties of Root through Petroleum Ether, Ethyl Alcohol and Water Extracts

Properties of Extracts	*From Different Solvent Fraction of Roots*		
	Petroleum Ether	*Ethyl Alcohol*	*Water*
State	Semi Solid	Solid	Solid
Colour	Brown	Dark Yellow	Dark Brown
Taste	Pungent	Pungent	Sweetish Pungent
Odour	Specific	Specific	Specific
Yield (%)	2%	5.62%	9.50%
pH	4.7	6.4	5.1
Refractive index	1.31	1.31	1.37

Physical state of material is a property, which play an important role for identification. The petroleum ether extract was semisolid while ethyl alcohol and water extracts were solid. Petroleum ether extract was brown in colour, ethyl alcohol extract was dark yellow and water extract show dark brown colour. All the three extracts are pungent in taste and shows the specific odour. Yield of the extracts exhibit the solubility of material into the solvents. The minimum yield of chemical constituents in the plant was obtained from the petroleum ether extract and maximum yield in water extract, because water is a highly polar solvent. The yield of petroleum ether extract obtained was low in quantity *i.e.* 2 per cent as compared to ethyl alcohol extract *i.e.* 5.6220 g and water extract 9.5020 per cent. The root was more soluble in water in comparison to petroleum ether and ethyl alcohol. The pH is the parameter to exhibit the acidity or alkalinity of the solution.

Table 35.2: Qualitative Phytochemical Tests of Roots

Sl.No.	Test	Petroleum Ether	Ethyl alcohol Extract	Water Extract
1	Tests for Sterols			
(a)	Testsolution + Conc. H_2SO_4	+	+	–
(b)	Test solution + Sulphur	+	+	–
(c)	Salkowski Test	+	+	–
2	Test for Saponins			
(a)	Haemolytic Test	–	–	+
(b)	Foam Test	–	–	+
3	Test for Proteins			
(a)	Xanthoproteic Test	–	+	+
(b)	Millon's Test	–	+	+
(c)	Biuret Test	–	+	+
(d)	Ninhydin Test	–	+	+
4	Test for Alkaloids			
(a)	Dragendroff's Test	–	+	–
(b)	Mayer's Test	–	+	–
(c)	Wagner's Test	–	+	–
5	Test for Carbohydrates			
(a)	Barfoed's Test	+	+	+
(b)	Benedict's Test	+	+	+
(c)	Molisch's Test	+	+	+
6	Test for Flavinoids			
(a)	Shinoda Test	–	+	–
(b)	Ferric chloride Test	–	+	–
(c)	Lead acetate Test	–	+	–
(d)	Zn-HCl reduction Test	–	+	–

+ve: Shows positive result, –ve: Shows negative result.

The refractive index is helpful to identify the organic substances. The petroleum ether and alcohol extracts gave the same refractive index *i.e.* 1.310 while water extract showed 1.370.

Test for the different chemical compounds from the all of three extracts (petroleum ether, ethyl alcohol, and water) gave positive and negative results for various compounds. All the three extracts gives positive result for carbohydates. Sterols are present in the petroleum ether and ethyl alcohol extracts of the root while water extract gave negative test for the sterols by sulphuric acid, sulphur and salkowski tests. Alkaloids are present in ethyl alcohol extract of root as shown by the dragendroff's test, Mayer and Wagner test. While saponins are present only in water extract of root by Haemolytic test and foam test. Flavinoids and proteins are present in the ethyl alcohol extract of extracted material by sinoda, ferric chloride, lead acetate, zinc chloride HCl reduction test and xanthoprotic, millon's, biuret and ninhydrin test respectively. The terpenes are present in the petroleum ether extract of root. The terpenes, fatty acids, alkaloids and sugar components have previously identified.

References

Arora, J.P.S., Singh R.P., 1999. *Numerical Physical Chemistry, Physical Chemistry, Vol. 1.* Premier Publishing House, M. Nagar, U.P., p. 458–459.

British Pharmacopoeia, 1968. p. 1266–1268.

Chopra, R.N. Nayer, S.L. and Chopra, I.C., 1956. *Glossary of Indian Medicinal Plants.* CSIR, New Delhi, p. 2.

CSIR, 1976. *The Wealth of India: A Dictionary of Indian Raw Materials*, Vol. X, CSIR, New Delhi.

Indrayan, A.K., Neeraj Kumar, Sharma, S. and Sharma, V., 2004. *Indian Drugs*, 41: 339–344.

ISI, 1954. IS: 584 (Part–I), Indian Standards Institution, New Delhi.

Kirtikar, K.R. and Basu, B.D., 1975. *Indian Medicinal Plants*, 2nd edn., 1: 314–315.

Nadkarni, K.M., revised by Nadkarni A.K., 1976. *Indian Materia Medica*, 3rd edn., 1: 8.

Sharma, P.V., Ahmed, Z.A. and Sharma, V.V., 1988. *Ind. Drugs*, p. 26, 333.

Sharma, P.V., Ahmed, Z.A. and Sharma, V.V., 1989. *Phytochemistry*, p. 28, 3525.

Medicinal Plants: Conservation, Cultivation and Utilization (2007) *Pages 273–280*
Editors: **A.K. Chopra, D.R. Khanna, G. Prasad, D.S. Malik and R. Bhutiani**
Published by: **DAYA PUBLISHING HOUSE**

Chapter 36

Comparative Growth Pattern in Nine Cultures of Ash Gourd

Miti Rani and R.K.S. Rathore
Department of Botany, RBS College, Agra

ABSTRACT

Observations on nine cultures of Ash gourd (*Benincasa hisipda* Cogn.) at RBS College Experimental Farm, Khandari, Agra revealed interesting variations on growth parameters such as seed germination percentage, appearance of tendrils, branching pattern, vine length, total number of nods/leaves per plant, flowering behaviour, ratio between female and male flowers per plant, fruit bearing capacity, fruit storability, comparative seed size and its bearing on seed germination percentage etc.

The overall performance of nine cultures revealed that Coimbatore Local has maximum fruit bearing capacity followed by Agra Local and IVAG-13. Mature fruits of Coimbatore Local were stored, under ambient conditions, for seven months with only 20 percent loss in fresh fruit weight.

Introduction

Ash gourd (*Benincasa hispida* Cogn.), a member of Cucurbitaceae is variously known as Petha, Pani-Kumrha, Kalliyama, Ellaveri etc. It is supposed to have originated in Indo-Malaysian region. China is cultivating Ash gourd crop from the very ancient times but it is difficult to say when its cultivation started in India (Anonymous, 1988). Geographically it is found growing in China, Japan, Polynesia, Eastern Australia, Malaysia and India. It has only recently been introduced into European countries, (Peter, 1998). Young fruits of Ash gourd are used as vegetable. It is a year-round vegetable and harvested three times in a year in one part of the country or the other. The fruit pulp of semi-ripe and ripe fruits is made into mash cakes and cooked in sugar syrup (chashni) to make petha sweet. Ash gourd fruit pulp is also used as a substitute in tomato ketchup. The young leaves are sometimes used as spinach. According to Kirtikar and Basu (1935) various plant parts of Ash gourd are valued in Indian medicine. The juice is cooling. The decoction of fruit is styptic, diuretic laxative and nutritious. It is given to cure internal hemorrhages and diseases of respiratory tract. It is also popular as an antidote for alcoholic poisioning and antimicrobial activity. The ash of fruit rind is applied on painful swelling. The seeds and their oil are considered antihelmintic and prescribed in cases of roundworm and tapeworm infestation. The juice of ripe fruits is considered useful in haemoplysis and pthisis. Petha fruit is said to be good for patients having weak nervous system.

Having so many uses and adding to the fame of Agra, it was considered worthwhile to conduct botanical investigations in Ash gourd plant. Morphological characterization of nine cultures of Ash gourd has been completed by the present author (Miti Rani, 2002).

Material and Methods

Seeds of Ash gourd collected from Agra, Varanasi and Coimbatore Local were planted at RBS College, Botanical Garden and Research Farm, Khandari, Agra during Crop season 2002-2003. This germplasm was named as Agra local, IVAG-4, IVAG-5, IVAG-6, IVAG-13, IVAG-16, IVAG-27, IVAG-67-2 and Coimbatore local.

A well-prepared field of area 6 × 8 was divided into nine raised beds. Beds were intersecting with water channels of 30 cm width and 10 cm depth. Six pits of 30 cm diameter were prepared (Three on each side of the water channel) adding 1.5 kg FYM and 5 gm Forate granules in each pit to take care of termites and nematodes, (Seghal *et al.*, 2000). Twenty-four seeds from each culture were counted and measured for seed size. These seeds were soaked overnight before sowing in 0.2 per cent aqueous solution of Therum to protect the seedlings from fungal infection. The seeds were sown nearly 2 cm deep in the soil and first light irrigation was given seven days after sowing. Thereafter irrigation and weed management were taken up as and when required. The germination percentage of seeds for each culture was calculated on the basis of observations recorded up to 14 days after sowing. The experimental field was visited every day by the investigator till the fruit harvesting and various parameters of growth pattern were recorded and presented in Table 36.1.

Results and Discussion

General Plant Morphology

Ash gourd plants are viny in habit (Plate 36.1) with stout, angular, hispid stems, 5-7 lobed reniform petiolate leaves. Both male and female flowers appear on the same plant. The flowers are large, stalked, solitary in leaf axils, corolla yellow in color, 6-9 cm in diameter. Pedicel densely hispid, 5-15 cm long in male flowers and 2-4 cm in female flowers. Floral parts pentamerous except gynoecium, which is tricarpillary with proliferated parietal placentation and inferior ovary. The fruits at later stages of development get a waxy deposition on their rind. The average seed size of nine cultures was measured and resented in Table 36.1.

Germination

Seeds of Coimbatore Local and IVAG-13 cultivars were first to sprout. It was followed by IVAG-16 and IVAG-6 with Agra Local. Maximum seed germination percentage (93.3) was observed in IVAG-13 followed by IVAG16 (75) and Coimbatore local (70). IVAG-27 showed poorest (20) seed germination percentage and IVAG-4 with twenty-five and Agra Local with thirty percent seed

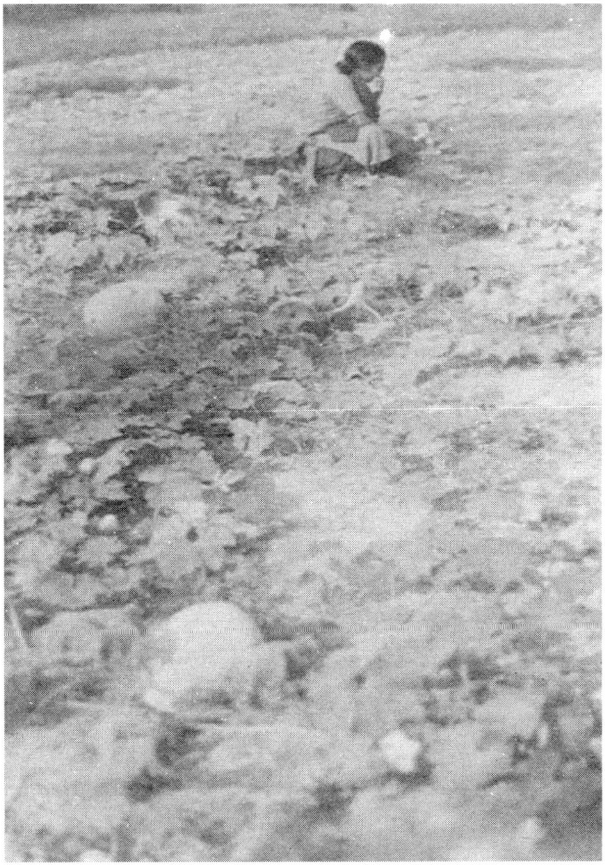

Plate 36.1: Ash Gourd Crop in the Experimental Field, Khandari Farm, Agra

germination also remained poorer seed germinating cultures (Table 36.1 and Figure 36.2) For IVAG-13, it appears that smaller seed size of this genotype has favored better germination and IVAG-27 having largest seeds among nine cultures has poorest seed germination (Figure 36.1). However, the criterion of seed size does not apply so accurately on seed germinability percentage in Agra Local and Coimbatore Local. According to Gutterman (1992) the influence of day length and red and far red light during storage of post harvest *Cucumis* fruit also determine the seed germinability. Since the seeds of nine cultures of Ash gourd sown in our experimental field originated from three locations, environmental influences during seed maturation and storage might have also played their roles.

Appearance of Tendrils

The tendrils generally appear on Ash gourd vines in between three to seven weeks of germination. The first tendril is invariably undivided and thereafter bi-tri-, tetra-or even pentafid tendrils appear at subsequent nodes. Agra local showed first tendril to appear on 9th or 10th node whereas IVAG-5 developed it on 12th or 13th node. In rest of the cultures the first tendril appeared on 10th or 11th node.

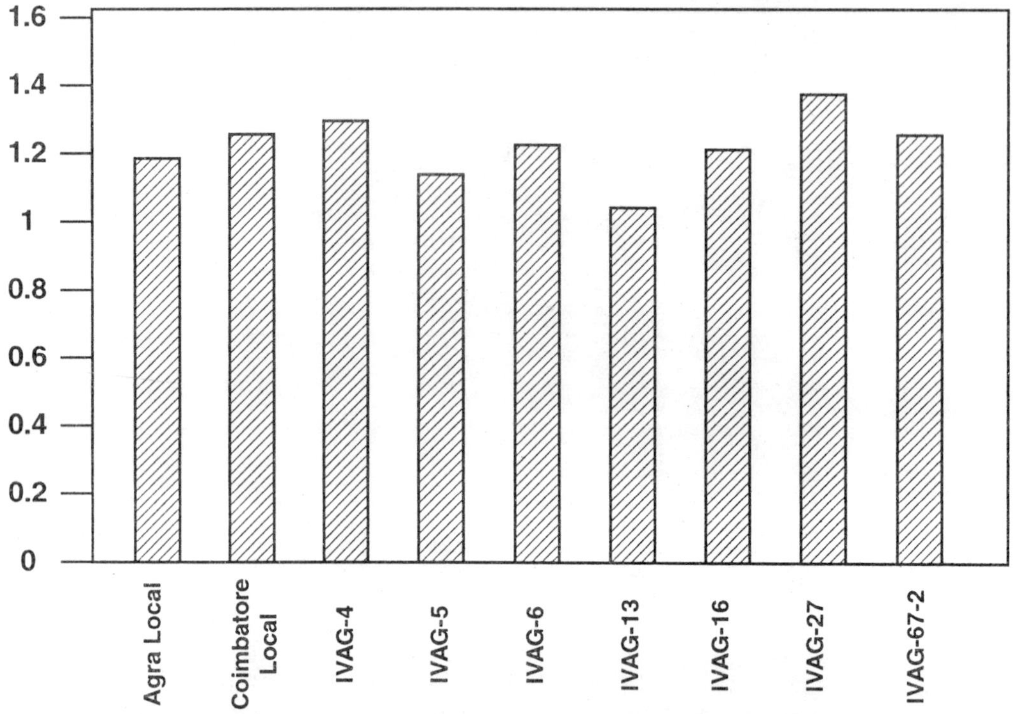

Figure 36.1: Variability in Seed Size of Different Genotype of *Benincasa hispida*

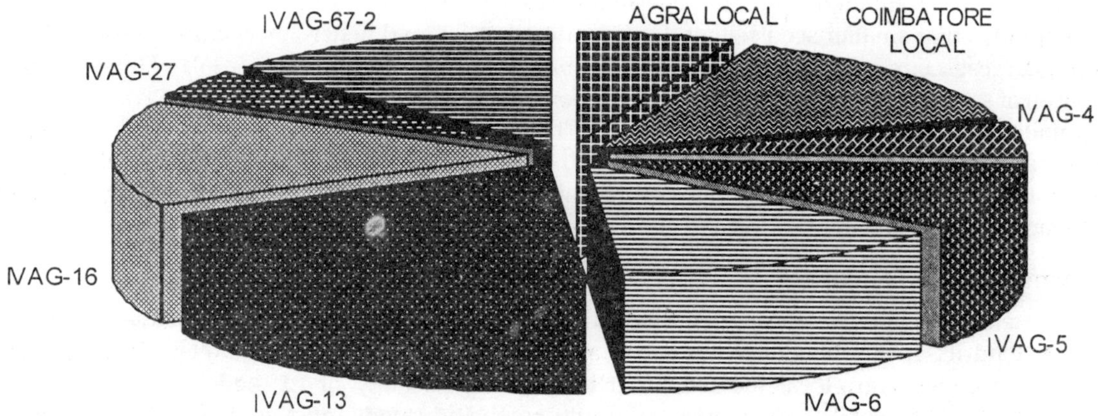

Figure 36.2: Variation in Germination Percentage in Seeds of *B. hispida*

Branching Pattern

Ash gourd vines of nine cultures under present investigation showed a differential branching pattern. Thus number of primary and secondary branches was recorded for each culture. Genotypes IVAG-5, IVAG-6, and IVAG-16 did not bear secondary branches whereas IVAG-67-2 with maximum number of secondary branches showed tertiary branch also. Maximum number of primary branches (9-10) were observed in IVAG27 and minimum (2) in Agra local. Likewise IVAG6 with three primary branches and Coimbatore local with four primary branches are considered less branching type and IVAG27 with maximum primary branches and IVAG67-2 having maximum secondary branches are profusely branched vines.

Vine Length

Length of vines for each culture was measured in meters, on the basis of length of the main branch at the time of crop harvesting. Longest vines (6.83 m) were recorded in IVAG6 followed by IVAG-16 (6.64 m) and IVAG-13 (5.69m) whereas shortest vines were those of IVAG-67-2 (2.71m), Agra Local (2.83m) and IVAG5 (3.07m) (Figure 36.3)

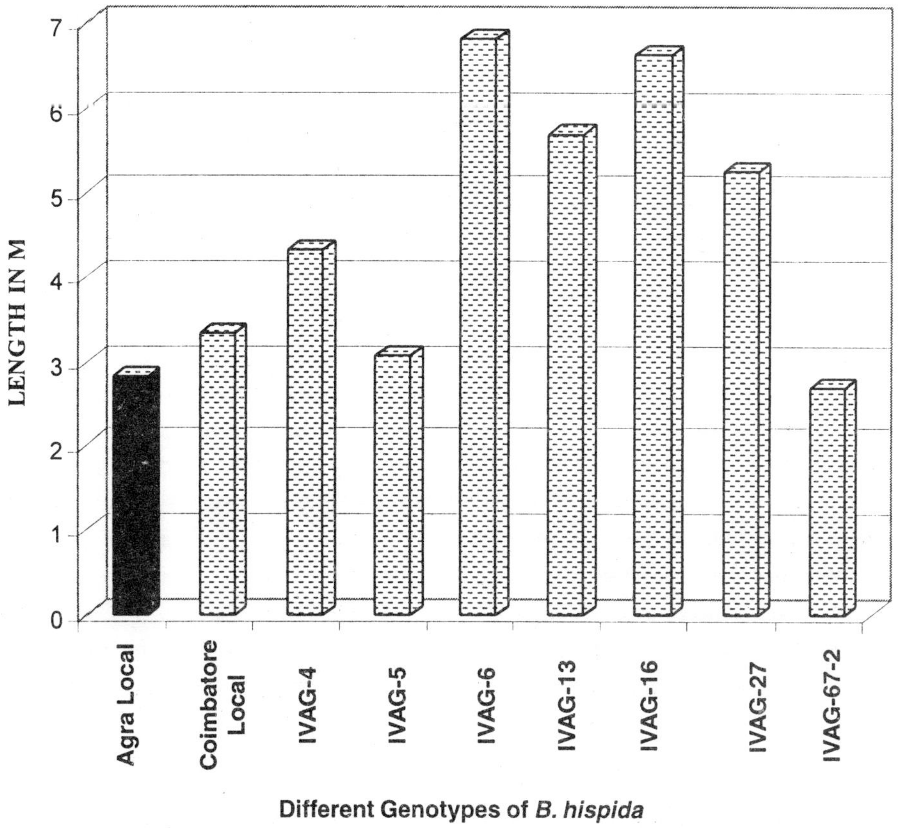

Figure 36.3: Variation in Vine Length in Meters

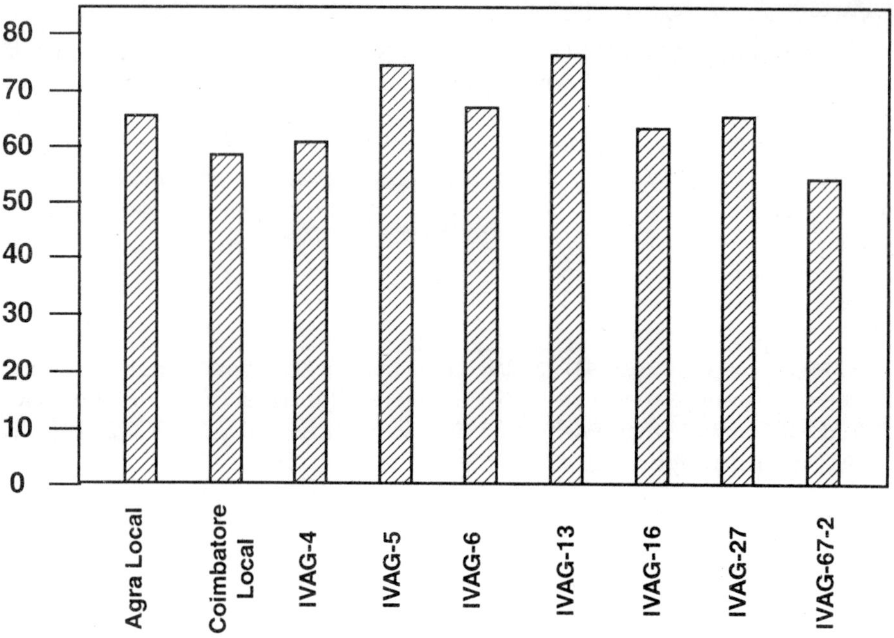

Figure 36.4: Total Number of Leaves/Nodes on Main Vine

Table 36.1: Comparative Growth Parameters in Nine Culture of Ash Gourd

Sl.No.	Characters	Cultivars								
		Agra Local	Coimbatore Local	IVAG-4	IVAG-5	IVAG-6	IVAG-13	IVAG-16	IVAG-27	IVAG 67-2
1.	Length of Seeds in cm	1.22	1.28	1.32	1.16	1.26	1.04	1.24	1.42	1.26
2.	Germination percent	30	70	25	50	65	93.3	75	20	66.6
3.	Appearance of first tendril (in node no.)	9-10	11	10	12-13	10-11	10-11	9-10	10-11	11
4.	Total length of main vine in meters	2.83	3.33	4.33	3.07	6.83	5.69	6.64	5.25	2.71
5.	Total number of primary branches	2	4	3.5	5.5	3	4.3	5	9.5	8
6.	Total number of Secondary branches	4	2.5	1.5	-	-	1.0	-	1.5	11.5
7.	Total number of Nodes/Leaves on main vine	62	55	58	71	64	73.5	60	63	51.5
8.	Total number of Nodes/Leaves per plant	103	112	93	93	88	120.84	97.97	185	150.5
9.	Days taken to first male bud appearance	42	43	47.5	77.5	58	44.5	54	55	55
10.	Days taken to first female bud appearance	67.5	54	64.5	86	71	60.5	79	66.5	67.5
11.	Difference between days of I male and I Female bud appearance	25.5	11	17	8.5	13	16	24.75	11.5	12.5
12.	Total no. of male flowers per plant	60.5	52	33.5	23	54.5	59	39.25	65	86
13.	Total no. of female flowers per plant	6.5	7.5	2.5	5	5.5	6	4.5	5.5	5
14.	Ratio of female and male flowers per plant	1:9.3	1:6.9	1:13.4	1:4.6	1:9.9	1:9.8	1:8.7	1:11.8	1:17.2
15.	Ratio between total no. of leaves per female flowers	16:1	15:1	37:1	19:1	16:1	20:1	22:1	34:1	30 :1

Total Number of Nodes/Leaves per Vine

Each Ash gourd vine bears single leaf per node. Thus the number of nodes per plant tallies with the number of leaves per plant. IVAG-27 topped the list of nine cultures in having maximum number of nodes/leaves (185) per vine. This was followed by IVAG-67-2 with 150 nodes and IVAG-13 with 121 nodes. When examined on main branch of each vine highest number of nodes/leaves were fond in IVAG-13 followed by IVAG-5. Minimum number of nodes/leaves on main branch was found in IVAG67-2. However this was compensated by producing maximum number of secondary branches.

Flowering Pattern

Generally male flowers appear first on all the cucurbitaceous plants to ensure pollination of female flowers. In Ash gourd it took 42 to 77.5 days after sowing to appear first male flower bud in various cultures and 54 to 86 days after sowing for first female flower bud to appear. Agra Local and Coimbatore Local were first to develop male flower buds within 42 and 43 days of sowing respectively whereas IVAG-5 took as many as 77.5 days to develop first male flower bud. For first female flower bud to appear with in 54 days of sowing was Coimbatore Local and IVAG-5 took 86 days to develop it, when compared for the interval of days between appearance of male and female flowers buds on the same vine, Coimbatore Local (11 days), IVAG-27 (11.5 days) and IVAG-67-2 (12.5 days) have narrower gap than Agra Local (25.5 days) and IVAG-16 (24.75 days) (Table 36.1)

Culture IVAG-67-2 is noted for highest number of male flowers (86) per plant and IVAG-5 for lowest number of male flowers (23 only) per plant. Likewise highest number of female flowers per plant (7.5) was noted in Coimbatore Local followed by Agra Local (6.5) and IVAG-13 (6 female flowers per plant). Lowest number of female flowers (2.5) was recorded in IVAG-4.

When compared for the ratio of female to male flowers in each genotype, it was found lowest (1:1.46) in IVAG-5 followed by 1:6.9 in Coimbatore Local and 1:8.7 in IVAG-16. Culture IVAG-67-2 had highest female: male flower ratio *i.e.* 1:17.2 followed by 1:13.4 in IVAG-4 and 1: 11.8 in IVAG-27.

After assessing the overall performance of nine cultures at our experimental farm it is concluded that Coimbatore Local has maximum fruit bearing capacity followed by Agra Local and IVAG-13. Mature fruits of Coimbatore Local were stored under ambient conditions for seven month with only 20 percent loss in the fresh fruit weight.

Acknowledgements

The author is grateful to Dr. R. K. S Rathore, Deptt. Of Botany RBS College, Agra for suggesting the topic and guiding throughout the course of this study. The seeds of seven cultures of Ash gourd obtained from Dr. Sudhakar Pande, Scientist, of Indian Institute of Vegetable Research, Varanasi and Coimbatore Local from Dr. (Mrs.) T. E. Sheeza, Scientist, CARI PortBlair. Both these persons' help in providing the quality seed research material are being gratefully acknowledged. I am also thankful to the Principal, R. B. S. College, Agra for providing field and laboratory facilities to carryout this work.

References

Anonymous, 1988. *The Wealth of India: Raw Materials*, 2(B): 104.

Gutterman, Y., 1992. Influence of day length and red or far red light during the storage of post harvested ripe *Cucumis* fruit, on the germination of seeds. *Journal of Arid Environments*, 23: 443–449.

Kirtikar, K.R. and Basu, B.D., 1935. *Indian Medicinal Plants.* Lalit Mohan Basu Allahabad, 4 Vols. 2nd edn.

Peter, K.V., 1998. *Genetics and Plant Breeding of Vegetables*. Directorate of Information and Publication of Agriculture, Indian Council Agricultural Research, Krishi Anusandhan Bhawan, Pusa, New Delhi.

Rani, Miti, 2000. Morphological characterization of nine cultures of Ash gourd (*Benincasa hispida* (Thunb) Cogn. *J. Agri. Sci. Res.*, 38(122): 94–96.

Sahgal, Mukesh, Gaur, H.S. and Singh Ramvir, 2000. *Bhartiya Fasalon Ki Pramukh Sutrakrami Beemariyan Evam Unaka Prabandhan*, ICAR Bulletin on All India Coordinated Research Project on Plant Nematode Control methods: Division of Nematology, IARI, New Delhi.

Medicinal Plants: Conservation, Cultivation and Utilization (2007) *Pages 281–298*
Editors: A.K. Chopra, D.R. Khanna, G. Prasad, D.S. Malik and R. Bhutiani
Published by: DAYA PUBLISHING HOUSE

Chapter 37

Medicinal Plants of Rigveda

Deepika Chauhan, Navneet and Prabhat
Department of Botany and Microbiology, Gurukula Kangri University, Haridwar – 249 404, India

ABSTRACT

Vedas are the light house for the entire humanity. The light of the Vedas is the foundation of world. Vedas promote universal brotherhood, human welfare and universal prosperity. Vedas have a wider spectrum of knowledge embedded in them, as they can rightly be declared to be the true repositories of all eternal and true knowledge. To say that the Vedas contain only the spiritual and religious material, will be the travesty of truth. From the time immemorial, Vedas have been supposed to be treasure-house of all knowledge and were declared as the only source head of every thought and action. Maharishi Dayananda, the greatest vedic scholar of this age, wrote in most unambiguous terms. "Vedas are the respositories of all true knowledge".

Our ancient medical system which is still in vogue as ayurvedic system, originated and developed from Rigveda and many facts of life and culture, education and bearing, economy and polity as well as custom and tradition have roots in Rigveda. According to Vedas the causatative agents of disese are organisms and poisons.The germs, organisms and insects are five types, *i.e.* visible (drasta), invisible (adrasta), creeping insects (kururu), living in beds etc. (algandu) and moving fast (salune). There are two types of germs: Durnama and Sunama. Durnama cause disease hence must be destroyed. Sunama nourish the body, hence must live there. Rigveda widely deals with the medicine and herbs, their healing properties and their importance. Herbs are the important source of curing disease. On the basis of their healing properties and their importance. Medicines were prepared form the extract of these herbs. The extracts of herbs have been described as the source of longevity. In Rigveda hundreds of herbs were used as medicine.

Introduction

Popular tradition says that there are four Vedas–the Rig, the Yajur, the Sama and the Atharveda. Oodox opinion limits the number to the first three. The Atharveda has little common with the other and the language indicates a latter era. These Vedas represents the several schools of vedic thoughts founded respectively by paila, vaisampayana, jaimini and sumanta. Each veda consist of two parts, the mantra and the brahmana. The first consists of the second is a collection of rules prescribing the method and plan of the various rituals and ceremonies at which the mantras are to be recited, together with illustrative remarks explaining the origin and purpose of each rite. Of the Samhitas the most copious is Rigveda. The Yajur veda deals largely with sacrificial liturgy.

The Rigveda form the full content of the worship of the Vedas and that a study of that veda will help the incurring student to have a fair knowledge of the social and religious institutions. The rigveda samhita consist of the 1017 hymns of different lengths they were apparently enchanted by several rishis at different sacrificial rites and during other ceremonies. Vedic scholar classify hymns in two different ways. One arrangement divides them into eight khandas or Ashtakas and each Ashtakas into eight adhyas or chapters. The other plan divides the suktas or hymns into ten mandalas or cycles. The foundation stone that India contributed to civilization, the Vedas is said to embody the regulations, the laws of the universe as seen by the gifted poet, prophets, or seers the sis, to be the Indians. The authority of the Vedas is supreme and final point the Vedas was given to man at the earliest stage, when the biological species was sufficiently evolved to receive the divine inspiration. it continued to inspire human literature for millenniums of years. In India most ancient human's literature that we possess now is that of the books known as the Brahmanas, but they were also written thousands of years after the divine revolution. These Brahmanas all without exception, accept the authority of Vedas.

The Indian tradition tells us the Vedas originally excited as a single unit, and that it was only latter on that they were classify into sakhas for sacrificial purposes by vyasas. Diligent researches in carefull scrutinizes have led the scholars and the critics of the rigvedas to found the ostensible conclusion that the samhitas is a religious work that is historical work and so on.

Every Hindu believes that his religious practices and rites are based upon the Vedas. The Vedas relate to the worship of the Devas. This worship comprehends offerings, prayers and praises. The offering to the Vedas consisted of oblation and liberation: Ghee poured on the fire, and Juice of the soma plant. The hymns recited the glories of the Deva invoked, and describe that power, the goodness and even the personal beauty of the Deva addressed. They also rehearse the past bounties and explits of the Devas. The Devas are implored to bestow blessings on the man who has instituted the ceremony in which these hymns are recited. The blessings prayed, for the most part, of the a temporal nature wealth of cattle and horses an grains, and protection against enemies. It is also assured that the Devas derive much benefits from the offerings made to them and that the praises addressed to them augment their power for good.

The Vedas are the permeable source of knowledge, which paved the way for the advent to world culture and world civilization. The significance of the Vedas is discernible in the entire Indian heritage. The Vedas are the treasures of knowledge and the origin of Dharma. The extension of the basic knowledge emanated from the Vedas and they are the light house for entire humanity. The light of the Vedas promotes universal brotherhood, human welfare and universal prosperity. The Vedas have been at the root of cultural and social consciousness. The study and analysis of Vedas have shaped various cultures. The Vedas have refined not only the Indian culture but also the world culture. The west has benefited from the study of the Vedas as much as India.

Description of Plant

Sigru *(Moringa oleifera)*

आवदिन्द्रं यमुना तृत्सवश्रव प्रात्र भेदं सर्वताता मुषायत् ।
आजासश्रव षिग्रवो यक्षवश्रव बलिं शीर्षाणिं जभ्रुरश्व्यानि ।।

RV; 7.18.19

Sigru is a small or medium sized tree and attains the height of about 10m. It is found wild in the sub Himalayan tract and is also cultivated throughout India. Root, bark, fruit, flower and seeds are used as medicine.

This is a green and woody plant. This plant bears a white yellowish flowers.

Phytochemistry

Preliminary chemical investigation of *M.oleifera* bark revealed the presence of steroids and terpenes and absence of alkaloids, saponin, tannins and mucilage. The hexane extract of the bark yielded a triterpenoid–bayrenol *Moringa oleifera* leaves on ethanoic extraction yielded a number of amino acids, viz, aspartic acid, glutamic acid serine, glycine and, theonine, α–alanine, valine, leucine iso-leusine, histidine, lysine, arginine, phenylaneine, tryptophan, cystine and methionine. The ether extract of leaves yielded α and β carotene. Latter nine amino acids in the flower, eight in the fruits and seven each in the protein hydrolysate of flower and fruits of *M. oleifera*.They were identified as alanine, arginine, glutamic acid, glycine, cerine, threonine and valine. These amino acids were common in all the parts tested, where as aspartic acid was present in the flower as well as the fruits and lycine occurred only in the flower. The flower contain both sucrose and D–Glucose where as the fruits showed the presence of sucrose only.

Pharmacology

The roots are carminative and stomachic, abortiacient, cardiac tonic and also use in paralytic conditions and intermittent fever. They are also useful as rubefacient, in spasmodic affections of the bowels, hysteria and flatulence as well as in epilepsy. Root bark is used as fermentation to relive spam. Bark is considered to be an abortifacient. Seed oil is applied extremely in rheumatism. Leaves are emetic and their juice with black papers is used in headache. The poultice of leaves is use in reducing glandular swellings.

Durva *(Cynadon dactylon)*

यं त्वमग्ने समदहतस्तमु निर्वापया चमत बमदज ।
कियास्व्वात्र रोहतु पाकदूर्वा व्यल्कशा ।।

RV; 10.16.13

Description

It is perennial and creeping herb with underground rhizome. Culms are decumbent–ascending and nodes are glabrous. Leaves are linear sub late and scabrid on the upper surface margin. Ligules are minute, scarious, erose and ciliate rim. The sheaths are composes, keeled, and glabrous exept hairy throat. Spikes are 2-4 and 1.5–3.0 cm × 0.1–2 cm spikelets are 0.02 cm × 0.1 cm. lower glume is linear lancelets, acute, 1 nerved and 0.1 cm long. Upper glume is about 0.1 cm long. Lemmas are 3 nerve, bidentate, mucronate and ciliate on the keel in the upper half. Pleasures 2–keeled and 0.1 -0.2 cm long. Stamens are 3 grains oblong and free within the glumes. Flowering is during July–September and fruiting October–December.

Phytochemistry

No information is available.

Pharmacology

The decoction of its root is diuretic and is used in dropsy and in secondary syphilis. An infusion of the root is used for stopping bleeding from piles and crushed roots mixed with curd used in chronic gleet. The juice of the plant is said to be astringent and is used externally to fresh cuts and wounds and internally as diuretic. It is used in dropsy and anasarca, hysteria, epilepsy, insanity, in chronic diarrhea, dysentery.

Kusha (*Desmostachya bipinnata*)

शरास चमत बमदज कुशरासो दर्भास चमत बमदज सैर्या उत ।
मौञ्ज अदृष्टा बैरिणा चमत बमदज साकं न्यलिप्सत ॥

RV; 1.191.3

Description

It is tufted and perennial grasses with a thick root stock, culums are erect and nodes are glabrous. The leaves are liner, narrowed into a filiform tip and 0.1-0.3cm broad.The sheaths are glabrous with hairy throut.The panicles are 45.0 cm, 1.0-2.0cm. The spikes are crowded and 1.0-3 cm. The spikelets are purple brown, biseriata and 3-4 flowered. The lower glume is keeled, mucronate, 1-neved and 0.5-0.07cm long and the upper glume is 0.1cm long. The lemmas are subacute with scabrid keeled, and 3 nerved. The paleas are 0.13cm long stamens are 3 and the anthers are.08-0.1cm long Grains are 0.05-0.06cm long, obliquely ovoid, trigonous and laterally compressed.

Phytochemistry

The leaf culms yield pectose, lignin, cellulose and ash.

Pharmacology

The roots are bitter, sweet, cooling diuretic, emollient, galactagogue and astringent and are used in asthma, jaundice, vitated conditions of pitta and hyperdipsia. The culms are, diuretic, stimulant and are used in diarrhea, dysentery, leucorrhoea, skin diseases, stones, memorrhagia and thrst.

Vamsa (*Bambusa arudinacea* Roxb)

ओचित्सरवायं सरव्या वव त्यां तिर चमत बमदज पुरु 'चिदर्णवं जगन्वान् ।
थ्पतुर्नपातमा दधीत वेघा अधि क्षमि प्रतरं दीघ्यान चमत बमदज ॥

RV; 1.10.1

Description

It is a tall bamboo with crowded culms arising from branching roots stock.Culms-sheath are rounded at apex and hairy with dark-brown hairs on the back and glabrous within.The leaves are linear or linear-lenceolate and glabrous or hairy beneath.The inflorescence is an enormous panicle, often comprising of the whole culm. The spikletes are lanceolate and acute. Grains are ending in a shoret beack and about 0.5-0.8cm long.

Phytochemistry

The roots contain cyanyenetic glucoside, benzoic acid, resin and waxes. Besides, cholin, betain and enzymes have also been reported from the plant.

Pharmacology

The leaves are emmenagogue and are used in haematemesis. Dastur (1962), stated that a decoction of its leaves is given to India after childbirth and as anthelmitic, these are particularly useful for threadworm. The juice of leaves with aromatics is given in blood, vomiting and an infusion of the leaves given internally for gonorrhoea.

Aratu (*Oroxylum indicum*)

अयं दशस्यन्नर्येभिरस्य दस्मो देवेभिर्वरुणो न मायी ।

अयं कनीन ऋतुपा अवेधमिमीतारस् यातुष्पात् ।।

RV; 8.46.27

Description

A small to medium sized deciduous tree, grows throughout greater part of India at, 200m. except in western drier areas.

Phytochemistry

Root bark, stem bark, fruits and seeds is used.

The ethanolic extract of *O.indicum* leaves gave baicalein and scutellarein, from the ether fraction, a flavone glycoside, identified as baicalein-6–glucronide, from the ethylacetate fraction, and two glucuronides identified as scutellrein-7-glucuronide acid baicalein-7-glucuronide from the aqueous mother liquor. The defatted leaves of *O. indicum* on extraction with choloroform yielded, a gummy solid yielding an anthraquinone, aloe–emdin.

The ethanolic extract of the stem bark of *O. indicum* on fractionation yielded oroxylin-A from the benzoic extractive; oroxylin-A, baicalein and scutellarein from ether extractive and scutellarein-7-rutinosid from the ethylacetate fraction. Chrysin and baicalein-7-glucronide also occurred in the mother liquor of ether and ethylacetate fraction.

Pharmacology

The decoction of *O. indicum* bark showed good diuretic activity in rats, comparing favourably with potassium acetate and being more potent then urea. The ethanolic extract of the fruits of *O. indicum* showed spasmogenic action on isolated guinea pig ileum, whereas the root and stem as well as the stem bark extracts had no such effect. The plant was devoid of antibacterial, antifungal, antiprotozol, anthelmintic, antiviral hypoglycaemic and anticancer activities. It has no effect on CNS and CVS.

Kimsuka (*Butea monosperma*)

सूकिशुकं शल्मलिं विरूपं हिरण्यवर्ग सुवृतं सुचम् ।

आ रोह सूर्ये अमृतस्य लोकं स्योनं पत्ये वहतुं कृणुष्व ।।

RV; 10.85.20

Description

It is a moderate sized deciduous tree upto 15cm high and 1.5-1.8m girth. The bark is fibrous, bluish-grey or light brown and exuding a ruby red vitreous gum. The leaves are pinnately 3-foliate, large, unequal and 10.2-20.4cm. The flowers are 3.8-5.0cm. long and orange –red and are fasicled on rigid axillary and terminal racemes.The pods are silvery-white and broad. The seeds are flat, elliptic reddish grey and 3.2cm. across. Flowering is in February-March and fruiting during April-May.

Phytochemistry

The flowers contain butin and its 7-glucoside and 3β-D-glucoside, butein, isomonopermoside, coreopsin, sulphurien, palastrin, butin and isobutein.The gum from bark contain leucocyanidin and its tetramer (procyanidin), riboflavin and thiamine. Glycine, a glycoside and an aromatic hydroxy compound have been seprated from the roots of the plant unsponifiable matter of seed oil contains α-amyrin, β-sitosterol and its glucosides.The fatty acid composition of the seed oil comprises of myristic, palmitic, stearic, arachidic, behenic, lignoceric, olic, linleic and linoleic acids.The seeds contain palasonic, aleuritic and jalaric acid, laccijaric acid and its derivatives, cantharic n-heneicsonic acid and nonospermin.

Pharmacology

The seeds are anthelmintic, acrid, bitter, aperient and rubefacient. The seeds are used in flatatulence and piles. A decoction of seeds is given in gravel and paste of powdered seed with lemon juice is applied in herpes and as a cure of ring worms and also for cooling effect. Fine powder of seeds along with *Acorus calamus* rhizome or mixed with juice of *Cyperus rotundus* rhizomes is used as a cure for delirium.The flowers are diuretic, depurative, astringent and aphrodisid.

Haridra or Haridrava (*Pinus deodara*)

शुकेषु मे हरिमाणं रोपणाकासु दध्मसि ।
अथो हारिद्रवेषु मे हरिमाणं नि दध्मसि ।।

RV; 1.50.12

The generic name Pinus has been derived from Greek word pinos, used by Theophrastus for a pine tree.

Description

It is large tree with systematical branches high upon the trunk and forming a round head of light foliage and reaching up to 30 m in height. Normally, it is evergreen but becomes completely or partially deciduous in dry season. The bark is dark grey and deeply fissured. The leaves are 20-30 cm long, arranged in form of cones which are 1.5 cm long. Female cones are 10.0–20.0 cm × 7.5-12.0 cm, ovoid and are solitary or 2-5 together and woody. The seeds without wings are 0.7-1.3 cm × 0.5-0.6 cm and winged; wings are membranous and long.

The cones formation is started in January next year during June–July its cones become old and in next summer, burst and seeds are shed out. About 26 months are spared to complete the whole process. The dry cones remain long on the tree.

Phytochemistry

The plant contains α–and β–Pinene and careen. These needles of plants are good source of vitamin C and E and carotenes. The heart wood contains stilvene and flavonoids namely pinosylvin, pinocemvrin and pinovanksin.

Pharmacology

The wood is stimulant, diaphoretice, and is useful in the burning of the body, cough, fainting and ulceration. The wood is said to be beneficial in snake-bite and scorpion-stings also. The oleoresin is considered to by anodyne and diuretic and is beneficial in coryza, and oedema. This is adviced to be given in the doses of 1.8–5.4 gm four times daily in gonorrhoea. It is expectorant and useful in chronic bronchitis and is specially recommended in gangrene of lungs, also given as carminative in flatulent colic and to arrest minor hemorrhages in tooth socket and nose. Externally, it is used as a ruvefacient in rheumatic affection and for deep seated inflammation, especially of abdomen and applied as a plaster to be bubos and absence for suppuration.

Muja (*Saccharum munja*)

वर्धी वृत्रं मरुत इन्द्रियेण स्वेन भामेन तविषो वभृवान् ।

अहमेता मनवे विन्द्र चमत बमदज सुगा अपाकर वज्रबाहु ॥

RV; 1.161.8

It is a tall perennial grass with erect culms. The leaves are linear, somewhat glaucous beneath, scabride on the margin and upto 2 cm broad. The pennical is dense and wide, while villous upto 100 cm long with whorled branches. Sessile spikelets are lanceolate, acute, 0.5 cm long and 2–nerved. The pedicelled spike lets are similar to sessile spikelets flowering and fruiting is during October–January. Stamens and roots are used.

Phytochemistry

The stem is considered as refrigerant and aphrodisiac. These are useful in burning sensation, blood problems, thirst, erysipelas and urinary complaints. The roots are used as diuretic and demulcent.

Madhuka or Mahuva (*Madhuka indika*)

सूर्ये विषमा सजामि तिं सुरावतो गृहे ।

सो चित्रु न मराति नो वयं मरामारे अस्ययोजनं हरिष्ठा मघु त्वा मघुला चंकार ॥

RV; 1.192.10-13

Description

It is a large deciduous tree with about 17m. height. The bark is grey or blackish with shallow wrinkle and vertical cracks. Young branches, leaves and petioles are pubescent or tomentose. The leaves are clustered at the ends of branches, 12.5-17.5cm × 7.5-10.0cm, elliptic or oblong-elliptic and shortly acuminate base. The flowers are many, at the ends of the branches and are borne on droping pedicels. The calyx is coriaceous and densely rusty-tomentose.The corolla is yellowish-white and early caducous. Stamens are 20–30 and anthers are hispid a the back with stiff hairs.The fruits are ovoid, fleshy and green berries and about 2.5-5.0 cm long. The seeds are 1-4. Flowering is during April –May and fruiting in June–July.

Phytochemistry

Isolated leucodelphindin from the bark of the plant.The fruits contain vitamin A and C, ethylcinnamate, sesquiterpene alcohol, α-terpenol, 3β-monocaprylic ester of erythrodiol and 3β-capryloxy oleanolic acid and α and β-amyrin. The seed-oil has arachidic, linoleic, olic, myristic, palmitic and steric acid.

The flower contain L-arabinose, D-galactose, glucose, D-glucuronin acid, fructose, maltose, L-rhamnose, D-xylose, biotin, folic acid, isositol, niacin, pantothenic and riboflavin, thiannin, amylase, catalase, emulsion, invertase, maltase, oxidase, malic acid and sussinic acid, anthocyanin, betaine acid and protein.

Pharmacology

The seeds are laxative and are used in piles and constipation. The gummy juice of the seed is applied in rheumatism and skin-diseases. The residual cake mowrah meal, obtain after the extraction of the oil from the seeds is said to be used as fish poison and as worm-killer for lawns. The decoction of the bark is also used as astringent, emollient, hypoglycaemic and tonic and their powder is used in bleeding gums, stomachache, tonsilitis and diabetes. Besides, the stem-bark also possesses some insecticidal properties.

Asvavati, Udojasa, Urjayanti (*Ficus religiosa*)

असबत्थे वो निषदनं पर्णे वो वसतिष्कृता ।
गोभाज इत्किलासथयत्सनवथ पूरुषम् ।।

RRV; 10.97.7

Description

It is a large or medium-sized deciduous tree with speading branches of about 10-12m thick. Bark is grey with brownish specks, smooth and 1.3cm thick.Trunks are irregularly shaped. The leaves are alternate, 10.0–17.5 cm × 7.5–12.5 cm, broadly ovate or rotund, caudate and long petioled. Male flowers are very few and sessile, sepals 3, stamen 1 and filament short Female and gall flowers, sepals 5, style short and lateral. Fruits are sessile in axillary pairs, depressed-globose, 1.3 cm across and dark purple when ripe.

Flower is during summer and fruiting in rainy season.

Phytochemistry

The bark contain β-sitosteryl-d-glucoside and vitamin K, n-octacosanol, methyloleanolate, lenosterol, stigmasterol and lupin-3 one have been reported from its stem bark.

Pharmacology

According to Chopra *et al.* (1956), the bark is astringent and is used in gonorrhoea. Pulverised bark is applied externally on unhealthy ulcer and wounds to promote granulation and found very efficaceous when rubbed with honey to apthous sores of children. The dried bark in powdered form is used in and fistula and in the form of a paste, as an absorbent in inflammatory swelling.Tender and fresh leaves are beneficial when used alongwith butter fat to cover the inflammatory ulcers. The oil medicated with its leaves is used as ear drops in ear ache. The leaves and its twigs are also considered as laxative.The seeds are laxative and in powder form these are given for three days during menses as to sterilized women. Besides, various parts of the plant are used in otitis media, suppurativa, mouth sores, atrophy, emaciation or cachexy, rheumatism, smallpox, carbuncle, mucus in urine, spermatorrhoea, gravel, cholera and rinderpest.

Table 37.1

Name of the Vedic Plant	Botanical Name of the Vedic Plant	Family of the Vedic Plant	References
ASVAVATI,UDOJASA,URJAYANTI	*Ficus religiosa*	Moraceae	RV; 10.97.7
JIVANTI	*Leptadenia reticulata*	Asclepiadaceae	RV; 5.78.9
VISANAKA	*Gymnema sylvestre*	Asclepiadaceae	RV; 6.16.20 RV; 9.96.8
SIGRU	*Moringa oleifera*	Moringaceae	RV; 7.18.19
HARIDRA(HALDI)	*Curcuma longa*	Zingiberaceae	RV; 1.50.11-12
ARATU/ARADU			
ARALU	*Oroxylum indicum*	Bignoniaceae	RV; 8.46.27
ASVATTHA	*Ficus religiosa*	Moraceae	RV; 1.138.8 RV; 10.97.5 RV; 1.35.8 RV; 1.164.4
UDUMBARA	*Ficus glomerata*	Moraceae	RV; 10.14.12
KARUNJA	*Pongamia glabra*	Leguminacae	RV; 1.53.8 RV; 10.48.8
KARSMARYA or KASMARYA	*Gmelina arbora*	Verbanaceae	RV; 6.48.1-7
KIMSUKA	*Butea monosperma*	Leguminaceae	RV; 10.85.20
KHADIRA	*Acacia catechu*	Leguminaceae	RV; 3.18.19 RV; 3.15.19 RV; 3.53.19
PALASA	*Butea frandosa*	Leguminaceae	RV; 10.97.5 RV; 4.2.7-4
MADHUKA (MAHUVA)	*Madhuka indica*	Sapotaceae	RV; 1.191.10-13
VIBHITAKA or VIBHIDAKA	*Terminalia bellerica*	Combretaceae	RV; 7.86.6 RV; 10.34.1
SALMALI	*Bombax ceiba*	Bombacaceae	RV; 7.50.3 RV; 10.85.20 RV; 3.53.22
SIMSAPA	*Delbergia sisso*	Leguminoceae	RV; 3.53.19 RV; 3.15.9
HARIDRA or HARIDRAVA	*Pinus deodara*	Pinaceae	RV; 1.50.12
AVAKA	*Blyxa octandra*	Hydracharitaceae	RV; 10.68.5
URVARU (KHAIR)	*Cucumis sativus*	Cucurbitacae	RV; 7.59.12
PUDARIKA	*Nelumbo nucifera*	Nympheaceae	RV; 10.142.8 RV; 10.107.16 RV; 7.33.11 RV; 8.72.11 RV; 6.16.13
MADHUVATI	*Vitis vinifera*	Vitaceae	RV; 10.16.3
ARJUNA	*Terminalia arjuna*	Combretaceae	RV; 1.122.5 RV; 3.39.2 RV; 7.55.2

Contd...

Table 37.1–Contd...

Name of the Vedic Plant	Botanical Name of the Vedic Plant	Family of the Vedic Plant	References
KASA	*Sacchraum spontaneum*	Gramineae	RV; 10.100.10
KUSA	*Desmostachya bipinnata*	Gramineae	RV; 1.191.3
DURVA	*Cynadon dactylon*	Gramineae	RV; 10.16.13 RV; 10.134.5 RV; 10.142.8
BHANGA	*Cannabis sativa*	Cannabiaceae	RV; 9.61.13
MUNJA	*Sacchrum munja*	Gramineae	RV; 1.161.8 RV; 1.191.3
VAMSA	*Bambusa arundinadea*	Gramineae	RV; 1.10.1
YUVA	*Hordeum vulgare*	Gramineae	Rv; 1.23.15 RV; 1.66.3 Rv; 1.117.21 RV; 1.44.11 RV; 1.135.8 RV; 1.176.2 RV; 2.5.6

Khadera (*Acacia catechu*)

अभि व्ययस्व रवदिरस्य सारमोजोधेहि स्पन्दने शिंपायाम् ।
अक्ष वीड्डो वीड्डयस्व मायामादस्मादव जीहिपो न चमत बमदज ॥

RV; 3.18.19

The generic name *Acacia catecha* has been adopted from Greek word Akis a sharp paint, fefering to the thorns of the plant.

Description

It is moderate-sized tree with thorny branches. Bark is rough, dark grey or grayish-brown and about 1.2cm thick exporting in long narrow strips. The leaves are 10.0-17.5cm long, pinnate with a pairs of recurves pirckles at base of rachis and pinnae 40-80, leaflets are 60-100 small and ligulate. Flowers are pale-yellow in axillary cylindrical spikes. The pods are thin, glabrous, lustrous, straight, star-shaped, dark brown and orbicular.

Flowering is in rainy season and fruiting during November–January.

Phytochemistry

Catechu contain 2-12 per cent catechins 25-23 per cent phlobatannin, 20-30 per cent gummy matter, quercitrin and querchitin. The Acacia tree has epicatechin that is distinct from catechin in gum gambhir. Epicatehin from white acellular crystals which are soluble in hot water and alcohol and given a green colour with ferric salts. Catechutannic acid is an amorphous, phlobatannin, which is form epicatechin by loss of the elements of water, it redily yields the phlobouphene catechu–red.

Pharmacology

A flavonoid from the plant was found to have significant anti-inflammatory effect. No significant neuropharmalogical effects were seen Alkaloids show mild hypotensive effects. The astringent principles of the plant have a protine precipitating activity on mucosal surfaces and in wounds and ulcers. Catechu is widely used as a component of the beetel leaf chewed in India. It is used for the local treatment of otitis and otorrhoea. It is also useful indental, oral, throut and tonsillar infections, and as an astringent for reducing oozine ulcers and wounds. The extract in also indermatoses-locally systematically.

Karanja (*Pongmia pinnata*)

त्वं करज्ञ्मुत पर्णयं वधीस्तेजि ठयातिथिग्वस्य वर्तनी ।

त्वं शता वृंदस्याभिनत्पुरोऽनानुद चमत बमदज परिषूता ऋजिना ॥

RV; 1.53.8

Pongmia pinnata is known as karanja in Sanskrit. Two species of Karanja *viz.*, urkara karanja (*P. glabra), kanta-karanja or cirivivah karanja (P. pinnata) ha*ve been found in India. The plant are common throughout India. They are planted along road side as an Avenue tree and also distributed in Eastern Asia, Himalaya, Sri Lanka, Burma, Malaya, Northern Australia and Polynesia.

Description

P. pinnata bark is grayish, green or brown, smooth and covered with tubercles, leaves, imparipinnate, leaflets 5-7, ovate or elliptic, flower, lilauce, or white tinged with pink or violet, fragrant in axillary racemes, pods compressed woody, indehiscent, yellowish grey when ripe, varying in size and shape, elliptic to obliquely, oblong 4.0 -5.0 cm broad with a short curved beak, seed usually 1, rarely 2, elliptical or reniform, 1.7-2.0 cm. long and 1.2–1.8 cm broad wrinkled with reddish, brown leathery testa. The harvest season extends in generally obtained from November–December to May–June. The pods are collected and the shells removed by hand.

Phytochemistry

The oil resembles ground nut oil in composition. The fatty acid composition of the oil shows the following ranges of values: palmitic, 3.7-7.9; stearic, 2.4-8.9; aracihidic, 2.2-4.7, behenic, 4.2-5.3; legnoceric, 1.1-3.5, oleic, 44.5-71.3, levolic, 10.8-18.3 and eicoenoic, 9.5-12.4 per cent and traces of docorrenoic and tetracosemic acids. The un-saponifible matter contain β sitosterol. Karanjin and ponganol compounds isolated from *P. pinnata.* Karanj is highly toxic to fish, pong mol exhibit comparatively mild toxicity. The flowers contain an aliphatic. Waxy matter, free kaempferol, pongamin, γ-site sterol glucoside, guercetin, negoglbrin and glabrosaponin. The stem bark contains two closely related derivatives, kananjin and dimethoxy karanj in feebly toxic to fish. The root bark from Australia been reported to contain Karanj and pongapin and smaller amount of two linear furamo flavones, pinnata and gumatin which are isomeric with karanjin and pongupin respectively. The roots admixture part extract contain anticancer alkaloid as pacitaxol, fluorophenylanine.Vinblastin sulphate and vincristin sulphate, teniposide and oetoporide derivative compounds.

Pharmacology

In Ayurveda, karanja in highly valued for the treatment of many diseases. It is applied in scabies, herpe's, leucoderma, dyspepsia with sluggish liver.The galactaggue juice of leaves is prescribed in flat ulcers, dyspepsia, diarrhea. Cough and used in leprosy and gonorrhea. Roots juice is used for cleaning foul ulcers, gonorrohoea and flat ulcers sores, decoction of fresh bark is used in beriberi. The decoction of flowers juice used for diabetes. The seed are also used to treat painful, rheumatic joints, skin disease leprous sores. Root admixture extract found exclusive anti-cancer compounds.

Karanj has been used extensively by our Rishis and practioners of Ayurveda since time immemorial.

Madhuvati (*Vitis vinifera*)

अपो वा गच्छयदि तत्र ते हितमोषधीषु प्रति तिष्ठा शरीरै : ।
अजो भागस्तपसा तं तपस्व तं ते शोचिस्तपतु तं ते अर्चि ॥

RV; 10.16.3

Description

It is a large woody climber bitid tendrils. The leaves are globorous above, clothed beneath with grey deciduous tomentum, suborbiculear, cordate and more or less deeply 5-lobed. The flowers are pentamerous and green and are borne in umbel-like cymes, which form large pyramidal compound panicles. The fruits are subglobose berries with 1-5 seed. But the fruits realy come to perfection due to heavy rainfall which usually takes place before these have properly ripened.

Phytochemistry

The mature fruits contain malic, tartaric acid, cemic acid, which the oxalic acid has been reported from its unripe fruits.

Pharmacology

Grapes, juice, sap, leaves, dried fruits and ashes of the wood are used. The grapes are demulcent, laxative, refrigerant, stomachic, diuretic and cooling. These are considered very useful in chronictic and bronchitis, heart-disease, brights disease and gout. The juice of the unripe grapes is astringent and is used in throat affection. Straind grape juice, one tea spoonful is given to children for constipation. The juice is also good for thrush in children and that of sour grapes is useful for bruise and sprains the sap of the young branches. The leaves are astringent and are used in diarrhea. Dried fruits, known as Munakka are cooling demulcent, sweet, laxative and stomachic.

Kasa (*Saccharum spontaneum*)

यव्दाग्वदन्तेविचेतनानि राष्ट्री देवनां निषसाद मन्द्रा ।
चतस्त्र ऊर्ज दुदुहे पयांसि क्क स्विदस्याः बमदज परमं जगाम ॥

RV; 10.100.10

Description

It is perennial gregarious grass with glaborous and erect culms. The leaves are linear-filiform, glaucous beneath, often redued to midrib, scabrid on the margin and 0.1-0.4cm broad. The sheaths are auriculate and glabrous except hairy throat. Pedicels are ciliate and.2-0.3cm long sessile spikelets are liner-lanceolate and 0.3–0.4cm × 0.04.005 cm flowering and fruiting is during September-December.

Phytochemistry

The plant has been reported to contain calcium oxalate.

Pharmacology

The root and whole plant is used. The roots are diuretic and a decoction of roots with that of Gokshra and Mishri is given to remove urinary bladder calculi. The plant is considered as laxative and aphrodisiac. An extract of the plant is given in burning sensation, phthisis, blood disease, vesical calculi, bilousness and haemorrhagic diathesis.

Bhanga (*Cannabis sativa*)

उपो पु जातमप्तुरं गोभिर्भं परिष्कृतम् ।
इन्दुं देवा अयासिट्ठुः ॥

RV; 9.61.13

Description

It is a tall annual herb about 1.2-4.9M high with angular stem. The leaves are palmate, alternate or lower one opposite and 5.0-0.20.0cm long, the lobes of the upper leaves are 1-5 and in lower 5-11, liner lanceolate, sharpely toothed, long-pointed and narrowed at base. The flowers are small, greenish and unisexual. The males are born in long dropping panicles and female in short axillary spikes. The achenes are 3cm aross, ovate and flat and are enclosed in persistent perianth. Flowering and fruiting is during March–May.

Phytochemistry

The plant contains cannabinol, tetrahydrocannabinol, cannabidiol, cannabichromene, 1-dehydrotetrahydrocannabinal and acid other phenolic compounds along with eugenol, guaicol-sequiterpenes, hydrocarbons, piperidine, amino acid prenylated and c-glycosylflavonoids.

Pharmacology

The seed, leaves, dried flowering or fruiting tops of the female plant and resinous exudates are used for medicinal purposes.

The plant is considered as a tonic analysic and antiseptic and is useful in gonorrhoea, menorrhagia, diarrhoea, holera, hydrophobia, tetanus and rheumatism. The leaves are used in ear troubles and their juice is upplied on cuts after mixing with sugar. The juice of leaves is also used to destroy worm and vermin. The crushed leaves are applied on skin in skin diseases.the chronic use of cannabis useful in patients of diabetic hypertension the leaves are also used as snuff and are given internally about 5gm per day to relieve pain and swelling.

Pundarika (*Nelumbo nucifera*)

अभ्यारमिदद्रयो निषित्कं पुघु । अवतस्य विसर्जने ॥

RV; 10.107.16

Description

It is an attractive perennial herb with creeping rhizome. The leaves are orbicular, glaucous, floating, pettate and 60-90cm in diameter, petiole is very long and smooth or pickly. Flowers are solitary, bisexual, regular, large, rosy, white or rarely yellow and 10.2-25.4cm across. Sepals are 4-5 and caducous. Petals are many seriate, canducous. Stamens are many-seriate carpels are irregularly scattered and ovules 1-2 fruits are torus, spongy, rop-shaped and 5.0-10.0cm in diameter. Seeds are elongated, spherical, smooth, black and exalbuminous.

Phytochemistry

The plant contains a number of alkaloids, roemerine, nuciferin, dehydronciferine, anonoine, dehydrounonaine, N-methylisocoulaurine, prouciferine, N-nornuciferine, Ni-methyloclaurinc, oxoushinsunine, armepavine, N-norarmepavin, asimilobine, lirindine, liensinine, isoleinsinine, neterine and nelumnine and β-sitosterol, glucose, pemitic acid and 10–monoacosanol.

Pharmacology

The juice of its tender leaves mixed with sugar is given in elephantiasis. Powdered rhizomes are prescribed for piles as demulcent and beneficial also in dysentery and chronic dyspepsia. The rhizome extract possesses antipyretic activity also. The flowers are cooling and astringent and are used in cholera, diarrhea, fever and liver disease and their decoction is used as cardiac tonic.

Yuva (*Hordeum vulgare*)

तम्र्दरं न पृणतायवेनेन्द्रं सोमेभिरत्तदपो वो अस्तु ।
अस्मभ्ंय तहृसो दानाय राधः समर्थयस्व बहु तें वसव्यम् ॥

RV; 1.23.15

Description

It is an annual erect, stout and tufted grass about 5-12 m height. Leaves are few and linear–lanceolate, upper one close to the spikes; sheath is striate and ligules short and membranous. The spikes are terminal, linear–oblong, compressed, 5-6 cm long and densely flowered. The spikelets are sessile and arranged on two sides of a flattened rachis; all fertile or lateral ones barren and sometimes rudimentary. The glumes are 2, small, narrow, short–awned and enclosing thre spikelets, lemma lanceolate and lodicules 2. The fruit is a caryopsis and elliptic, 9.0 cm long, short pointed, smooth free or adherent to palea or both to lemma and palea and groove on the inner face.

Phytochemistry

The seeds contain ubiqinones, proanthocyanidins, and chrysoeril. The barky grits contain pangamic acid. The stem and leaves contains flavones and cyaogenic glucoside besides, glycosides of horatines A and B are found in seeding.

Parts Used

The grains are used.

Pharmacology

The grains are demulcent and easy to digest and are used in the dietary. An ethyl alcohol (50 per cent) extract of the plant is antiprotozol and antiviral. The sutter, powder of the parched grain is much employed in the form of a gruel in case of painful and aortic dyspepsia, the sattu is alos given to reduce sugar level in urine to diabetic patients. The ashes of the stalks are used for indigestion.

Vibhitaka(*Terminalia arjuna*)

प्रातर्यावाण रथ्येव वीराजेव यमा वरमा सचेथे ।
मेने इव तन्वा३ ुम्भमाने दम्पतीव तुविदा जनेपु ॥

RV; 10.34.1

Description

It is a large tree often with buttressed trunk, smooth grey bark and drooping branch lets about 20–25 m high. The leaves are usually sub-opposite, oblong of elliptic-long, pale dull green above and pale-brown beneath, 10.0–20.0 cm long and hard. The flowers are yellowish-white and are borne in shortly panicled-spikes. The fruits are 2.5–5.0 long drupes, ovoid or obovoid-oblong, fibrous woody, glabrous and with 5–7 equal, hard, coriaceaus and thick narrow wings.

Phytochemistry

The fruits contain alicylic and amino acids an polyols, arachidic, stearate, cerasidin, hentriacontane, myristyl oleacte, mannitol, β-sitoserol, friedelin, methyl oleanolute, ellagic and gallic acids, arjunic acid arjunone and tannin. The root bark yields arjunic acid, 2, 3, 23–trihdroxyl–olean-12 en–28-oic acid, arjunolic acid and its saponin, arjunoside I, II, III, and IV and 8 hydroxyhexadecanoic acid.

Pharmacology

The fruits are used as tonic and deobstuent. Externally, the leaves are used as a cover on sores and ulcers and their juice is used in earache. The bark is antidysenteric, antipyretic astiringent, cardiotonic, lithotriptic, stypmptomatic hypertension. A decoction of the thick bark made with milk is given every morning on an empty stomach or its powder with milk gur as a cardio tonic.

Khira (*Cucumis sativus*)

व्यरबकंयजामहे सुगन्धिंत पुष्टिर्धवर्धनम् ।

उर्वारुकसिव बन्धनान्म त्योर्मुक्षीय माम तात् ॥

RV; 10.10.5-6

Description

It is slender and densely hespid annual herb. The leaves are large, simple, alternate, ovate-suborbicular, deeply cordate at base and 3-4 lobed. Flowers are large, yellow and monecious. Male flowers are large, yellow and monecious. Male flowers are clustered, bearing, anthers cohering, connective, crusted or above the cells. Female flower are solitary and cohered with bulbous–based haris. The fruits are large grayish–yellow hairs. The fruits are larger grayish–yellow or grayish–-white and 10.0-25.0 cm × 2.5–3.7 cm seeds are many acuminate at both ends, white and smooth.

Phytochemistry

The fruits contain an enzyme erepsin, proteolytic enzyme, ascorbic acid oxidase, succinic and malic dehydrogenases.

Pharmacology

The fruits are sweet, refrigerant, haemostatic, tonic and diuretic. These are useful in hyperdipsia, burning sensation, thermoplegia, fever, insomnia, cephalagia, bronchitis, jaundice, hemorrhages, strangury and general debiliy.

The seeds are astringent, sweet, retrigrant, nutritive, purgative, antipyretic, tonic and diuretic and are used in burning sensation, constipation, intermittent fevers, streengury, renal calculus, urodynia and general debility.

Simpsapa (*Dalbergia sissoo*)

स्वप्नेनाभ्युप्या चुमुरिधुनि च जघन्थ दस्युं प्र दभीतिभावः ।

रम्भी चिदत्र विविदे हिरण्यं सोमस्य ता मद इन्द्रैंकार ॥

RV; 7.50.3

Description

It is fairly large deciduous tree with grey bark up to 15-18m in height.The branches are downy, grey and spreading. The leaves are 3-5, alternate, imparimate, bifarious, roundish, acuminate and 3.5-

6.0cm×3.0–5.4cm. The flowers are sessile in axillary panicles shorter then leaves and yellowish white. The pod are 3.5–4.5cm long, 1–4, kindney shapped and flat.

Phytochemistry

Leaves contain flavone and sissotin. The flower yield 7, 4-di-methyltectorigenin isolated mesoinositol 7-methyltectorigen in and a new flavone glycoside from the immature pods. While reported isocaviunin, tectorigenin, dalbergin, biochanin-A and 7-hydroxy-4 methylocoumarin, from the mature pods. The heart wood contains dalbergin, oMe-dalbergenone, hydroxyl and oMe-dalbergenones, dalbergichromene, nordalbergine, isodalbergin, allyphenal of latifolin, dalbergiphenol, OH-terans-stilbene and biochanin-A.

Pharmacology

The leaves are considered bitter and stimulant and their decoction is used in gonorrhoea. The bark is alterative and dried barkis haemostatic and is effective in bleeding piles, menorrhoea and in varicose veins. The wood is alterative and is used in leprosy, boils and eruption and to alloy vomiting. The roots are considered astringent. The plant is also used in Unani-system of medicine. The drug in Unani called, Shishan, Katel, is used as counter-irritant, anrisyphitic and blood purifier. The mucilage of the leaves mixed with sweet oil is used in exeoriation.

Salmali (*Bombax ceiba*)

यच्छल्मलौ भवति यन्नदीषु यदोषधीभ्य चमत· बमदज परि जायते विषम् ।
विदेवा निरितस्तत्सुवन्तु मा मां पधेन रपसा विदत्त्सरुः ।।

RV; 10.85.20

Description

The plant is a large handsome and deciduous are large spreading, glabrous and deciduous leaflets are 5-7, lanceolate, acuminate, tapering below, 15.0-20.cm long and quitentire, petioles are longer the leaflets. The flowers are crimson coloured, axillary or subterminal, usually solitary of clustered and appearing before the leaves. Fruits are 5-valved capsules, valved are woody and 10.0-12.0cm. long seed are many, globose and pale black. Flowering is during spring and winter season.

Phytochemistry

Bose and Dutta, isolated L-arabinose, D-galactose, D-galcturonic acid and rhabinose traces from the gum. The partial hydrolysis yields aldobiuronic acid. Bose and Dutta, further isolated 2, 4, 6, and 2, 3, 4-tri, 2, 6-di-o-methyl-D-galactose and 2, 3, 4-tri-o-methyl-D-galacturonic acid from the hydrolysis of the gum. β-sitosterol and its glucoside are found in all parts of the plant. The root yields triacontanol and a new glycoside. Fresh petals of the flower have essential oil, hentriacontriacontanal, quercetin, β-sitosterol and its glucosides, kaempferol, glucosides of pelaryonidin and cyaniding, 3-biosides and flavones.

Pharmacology

Prtused flower, leaves, root, bark, seeds and young fruits are the parts used. The flower are astringent and cooling. The paste of flower and leaves is applied in cutaneous disesses. Besides this the leaves are also used as anti-inflammatory. The bark of stem is demulcent, emetic, styotic and tonic and its aqueous extract with the cured is used is to arrest blood-dysentery. The paste of the bark is used externally in cutaneous it is also used in gonorrhoea and syphilis, tuberculosis and in influenza. The young fruits are considered expectorant, stimulant and diuretic. These are useful in calculous affection, chronic inflammation and ulceration of kidneys and bladder.

Karsmarya (*Gmelina arborea*)

यज्ञायज्ञा वो अग्नये गिरागिरा च दक्षसे ।
प्रप्र वयमम त जातवेदस प्रिय मित्रं न शैसिषम् ॥

RV; 6.48.1-7

Description

It is an unarmed large deciduous tree about 20m high and pubescent with some white corky bark. The leaves are large, tawny tomentose. Underneath when young, cordate, ovate, accuminate and 10.0–20.0 × 7.5 -15.0 cm. The flowers are yellow tinged with browning terminal and axillary recemiform cymes. Inflorescence, calyx and corolla are toothed with dense soft and tawny tomentum. Fruits are ovoid of pyriform, smooth and 1.7–2.5 cm long drupex and orange–yellow when ripe. The seeds are oblong. Flowering is during February–April and fruiting April –July.

Phytochemistry

Arachidic, lauric, linoleic, myristic, oleic, palmitic and stearic acids are found in seed oil. The leaves contain β–sitosterol, apigenin, lutelin and quercetin. The heartwood contains β–sitosterol, ceryl alcohol, gonelinol, arborone arbonreol, 1-hydroxy–2–methyoxy–2, gmelanone, gmelofuran, 2–piperonyl–3-hydroxy methyl–1-4-4–hydroxyl -1,tetrahydrofuran, gummadiol, arbinose, galactose, glucose, rhamnose and xylose. The root contain β–sitosterol, umbelloferone, benzoic acid, and octacosanal.

Pharmacology

The fruits are refrigerant and their decoction is given in fever and bilious affections. The leaves are demulcent and their juice is useful in cough gonorrhoea, foetid discharge and maggot in ulcers.

The pastes of the leaves are applied on head forelieve headache. The roots are bitter, tonic, demulcent, laxative, refrigerant and stomaching and their decoction is given inanasaco fever and indigestion.

Haridra (HALDI)

शुकेषु मे हरिमाणं रोपणाकासु दध्मसि ।
अथो हारिद्रवेषु मे हरिमाणं नि दध्मसि ॥

Description

The plant is a perennial herb about 90-120 cm tall with short stem and tufted leaves. Primary tubers are at the base of aerial stem and are ellipsoidal and bearing many rhizomes. The rhizomes have distinct taste. Root are fleshy with ellipsoidal tubers. The leaves are 25-40 cm × 10-15 cm linear, acuminate, ascending and pubescent beneath. The inflorensence is produced on short leaflets peduncles, consists of cone-shaped collection of numerous ovate bracts and an bout 10-18 cm long and 5 cm broad. The flowers are pale–yellow and are borne in pairs in the axils. The seeds are black and shining with large, lace rate and white aril.

Phytochemistry

The rhizomes contain curccumin, zingiberine, p-rolynethyl carbinol and curcuminoids.

Pharmacology

The rhizomes and leaves are used. The rhizomes are aromatic, stimulant, carminative, and alterative, blood purifier, antiperiodic and tonic. Externally, those are applied to sprain and on wounds. Fresh juice often rhizome considered anthelmintic and is used as antiparastic in many skin affections. Its decoction is used on ingredient for stomachic preparations.

References

Arvindo, S. *On the Veda*. Printed at Shri Arvindo Ashram Press, Pondichert, India.

Divedi, K.D., 1999. *A Cultural Study of Atharvaveda*. Vishvabharti Research Institute, Gyanpur (Badhoi, U.P., India).

Iyengar, S.P., 1983. *Righved Samhita*. The Soumya Press, Madras.

Kaushik, P. and Dhiman, A., 2000. *Medicinal Plants and Raw Drugs of India*. Bishan Singh and Mahendra Pal Singh, Dehradhun.

Nath, N., 1965. *Age of Rigveda*. Pharma K.L. Mukhopadhyay, Kolkata.

Priyavarat, S., 2003. *Dravyagun Vigyan*, Chokhamba Bahartiya Aacadamey, Varanasi Vol. 2.

Shashtri, S.S.P. *Vidyalankar: Righved Samhita*. Veda Pratishthana, New Delhi.

Shastri, P.S., 1988. *Regveda of Aesthetics*. Vidya Prakashan, New Delhi, India.

Srivastava, S.K. and J. Vidhyalankar, 1988. *Classical writings on vedic and Sanskrit Literature*. Dr. Virendra Arora on behalf of Swami Sradhanand Anusandhan Parkashan Kendra and Printed by New Educationals, Shahadra, Delhi.

Medicinal Plants: Conservation, Cultivation and Utilization (2007) *Pages 299–301*
Editors: **A.K. Chopra, D.R. Khanna, G. Prasad, D.S. Malik and R. Bhutiani**
Published by: **DAYA PUBLISHING HOUSE**

Chapter 38

Utilization and Conservation of Medicinal Plants

Sudha Dubey and Jyotsana Bhoraskar
Holkar Science College, Indore

Introduction

In developing countries, where people are closely connected to traditional practices and livelihoods, more than 80 per cent of the population continues to rely on plants for their medicinal needs. Developed countries on the other hand tend to regard "traditional knowledge" as nothing more than "old wives' tales." But according to a 1985 survey conducted for the World Health Organization (WHO), in developed countries, approximately 74 per cent of the pharmaceuticals derived from higher plants were developed by chemists researching ethnomedical uses of these same plants. It seems likely that new pharmaceutical drugs remain to be discovered from novel compounds in traditionally used medicinal plants that have not yet been adequately investigated.

On a global scale, markets for such traditional modalities as Ayurvedic and Chinese medicine are well-established. These ancient bodies of knowledge and their *materia medica* are rapidly expanding into developed countries and the past two decades have witnessed a renaissance of alternative and complementary therapies throughout the world.

While traditional healthcare systems may differ greatly among cultures, they share several salient characteristics. First, market demand in traditional systems rarely exceeded natural supply, due to several factors. (*Editor's note*: One often-cited exception is the decimation and extinction of the traditional abortifacient and aphrodisiac plant *sylphyium*, derived from a member of the genus *Ferula*. This plant from northern Africa in what was previously called Carthage, now known as Tripoli, was in high demand for its root which was used in Greek medicine in classic times).

A combination of low population densities, localized markets, and limited technological advances usually kept the harvest of wild species within sustainable levels. Many traditional cultures still rely to a large extent on wild-harvested medicinal plants, supplemented by cultivation in kitchen or house gardens, scaled to the needs of an extended family. Due to a need for a variety of medicines, collection of plant resources often spreads over diverse terrains and microclimates. Now, however, rapid population growth and the resulting increased demand exert pressure on limited raw/wild materials and overwhelm this traditional balance. The pursuit of short-term gain may rapidly overtake the practical and ecological limits of harvesting from the wild before sound, sustainable alternatives can be developed. Future efforts in this area will follow the guidelines recently established by the WHO for Good Agricultural Practices for medicinal and aromatic plants (MAPs), including the sustainable collection of wild MAPs.

A second characteristic shared among traditional medicine modalities is that treatments are often long term and directed at chronic problems rather than acute symptoms. Examples include treatments such as St. John's wort (*Hypericum perforatum* L., Clusiaceae) for mild to moderate depression or milk thistle [*Silybum marianum* (L.) Gaertn., Asteraceae] formulations to promote healthy liver function.

In some cultures, knowledge of how to use plants medicinally is widely shared by all members of a community and transmitted through oral traditions or embodied in common practices, such as "herbal simples" commonly grown in kitchen gardens. In other communities, such knowledge is carefully guarded by respected healers trained in plant identification and use. Ethnomedical information, clearly, may be transmitted from one generation to another in many different ways. In some cultures, the knowledge of using medicinal plants has been reduced to a thinly spread residue of folk medicine, weakened by colonialism, and abandoned by younger, Westernized generations as "the old ways."

Traditionally Used Medicinal Plants Endemic to the Mascarene Islands

In the Mascarene Island group, peoples on the main islands of Mauritius and Rodrigues have managed to maintain much of their traditional herbal medicine lore. However, these small islands–1,400 miles east of Mozambique and some 200 miles north of the Tropic of Capricorn in the West Indian Ocean–are under increased pressure from a growing population and dwindling habitat. It is postulated that some 250,000 species of flowering plants exist worldwide and that 90 per cent are already known to science. But even today, major expeditions to the tropics continue to discover new species. Unfortunately, the flora of the tropics, like the fauna, is faced with serious threats to its very survival. On the island of Madagascar well over half of the original forest cover has been removed or seriously disturbed. (Madagascar is an island in the West Indian Ocean off the south-eastern coast of Africa where 80 per cent of the flowering plants are believed to be endemic; that is, not found anywhere else.) In Rodrigues, where more than 55 per cent of the flora is endemic, 30 per cent of the flora is seriously threatened with extinction. Many of these plants are medicinal. Scarce and slow-growing forests species, especially the endemic species, are particularly vulnerable to over-exploitation.

While some native plant species in Rodrigues–like those on Mauritius and another island in the archipelago, Reunion–are threatened with extinction, the islands' biodiversity seems high in terms of the sheer numbers of native species. Of the 486 species that characterize the archipelago, 160 are endemic to Reunion, 150 to Mauritius, and some 40 to Rodrigues. This corresponds to around 30 per cent of the indigenous flora of each island.

Promoting Phytomedicines

People in Mauritius still rely on herbal medicine, and work is underway at the University of Mauritius to validate some of the ethnobotanical information available locally. This work produced an ethnobotanical study on the following major ailments: urinary tract infections, diarrhea, dysentery, conjunctivitis, and wounds/boils/abscess/skin infections. The study examined 35 species and made the following observations:

1. There is a good correlation between the uses of some plants and their efficacy to treat some of the diseases;
2. For other plants, however, there was no conclusive evidence of any efficacy;
3. The best results were obtained with endemic plants; and
4. For some plants the results were inconclusive.

Conclusion

Small islands like those found in the Indian Ocean are biodiversity hot spots. Unfortunately, many of the local people are not using the flora and the fauna in a sustainable manner, which is one reason why so many of the endemic plants are on the verge of extinction. Another reason is widespread deforestation, which threatens both native species and habitat. Ironically, the importance and the future potential benefits of biodiversity are clear. It is also clear that medicinal plants have provided a short cut towards obtaining bioactive molecules.

The degree of biodiversity on many of these islands is still unknown. They have not been adequately explored to determine their full potential, though preliminary testing has already given promising results. Therefore, conservation and sustainability must become part of a comprehensive plan to ensure the viability of these irreplaceable plants.

Medicinal Plants: Conservation, Cultivation and Utilization (2007) *Pages 303–317*
Editors: A.K. Chopra, D.R. Khanna, G. Prasad, D.S. Malik and R. Bhutiani
Published by: DAYA PUBLISHING HOUSE

Chapter 39

Antimicrobial Properties of Herbal Tooth Powders

Sanjay[1], Navneet[1], Murali Manohar[2] and Prabhat[1]
[1]Department of Botany and Microbiology, [2]Faculty of Engineering and Technology, Gurukul Kangri Vishwavidyalaya, Haridwar – 249 404

ABSTRACT

The use of plants or plant parts to clean teeth are in practice since long time. Medicinal plants *i.e.* hard, apamarga, khair, babul, plasha, majuphal, jamun, giloya, pepal, amla, neem, tulsi, kalimirch, pipli, karpoor, tomar, lavang, pudina, garlic, mulahethi, akarkara, nirgundi, chameli, miswak, zaitum etc are widely used in the ayurvedic tooth powders *i.e.*, MDH dant manjan, Vicco vajradanti, Gurukul payokil, Arodent manjan, Agro dent manjan etc. available in the market to cure the diseases like stomatits, tonsils, ulcer, pyorrhoea, dental caries, and bad smell. These tooth powders are so formulated that they must protect our teeth against tooth decay and bad breath. In the present study the antimicrobial properties of seven plants *i.e.* babul, mulahathi, harad, nirgundi, chameli, plasha, and amaltash used in different formulations of herbal tooth powders is discussed.

Introduction

Ayurveda is the ancient science of life. In Sanskrit language 'Ayuh' mean life and 'Veda' means knowledge. Ayurveda may now appropriately be spoken of as the "Science of living" thereby bringing out its practical implications (Kirtikar and Basu, 1975). It aims to bring about a union of physical, emotional and spiritual health. Ayurvedic medicine is more than a system of healing. In Ayurveda about 2,000 plant species are considered to have medicinal value for positive health and cure of human sickness (Purohit *et al.*, 2003).

In Indian mythology, Lord Brahma is said to have composed Ayurveda, even before he created the universe. When illness, disease become rampant on earth, sages learnt the science of healing from Lord Indra and recorded them in the scriptures. The 'Rigveda' mentions 67 plants having therapeutic effect 'Yajurveda' lists 82 plants *Atharvaveda* is the ancient literature of medicinal plants, there are 288 plants described in it (Purohit *et al.*, 2003). In Atharvaveda there are 114 formulations for treatment of various diseases. Medicinal plants have made a good contribution to the development of ancient Indian literature of the earliest treatises. The most ancient book 'Charak Samhita' contains several therapeutic or internal medicines, about 600 plants used in the formulation of drugs are described in it. It also deals with other branches of Ayurveda like anatomy, physiology pathology and treatment etc. Surgery has been described in 'Susruta Samhita'. It deals primarily with various fundamental principles and theory of surgery, more than 100 kinds of surgical instruments and 650 drugs with their uses have been described in it (Thakkar, 1994).

Natural products are being used by about 80 per cent of the world population primarily in the developing countries for primary health care. These are preferred because of less testing time, higher safety, efficacy, cultural acceptability and lesser side effects. The chemical compounds present in herbal products are a part of the physiological functions of living organisms and hence they are believed to have better compatibility with the human body (Khanna *et al.*, 1986).

Herbal medicine is the oldest form of healthcare known to mankind. Herbs had been used by all cultures throughout history. It was an integral part of the development of modern civilization. The plants provide food, clothing, shelter and medicine. Much of the medicinal use of plants seems to have been developed through observations of wild animals, and by trial and error. As time went on, each tribe added the medicinal power of herbs in their area to its knowledge base. They methodically collected information on herbs and developed well defined herbal pharmacopoeias. In the 20th century much of the pharmacopoeias of scientific medicine was derived from the herbal lore of native peoples. Many drugs commonly used today are of herbal origin. Indeed, about 25 percent of the prescription drugs dispensed in the United States contain at least one active ingredient derived from plant material. Some are made from plant extracts, others are synthesized to mimic a natural plant compound.

The World Health Organization (WHO) estimates that 4 billion people,80 percent of the world population, presently use herbal medicine for some aspect of primary health care. Herbal medicine is a major component in all indigenous peoples, traditional medicine and a common element in Ayurvedic, homeopathic, naturopathic, traditional oriental and Native American India medicine. WHO notes that out of 119 plants derived pharmaceutical medicines, about 74 percent are used in modern medicine in ways that correlated directly with their traditional uses as plant medicines by native cultures. Major pharmaceutical companies are currently conducting extensive research on plant materials gathered from the rain forests and other places for their potential medicinal value.

Substance derived from the plants remain the basis for a large proportion of the commercial medications used today for the treatment of heart disease, high blood pressure, pain, asthma, and other problems. For example, *Ephedra* is a herb used in traditional Chinese medicine for more than two thousand years to treat asthma and other respiratory problems. Ephedrine, the active ingredient in *Ephedra* is used in the commercial pharmaceutical preparations for the relief of asthma symptoms and other respiratory problems. It helps the patient to breathe more easily. Another example of the use of a herbal preparation in modern medicine is the foxglove plant. This herb had been in use since 1775. At present, the powdered leaf of this plant is known as the cardiac stimulant. Digitalis is being given to millions of heart patients and it keeps them alive worldwide. St. John's Wort is widely used in the treatment of mild depression without the need for Prozac, St. John's Wort does not have the side effects such as that of Prozac. There are some Ayurvedic herbs that are very useful for reducing cholesterol, diabetes etc. Similarly the popularity of *Ginseng* and *Ginkgo biloba* (ginkgo) is rising due to its beneficial effects (Bhattacharjee, 1998).

Herbal medicine can be broadly classified into various basic systems, Traditional Chinese Herbalism, which is part of Traditional Oriental Medicine, Ayurvedic Herbalism, which is derived from Ayurveda, and Western Herbalism, which originally came from Greece and Rome to Europe and then spread to North and South America. Chinese and Ayurvedic Herbalism have developed into highly sophisticated systems of diagnosis and treatment over the centuries. Western Herbalism is today primarily a system of folk medicine. Interest in the United States had been growing in the recent years from the reported success stories related with the use of herbs.

Dental diseases and gum diseases are the growing health problem throughout the world, especially in our country due to changing life style, dietary habits excessive use of sugar and other sugar products.

The composition of tooth powders formulation are given in Tables 39.1–39.7.

Table 39.1: The Ingredients of Vicco Vajradanti

Sl.No.	*Name*	*Botanical Name*	*Family*	*Part Used*
1.	Babul	*Acacia nilotica*	Leguminosae	Bark
2.	Jamun	*Syzygium cumini*	Myrtaceae	Fruit
3.	Laung	*Syzygium aromatica*	Myrtaceae	Fruit
4.	Manjistha	*Rubia cordifolia*	Rubiaceae	Root
5.	Dalchini	*Cinnamomum zeylanicum*	Lauraceae	Chhal
6.	Bor	*Ficus elastica*	Moraceae	Chhal
7.	Vajradanti	*Adhatoda vasica*	Acanthaceae	Flower
8.	Akhrot	*Juglans regia*	Juglandaceae	Chhal
9.	Khair	*Acacia catechu*	Mimosaceae	Heartwood
10.	Patang	*Caesalpinia sappan*	Leguminosae	Chhal
11.	Akarkara	*Anacyclus pyrethrum*	Compositeae	Root, bark
12.	Bakul	*Mimusops elengi*	Sapotaceae	Chhal, bark
13.	Kababchini	*Piper cubeba*	Piperaceae	Seed
14.	Antamul	*Tylophora indica*	Asclpiadaceae	Root
15.	Ajwain	*Trachyspermum ammi*	Umbellifera	Fruit
16.	Maiphal	*Quercus infectoria*	Fagaceae	Fruit
17.	Triphla			
	(a) Amla	*Emblica officinalis*	Euphorbiaceae	Fruit
	(b) Harad	*Terminalia chebula*	Combretaceae	Fruit
	(c) Behera	*Terminalia bellirica*	Combretaceae	Fruit
18.	Jeshthamadh			

Table 39.2: The Ingredients of Dabur Red Tooth Powder

Sl.No.	Name	Botanical Name	Family	Part Used
1.	Kalimirch	*Piper nigrum*	Piperaceae	Fruit
2.	Pippali	*Piper longum*	Piperaceae	Fruit and Root
3.	Kapur	*Cinnamomum camphora*	Lauraceae	Wood
4.	Tagar	*Valeriana wallichii*	Valerianceae	Root
5.	Laung	*Syzygium aromatica*	Myrtaceae	Fruit
6.	Tomru	*Zanthoxylum armatum*	Rutaceae	Root
7.	Pudina	*Mentha spicata*	Lamiaceae	Whole Plant
8.	Kasni	*Cichorium intybus*	Compositae	Seed
9.	Harad	*Terminalia chebula*	Combretaceae	Fruit
10.	Garlic powder	*Allium sativum*	Lilliaceae	Bulbs
11.	Dantmukta	*Tylophora indica*	Typhaceae	Root

Table 39.3: The Ingredients of MDH Dant Manjan

Sl.No.	Name	Botanical Name	Family	Part Used
1.	Bakul	*Mimusops elengi*	Sapotaceae	Bark
2.	Majuphal	*Quercus infectoria*	Fagaceae	Fruit
3.	Vaivadang	*Embelia ribes*	Myrinaceae	Fruit
4.	Samudriphen	*Argyreia speciosa*	Convalvulaceae	Root
5.	Supari	*Areca catechu*	Palmae	Wood
6.	Akhrot	*Juglans regia*	Juglandaceae	Chhal
7.	Godanti	*Vitis vinifera*	Vitaceae	Fruit
8.	Ama Haldi	*Curcuma amada*	Zingiberaceae	Rhizome
9.	Laung	*Syzygium aromatica*	Myrtaceae	Fruit
10.	Kalanjan	*Alpinia galanga*	Zingiberaceae	Seed
11.	Pipal	*Ficus religiosa*	Moraceae	Bark, Root
12.	Kapur	*Cinnamomum camphora*	Lauraceae	Wood
13.	Podina	*Mentha piperita*	Lamiaceae	Leaves
14.	Triphla			
	(a) Amla	*Emblica officinalis*	Euphorbiaceae	Fruit
	(b) Harad	*Terminalia chebula*	combretaceae	Fruit
	(c) Behera	*Terminalia bellirica*	combretaceae	Fruit
15.	Kalimirch	*Piper nigrum*	Piperaceae	Fruit
16.	Tomru	*Zanthoxylum armatum*	Rutaceae	Root
17.	Cloveoil	*Syzygium aromaticum*	Myrtaceae	Leaves
18.	Eucalyptus	*Eucalyptus citriodor*	Myrtaceae	Leaves
19.	Sainda Namak			
20.	Sonagera			
21.	Suhaga phula			
22.	Fatkri Bhasam			

Table 39.4: The Ingredients of Gurukul Payokil

Sl.No.	*Name*	*Botanical Name*	*Family*	*Part Used*
1.	Babul	*Acacia nilotica*	Leguminosae	Bark
2.	Pellitoery	*Ancyclus pyrethrum*	Compositae	Chhal, Root
3.	Akhrot	*Juglans regia*	Juglandaceae	Chhal
4.	Kapur	*Cinnanomum comphora*	Lauraceae	Wood
5.	Neem	*Azadirachta indica*	Meliaceae	Bark
6.	Kalimirch	*Piper nigrum*	Piperaceae	Fruits
7.	Bariyari	*Sodii chrorium*	Malvaceae	Wood
8.	Tomru	*Zanthoxylum armatum*	Rutaceae	Root
9.	Thymol	*Thymus vulgaris*	Labiatae	Leaves

Table 39.5: The Ingredients of Adrodent Manjan

Sl.No.	*Name*	*Botanical Name*	*Family*	*Part Used*
1.	Pudina	*Mentha spicata*	Lamiaceae	Wholeplant
2.	Khair	*Acacia catechu*	Mimosaceae	Heartwood
3.	Motha	*Cyperus rotundus*	Cyporaceae	Leaves
4.	Neem	*Azadirachta indica*	Meliaceae	Bark
5.	Bakul	*Mimusops elengi*	Sapataceae	Chhal, bark
6.	Laung	*Syzygium aromatica*	Myrtaceae	Fruit
7.	Jaiphal	*Myristica fragrans*	Myristiaceae	Fruit
8.	Apamarg	*Achyranthus aspera*	Amaranthaceae	Bark
9.	Adark	*Zingiber officinale*	Zingiberaceae	Fruit
10.	Nagkasar	*Mesua ferrea*	Guttiferae	Bark
11.	Baybhirang	*Embelia ribes*	Myrsinaceae	Bark
12.	Akarkara	*Anacyclus pyrethrum*	Compositeae	Bark and Root
13.	Jeera	*Cuminum cyminum*	Umbelliferae	Bark
14.	Kalimirch	*Piper nigrum*	Piperaceae	Fruit
15.	Choti Elaechi	*Elettaria cardamomum*	Zingiberaceae	Fruit
16.	Dalchini	*Cinnamomum zeylanicum*	Lauraceae	Chhal
17.	Potash Alum			

Achyranthes aspera (APAMARGA)

It is a common weed found throughout India upto 1000 m usually in dry area and along the road sides. It belongs to family Achyranthaceae. It is commonly called Apamarga, in Sanskrit as Kharamansari and English name as Prickly Chaff-Flower.

Table 39.6: The Ingredients of Agro Dant Manjan

Sl.No.	Name	Botanical Name	Family	Part Used
1.	Akarkara	*Anacyclus pyrethrum*	Compositeae	Root
2.	Dalchini	*Cinnamomum zeylanicum*	Lauraceae	Chhal
3.	Khair	*Acacia catechu*	Mimosaceae	Heartwood
4.	Supari	*Areca catechu*	Palmae	Fruit
5.	Tomaru	*Zanthoxylum armatum*	Rutaceae	Root
6.	Behra	*Terminalia bellirica*	Combretaceae	Chhal
7.	Kalimirch	*Piper nigrum*	Piperaceae	Fruit
8.	Ajwain	*Trachyspermum amini*	Umbelliferae	Fruit
9.	Til	*Sesamum indicum*	Pedaliaceae	Fruit
10.	Amla	*Emblica officinalis*	Euphorbiaceae	Fruit
11.	Harad	*Terminalia chebula*	Combretaceae	Chhal
12.	Laung	*Syzygium aromatica*	Myrtaceae	Fruit
13.	Bach	*Psoralea coryliforia*	Fabaceae (Leguminosae)	Root
14.	Chameli	*Jasminum grandiflorum*	Oleaceae	Leaves, Flower
15.	Pudina	*Mentha spicata*	Lamiaceae	Wholepart
16	Molshree			
17.	Sonagaru			
18.	Sainda Namak			
19.	Gajpear			

Table 39.7: The Ingredients of Himalaya Herbals (Dental Cream)

Sl.No.	Name	Botanical Name	Family	Part Used
1.	Dudima	*Euphorbia hirta*	Euphorbiaceae	Root
2.	Tomru	*Zanthoxylum armatum*	Rutaceae	Root
3.	Bakul	*Mimusops elengi*	Sapotaceae	Bark
4.	Triphala			
	(a) Amla	*Emblica officinalis*	Euphorbiaceae	Fruit
	(b) Harad	*Terminalia chebula*	Combretaceae	Fruit
	(c) Behera	*Terminalia bellirica*	Combretaceae	Fruit
5.	Nimba	*Azadirachta indica*	Meliaceae	Bark, Stem
6.	Nirgundi	*Vitex negundo*	Verbenaceae	Leaves
7.	Vaivadang	*Embelia ribes*	Myrinaceae	Fruit
8.	Tankana			
9.	Vaikrantabhasma			
10.	Ajamoda Satva			

Description

It is a stiff erect herb about 30-90 cm. high with erect and simple or slightly branched stem. Leaves are 3.8-12.5 cm × 5.0-7.5 cm, opposite, elliptic, obovate or suborbicular, usually rounded at apex and tomentose or velvety on both surfaces. Flowers are bisexual, greenish-white and are brone in long spikes which elongatic in fruits and reach upto 50 cm. in length. Fruit is an oblong urticle which is enclosed in the hardened perianth and disarticulating easily and carrying spinous bracteols with it. The seed are subcylindrical with a truncate brown apex. Flowering is in winter and fruiting in summer.

Phytochemistry

Betaine, achyranthine, hentriacontune, ecdysterone and two glycosides of oleanolic acid have been reported from the plant. Beside, the seeds are known to contain saponin A and B (Chatterjee and Pakrashi, 1991).

Pharmacology

The plant is considered pungent, purgative, diuretic and astringent and is used in dropsy and haemorrhoids. The decoction of the plant is useful in pneumonia, cough and kidney stones and ash of the plant is given in haemorroids. The dried plant is useful in colic and gonorrhoea and also acts as laxative. The ashes of the plant with water and Jaggery are effective in ascties and anasarca sesamum oil medicated with ashes of the plant is used as eardrops. Achyrol, leaf-extract is used in leprosy and the juice of the leaves is in eczema and leprosy. The leaves made into a paste with water are applied to bites of poisonous insects, wasps and bees etc.The root are given in stomach pain and their paste is applied to remove opacity of cornea and to wounds as haemostatic besides, their decoction in diarrhoea. The root paste is given to stop bleeding after abortion. Powdered roots mixed with honey are given internally in haemorrhoides. A pinch of root powder in combination with pepper powder and honey forms a good remedy for cough.

The seed-paste is applied against insect-bite. The seeds are rubbed with rice water and are prescribed to patients of bleeding piles and a powder of the seeds is soaked in butter milk is given in biliousners. Its flowers are ground and mixed with curd and sugar and are given in menorrhagia and the flower tops are used in treatment of rabies. Besides, decoction of the whole plant is diuretic and efficaceous in renal dropsies and in combination with that of kakajanga *(Leea aequata)* useful in insomnia (Chatterjee and Pakrashi, 1991).

Terminalia chebula (HARAD)

Terminalia chebula is found in greater part of India, North West Bengal, Punjab and Sikkim. It belongs to family combretaceae. It is commonly called in Hindi as Hard, Haritaki, in Sanskrit as Abhaya, Amruta and English as Chebulic myrobalan.

Description

It is a large deciduous tree with dark-brown bark, young branchlets, leaf buds and leaves are long and soft and with shining rust coloured, sometimes silvery hairy. Leaves are mostly suboppossite, distant, 7.5–15.0 cm. long, ovate or oblong ovate, acuminate and deciduous in the cold season. The flowers are dull white or yellowish with offensive smell and bisexual and are borne in spikes from the upper axils and in small terminal panicles. The fruits are 2.5–5.0 cm. long, obovoid, ellipsoid or ovoid glabrous and more or less 5 ribbed when dry. The nuts are hard and with a rough grooved surface. Flowering is during April–June and fruiting in January–March.

Phytochemistry

The plant has been investigated for its chemical constituents and found to contain a large amount of pentacyclic triterpenes, tannins, anthraquinones, chebulic acids, resins fixed oil, amino acids, fructose, succinic acid and beta sitosterol (Chevallier, 1996; Khurana, 1959; Reddy *et al.*, 1993). Fruits contain astringent substances chebulinic acid, tannic acid, gallic acid, the resin and a purgative principle of the nature of anthraquinone and sennoside are also present.

Pharmacology

The plant has been used in protected diarrhoea with hematoachezia and prolapse at rectum chronic cough with sore throat and hoarseness of voice (Jixian, 1997; Zhu, 1998). Chebulic myrobalans are used in fevers. Cough, asthma, urinary diseases piles, worms and rheumatism and scropion-sting. *Bala-harade* is highly useful in chronic diarrhoea and dysentery. Flatulence, vomiting, hiccup, colic and enlarged spleen and liver. Brayed with sugar and water it is used in ophthalmia. *Java harade* is used similarly. Cold *infusion* of it is used as a gargle in sore mouth and stomatitis, spongy and ulcerated gums. Brayed in rose water, it is a cooling application to swellings (Nadkarni, 1976).

Acacia catechu (KHAIR)

It occurs in drier regions of Sub Himalayan tract upto an altitude of 1200 m. from Punjab to North-Eastern States, Madhya Pradesh, Gujrat, Andhra Pradesh and Tamilnadu. It belongs to family Mimosaceae. It is commonly called in Hindi as Khair, in Sanskrit as Khadira and English as Catechu.

Description

It is a moderate sized tree with thorny branches. Bark is rough, dark grey or greyish brown and about 1.2 cm. thick exploiting in long narrow strips. The leaves are 10.0-17.5 cm. along, pinnate with a pair of recurved prickles at base of rachis and pinnae 40-80, leaflets are 60-100 small and ligulate flowers are pale-yellow in axillary cylindrical spikes. The pods are thin, glabrous, lustrous straight, star-shaped-dark brown and 5-6 seeded. The seeds are flat, dark-brown and orbicullar. Flowering is in rainy season and fruiting during November–January.

Phytochemistry

The air dried pulversied leaves of the plant yielded quercetin, poriferasteral, Beta-D glucoside poriferasterol and quercetin 3-0, arabinofuranoside, quercetin 3-0 rhamnoside and quercetin 3-0 glactoside (Sharma *et al.*, 1997). Dye extracted from the inner wood is a brittle compact substance of chocolate colour containing much tannin and an acid called catechuic acid. It has astringent taste, its 35 percent contains catechu, tannic acid. Catechuic acid or catechin, catechu red, tannin, gum quercetin. Catechu tannic acid, coccuss as a dark reddish brown powder which oxidises in the air (Nadkarni, 1976). A new bio-active flavone glycoside was isolated from the ethylacetate soluble fraction of the ethanolic extract of the stem of the plant. Its structure was characterised as 5, 7, 3, 4–tetrahydroxy. 3–methoxy flavone 7-0-Beta-D-glactophyronosyl, 1 to 4-0-Beta glucopyrnoside by various chemical degradation and spectral analysis (Navneet, and Shri Krishna, 2004; Yadav and Sodhi, 2002).

Pharmacology

Catechu is chiefly used in India as an ingredient of the packet of betel leaves chewed by the people. It is a valuable astringent given in doses of 5-15gms. alone or combined with cinnamon or opium in passive diarrhoeas and haemorrhages, either in powder or as *tincture* combined with other astringents, especially useful for children. Take powdered catechu and powdered cinnamon bark each 10 or 15 grams, mix them together in sufficient honey or syrup and make into four pills, or take of catechu powder three drachms and cinnamon bark powder one drachm, infuse both in half pint of boiling water for two hours, filter and administer in does of 1½ to 2 ounces three time a day. For adults 5 drops of laudanum may be added to each dose during administration but not for young children. A small piece of catechu with cinnamon and nutmeg, held in toothache, loss of voice etc. also in cases of mercurial salivation bleeding, ulcerations and sponginess of the gums. In toothache it is employed to stuff the hollow of the aching tooth (Nadkarni, 1976).

Jasminium grandiflorum (CHAMELI)

Jasminium grandiflorum is found in greater part of India particularly in Uttar Pradesh, Uttaranchal, Bihar and Bengal. It belong to family oleaceae. It is commonly called Chameli. In sanskrit as Jati, in Hindi as Chameli, Beng, Jati and in English as common Jasmine.

Description

A large twining shrub, considered to be a native of North West Himalayas, growing upto 600-1500 m, widely grown in Indian gardens. It is a large scandent and glabrous shurb with striate branches. The leaves are opposite and imparipinnate, leaflets are 7-11, rhomboid-oblong, the lowest larger than uppermost pair. The flowers are fragrant, white and tinged with purple outside and are borne in divaricate cymes. The corolla is 5-lobed, elliptic and obtuse or acute. The fruits are didymous and ovoid berries. The seeds are erect and exalbuminous. Flowering and fruiting is during March-August.

Phytochemistry

The leaves contain jasminine and salicylic acid (Chopra *et al.*, 1956). The flowers contain methylanthranilate, benzylcyamide, cinnamyl benzoate, geranylgeraniol and its acetate, geranyl linalool, 4-methylbenzoate, methyl dihydrojasmonate, methyllinoleate, methylpalmilate, methyl-N-methylantranilate, myrcene, trimethylpentadecanone, phytol and its acetate, vanillin, cis-3-hexanol and its benzoate and 2-vinypyridine. The oil from the flowers contain benzylacetate, benzylbenzoate, benzaldehyde, benzyl alcohol, eugenol, fernesol, geraniol, cis-jasmone, *dl*-linaloil,linayl alcohol, nerol, nerolidol,1-a-terpineol, indole, isophytol and its ester, methylanthranilate, benzoic acid, peresol, methyljasmonate and (5-pent-2-enyl) -5, pentnolide. Besides, (z,z,z)–3,6,9 dodecatrien -1-ol, and ester of (z) -3,5 hexadien 1-ol have been encountered in the plant (Chatterjee and Pakrashi, 1995).

Pharmacology

The flowers are cooling (Chatterjee and Pakrashi, 1995) and are used externally in headache and skin-disease and in weak eyes. Mahomedan writers mentioned that the flowers are used as a plaster to loins, genitals and pubes as an aphrodisiac (Nadkarni, 1976). According to the Behl *et al.*, 1993, oil from the flowers is applied as cooling agent externally and the roots are used in ringworm. The leaves are astringent (Dastur, 1962) and they are chewed as a treatment for ulcerations or eruptions in the mouth. The fresh juice of the leaves is applied to corns between toes. A bland oil prepared with the juice of the leaves is poured into the ear in otorrhoea (Chopra *et al.*, 1956). According to Bhasawar, 1965, leaves also possess antibacterial activity against *Staphylococcus aureus*. The flower is acrid, bitter, with a sharp taste, heating, emetic, alexiteric, vulnerary, useful in stomatitis and disease of the mouth, the head, the teeth and the eyes, very good in toothache, Suppurations, and earache, given in disease of the blood, leprosy, ulcers, biliousness, Ayurveda (Kirtikar and Basu, 1975).

Vitex negundo (NIRGUNDI)

Vitex negundo is found in greater part of India and East Asia, China to the Himalayas it belongs to family Verbenaceae. It is commonly called in Hindi as Nirgundi, in Sanskrit as Indrani, Shephali, and in English as Indian Privet.

Description

It is a deciduous shrub with thin grey bark. The branchlets underside of leaves or inflorescence are hoary with short grey pubescene. The leaves are 3-5 foliolate, leaflets are lanceolate, 2.5-10 cm × 0.7-3.2 cm, the lowest pair is smallest sessile or subsessile, the middle pair, if present, more or less distinctly petiolulate and the odd leaflet is largest with a 0.7-1.5 cm long petiole, entire or crenate, glabrate, dark-green above and palegreenish tomentose beneath. The flowers are small and bluish purple and are borne in lateral cymes forming on elongated terminal thyrsus and often compound at the base. The calyx-teeth are triangular. The corolla is bluish or purplish white and 5-lobed. The stamens are 4, didynamous and excerted. The ovary is 2-4 celled and 4-ovuled. The drupes are succulent and black when ripe. The seeds are obovate or ablong. Flowering is during June-August and fruiting in cold season.

Phytochemistry

Subramanian and Misra (1978), isolated 2 new leuconathocyanidins I and II from the stem-bark as Methyl ethers of leucodelphinidin and leucocyanidin 7-0 rhamnoglucoside. The seeds contains β-sitosterol, p-hydroxy benzoic and 5-hydroxyisophthalic acids, linopleic, palmitic, oleic and stearic acids, n-hentriacontane, n-pentatriacontane, n-nonacosane, n-tritriacontane, 3β–acetoxyolean-12-en-27-oic, 2α, 3α–dihydroxyolean-5, 12-dien-28-oic, 2β, 3α-diacetoxyolean-5, 12-dien 28-oic and 2α, 3β-diacetoxy-18–hydroxyolean, 5,12–dien -28–oic acids, 5,7,3–trihydroxy-6, 8, 4–trimethoxy flavone and a flavonoid-artematin, 6-hydroxy-4 (4-hydroxy-3-methoxyphenyl)-3-hydoxymethyl-7-Methoxy-3,4-dihydro-2–maphthaldehyde, 5β-hydro 8,11,13-abietatrien-6a-ol and lanostan-8, 25-dien-3 β-ol. The leaves yield β. siosterol, 5–hydroxyisophthalic acid, 3,4-dihydroxybenzoic acid, 2-p-hydroxy-benoxylmussaenosidic acid, carotene, glucononitol and vitamin c.

The root contains β-sitosterol, 3-formyl 4,5-di-methyl-8-oxo-5H-6,7-dihydronaphtho (2,3-b) furan and acetyl oleanlic acid, P-hydroxybenzonic acid, vaniclic acids and luteolin have been reported from the stem-bark (Chatterjee and Pakrashi, 1995).

Pharmacology

The leaves are vermifuge, aromatic, tonic (Chopra *et al.*, 1956), alterative anodyne, antiparasitic, discutient, antiinflammatory and antirheumatic (Chatterjee and Pakrashi, 1995). Rheaumatic patients are advised to have bath in water boiled with its leaves. A smoke of dried leaves is taken in headache and catarrh. The decoction of the leaves with long pepper is given in catarrh fever with heaviness of head and dullness of hearing and also as bath in the puerperal state of women. The juice of the leaves is used for removing foelid discharges and worms from ulcers (Behl *et al.*, 1993; Nadkarni, 1976). The juice of the leaves with cow's urine is administered in the doses of 25gm, every morning in the enlargement of spleen (Dastur, 1962). The dried fruit is vermifuge (Chopra *et al.*, 1956). The fruit is also used in the treatment of angina, colds, coughs, rheumatic difficulties etc (Duke and Ayensu, 1985). The fresh berries are pounded to a pulp and used in the form of a tincture for the relief of paralysis, pains in the limbs, weakness etc.

The root is expectorant, febrifuge and tonic (Chopra *et al.*, 1956). It is used in the treatment of colds and rheumatic ailments (Duke and Ayensu, 1985). It is harvested in late summer and autumn, and dried for later use (Bown, 1995).

The plant is said to be a malarial preventative and is also used in the treatment of bacterial dysentery extracts of the leaves have shown bactericidal and antitumor activity (Duke and Ayensu, 1985).

Butea monosperma (PALASH)

Butea monosperma is found in greater parts of India, Burma and Srilanka. It belongs to the family Fabaceae. It is commonly called "FLAME OF THE FOREST". In Sanskrit it is called as Palasha, Dhak or Palash in Hindi and in English as Butea Gum Tree. It is also referred to as a treasurer of the Gods.

Description

It is an erect, medium sized tree of 12-15m high, with a crooked trunk and irregular branches. The bark is ash coloured, it exudes a kind of red juice when injured. The leaves are 3 foliate, large and stipulate. Petiole is 10-15cm long. Leaflets are obtuse, glabrous above, finely silky and conspicuously reticulately veined beneath with cunnate and deltoid base. From February to April (when the tree is leafless), the tree looks most sensational, with a riot of orange and vermillion red blossoms covering the entire crow and looking truly like a tree of flame. The corolla is long with silky silvery hairs outside and bright orange red. Calyx is dark, olive green to brown in colour and densely velvety outside. Stamens are diadelphes, anthers uniform. Ovary 2 ovule, style fuliform, curved and stigma capitate. Young pods have a lot of hair a velvety cover. The mature pods hang down like peculiar legumes. The seeds are flat and curved. Seed coat is reddish brown in colour and wrinkled. Dhak flowers yield an orange dye. A preparation of the same is used as an insecticide. The seeds are used in Ayurvedic and Unani medicines.

Phytochemistry

The main constituent of the flower is butrin (1.5 per cent), butein (0.37 per cent), butin 7-glucoside and 3β-D-glucoside. The flowers contain coreopsin, isocoreopsin, isobutrin, sulphurein (glycoside), palasitrin and other two with monospermoside and isomonospermoside, flavonoids and steroids. Studies prove that isobutrin slowly changes to butrin on drying. The flowers of the species are used for producing natural, herbal dye, which gives brilliant fugitive yellow colour (Tewari *et al.*, 2001). The bright colour of the flower is attributed to the presence of chakones and aurones. Seed contains oil and unsaponifiable matter of seed oil contains α-amyrin, β -sitoserol and its glucosides (Asolkar *et al.*, 199). The fatty acid compositon of the seed oil comprises of myristic, lignoceric, oleic, arachidic, palmitic, stearic, behenic, linoleic and linolenic acid. The seeds contain palasonin, aleuritic acid, jalaric acid, laccijalaric acid and its derivatives, cantharic n-heneicosanic acid and nonospermin (Behl *et al.*, 1993). The composition of the leaves varies with the place of origin. Basically it contains minerals, calcium and phosphorus. The gum from bark contains leucoayanidin and its tetramer (procyanidin), riboflavin and thiamine. Glycine a glycoside and an aromatic hydroxy compound have been separated from the roots of the plant (Chatterjee and Pakrashi, 1992).

Pharmacology

Flowers have astringent, sweet, cooling, constipating, aphrodisiac, haemostatic, diuretic, febrifuge, depurative and tonic properties. They are used as emmenagogue and to reduce swellings. They are useful in vitiated conditions of pitta and kapha, diarrhoea, haemorrhoids, menorrhagia, stangury, fever, leprosy, skin diseases, hyperdispsia, haemoptysis, arthritis, burning sensation, bone fractures, eye infections and are very efficacious in birth control. Gum (*Butea Kino*) have astringent, constipating, haemostatic, aphrodisiac, depurative and tonic properties. It is useful in diarrhoea, dysentery, haemorrhoids, haemoptysis, haematemesis, diabetes, leprosy, skin diseases, ulcer, pharyngodynia, general debility, hyperacidity, dyspepsia and fever. Due to astringent, bitter, pungent, all terative, aphrodisiac and anthelmintic properties. Useful in tumors, bleeding piles and ulcers. The decoction is useful in cold, cough and fever. The leaves are astringent, anti inflammator and haemorrhoids. Seeds are purgative, ophthalmic, antihelmintic, rubefacient, depurative and tonic. They are useful in herpes, skin diseases, ringworm, opthalmopathy, epilepsy, roundworm, arthritis, flatulence, constipation, and diabetes. Roots are useful in elephantiasis and in curing night blindness and other eyesight defects. Also applied in sprue, piles, ulcers, tumors, and dropsy. It is given in conjunction with ginger in case of snake bite. *Butea monosperma* is renowned in ayurveda for helping to boost the skin natural long-term resistance to sun damage in a balanced topical skin formulation.

Green young shoots of 1-2cm. thicknesses are used as toothbrush in rural areas (Tewari *et al.*, 2001).

Cassia fistula (GOLDEN SHOWER)

Cassia fistula belongs to the family Caesalpiniaceae and grows in scattered areas of India, South Eastern Iran, Egypt, Sudan and Brazil. In Sanskrit it is known as Aragvadha, Swarnaka and Kritamala, Amaltas or Bandarlauri in Hindi and in English it is called as Golden Shower, Indian Laburnum or Purging Cassia. Now it is popularly planted as an ornamental tree. It illuminates the cities and forests with its beautiful, bright yellow flowers. *Cassia fistula* has been used widely in folk remedies and Ayurvedic medicine for hundreds of years. The pods, flowers, leaves and root bark are used.

Description

A fast growing medium sized deciduous tree, 6-9 m tall with a straight trunk and spreading branches. Stem bark is pale grey smooth and slender when young and dark brown and rough when old. Leaves alternate 20-40 cm long, paripinnate, long stalked stipulate petioles 6-9 mm long, 4-8 pairs of leaflets 5-15 cm long are seen distinctly stalked, oblong or ovate, with a silvery pubescence. Flowers are large fragrant, bright yellow in long axillary racemes. They are hanging in showering bunches of up to 40 cm long earning it common name "golden shower tree". They appear when the branches are bare just before the new leaves emerge.

Flowers bore on long, slender, smooth, pedicles. The blooms are followed by the production of two-foot long, dark brown, cylindrical, woody seedpods that persist, on the tree throughout the winter before falling to litter the ground. Calyx is composed of 5 nearly equal, oblong, obtuse, smooth sepals. The corolla consists of 5 petals, which are oval, unequal, concave, spreading and waved. Ovary is filiform, smooth, cylindrical, curved and 1-celled containing numermous seeds (Harvey *et al.*, 1898). Fruits are dangling transversally septate, dark brown to black and indehiscent when ripe. Inside each septum, a sweet, viscous, dark brown pulp surrounds one seed. Each fruit contains numerous seeds. The seeds are obversion, biconvex in cross section, ventrally flattened, 7.5 to 10.0mm long, 6.0 to 7.5mm wide and 2.5 to 3.0mm thick. The seed coat is light brown, smooth and shiny.

Phytochemistry

The leaves of *Cassia fistula* contain free rhein, glycoside and sennosides A and B. Anthraquinone glycosides are concentrated in the leaves about 1.75 per cent (Abo *et al.*, 2001). The pulp has a feeble, nauseous odor, a mucilaginosacharine taste (Harvey *et al.*, 1898) and consists mainly of sugar (about 60 per cent) with rhein, oil, fistulic acid and albuminoids. Pulp contains 1,8 dihydroxyanthraquinone derivatives (Khurana, 1959). Kaempferol, flavonoids, fistulin, triterpenes and a pronthocyanidin have been isolated from the flowers. In flowers anthraquinone glycosides are concentrated about 1.58 per cent at the age of peak flowering (Abo *et al.*, 2001). The bark of the tree is rich in tannins, it contains barbalion, rhein and leucope-largonidin trimer (Behl *et al.*, 1993). The benzene extract of powdered stem bark yielded lupeol, β-sitosterol and hexacosanol. From the alchoholic extract of the pods an anthraquinone (fistulic acid) was obtained and identified as 1,4–dihydroxy -6,7–dimethoxy, 2-methyl anthraquinone -3 carboxylic acid. Chemical evolution shows that pods contain free and combined (0- and c-glycosides) (Akireme *et al.*, 2000). The root and its bark contain fistucacidin, flavonoids and phlobaphenes (Behl *et al.*, 1993). In addition to all these, other compounds documented in the plant include rheinglucoside, galactomannan, oxyanthraquinone substances, emodin and chrysophanic acid.

Pharmacology

There are many *Cassia* sp. worldwide which are used in herbal medicine systems but this particular family of the plants used widely for their laxative actions. It is often used as a highly affective moderate laxative that is safe even for children. The seeds are used in the treatment of many ailments. It is useful in the skin disorders, jaundice, constipation, typhoid, swollen throat and biliousness. It has been used in traditional Ayurvedic medicine for the treatment of cardiovascular diseases. Seed appear to have anticancer, antioxidant and antibacterial properties. Leaves have antibacterial and anti inflammatory activity; they are used to treat boils, erysipelas, malaria, rheumatism, ulcers, burning sensation (while urination), cough, chest complaints, eye ailments, flu, and liver ailments. Juice and paste of the leaves are used to cure skin diseases, eczema, ringworm and can be used as blood purifier. Roots have strong purgative property and it is affective against blood dysentery, pain in ribs, tumor, intestinal worms, burning sensation, leprosy, skin diseases, syphillis, tubercular glands and in case of snake bite.

Cassia fistula bark extracts CFA (aq.) and CFM (methanolic) possess significant antibacterial, anti-inflammatory and anti-oxidant properties. *Amaltas* flowers have demulcent and lubricating properties. The fruit pulp is a soft laxative and acts as anti-pyretic, antibacterial and a diuretic agent. It can be used in heart and chest infection (as tonic), spleen disorder, tonsils, wound infection and in constipation. Fruit extract in combination with a permeating substance, such as diethyl sulfoxide may be effective in treating cutaneous leishmaniasis. The pulp is used to combat anthrax, blood poisoning, backwater fever, dysentry and malaria.

An ethyl alcohol extract of pods and of the stem-bark is considered hypoglycamic, antiviral, anticancerous and used in pimples, burns, syphillis and diarrhoea (Behl *et al.*, 1993). *Amaltas* is also used in liver disorders, upward flow of the abdominal gas, bronchitis, arthritis and some of the metabolic disorders.

References

Abo, K.A., Adevemi, A.A. and Sobowale, A.O., 2001. Microscopic evolution and seasonal variations of anthraquinone of cultivated *Cassia fistula* Linn. *Afric. J. of Med. Sci.*, March–June; 30(1–2): 9–12.

Akanmu, M.A. and Iwalewa, E.O., 2004. Toxicity potentials of *Cassia fistula* fruits as laxatives with reference to senna. *African journal of Biomedical Research*, 7(1): 23–26.

Akireme, A.A., Omobuwajo and Elujoba, 2000. Pharmacopieal standards for the fruits of *Cassia fistula* and *Cassia podocarpa*. *Nigerian Journal of Natural Products and Medicine*, 4: 23–26.

Asolkar, L.V., Kakkar, K.K. and Chakre, O.J., 1992. *Second Supplement to Glossary of Indian Medicinal Plants with Active Principles.* Part I. Publication and Information Directorate, C.S.I.R., New Delhi.

Behl, P.N., Arora, R.B., Srivastava, G. and Malhotra, S.C., 1993. *Herbs Useful in Dermatological Therapy.* CBS Publishers and Distributers, Delhi.

Bhandari, C., 1993. *Vanoushdhi Chandrodaya.* Part I–X. Chowkhamba Sanskrit Sansthan, Varanasi.

Bhattacharjee, S.K., 1998. *Handbook of Medicinal Plants.* Pointer Publisher, Jaipur.

Bhawasar, R.C., Guru, L.V. and Chadha, A.K., 1965. Antibacterial activity of some indigenous medicinal plants. *Med. Surg.*, 5: 11.

Bown, D., 1995. *Encyclopedia of Herbs and their Uses.* Dorling Kindersley, London.

Chatterjee, A. and Pakrashi, S.C., 1991. *The Treatise on Indian Medicinal Plants, Vol. 1.* Publications and Information Directorate, C.S.I.R., New Delhi.

Chatterjee, A. and Pakrashi, S.C., 1992. *The Treatise on India Medicinal Plants, Vol. 2.* Publications and Information Directorate, C.S.I.R., New Delhi.

Chatterjee, A. and Pakrashi, S.C., 1995. *The treatise on India Medicinal Plants, Vols. 1–4.* Publications and Information Directorate, C.S.I.R., New Delhi.

Chevallier, A., 1996. *Encyclopedia of Medicinal Plants.* D.K. Publishing, New York, p. 141–273.

Chopra, R.N., Nayar, S.L. and Chopra, I.C., 1956. *Glossary of Indian Medicinal Plants.* Publication and Information Directorate, C.S.I.R., New Delhi.

Das, B. and Das, R., 1994. Medicinal properties and chemical constituents of *Vitex negundo Linn. Indian Drugs*, 31(9): 431–435.

Dastur, J.F., 1962. *Medicinal Plants of India and Pakistan*, 2nd edn. D.B. Taraporevala Sons and Co. Private Ltd., Bombay.

Duke, J.A. and Ayensu, E.S., 1985. *Medicinal Plants of China.* Reference Publications, Inc.

Harvey Wickes Felter, M.D., and John Uri Lloyd, Phr. M., Ph.d., 1898. *Kings American dispensatory. Cassia fistula* (U.S.P.)–*Cassia fistula*. Illustrated by Bentley and Trimen. *Med. Plants*, pp. 87.

Holdrige and Poveda, 1975; Irwin and Burneby, 1982; Isely, 1975 and Little and others, 1967. Henriatte's Herbal Homepage Part II *Species Descriptions–Cassia fistula* L. pp. 366.

Jixian, G.U.O., 1997. *Pharmacopoia of People's Republic of China.* The Pharmaceutical Commission of P.R.C., Chemical Industry Press, Beijing, China, pp. 61.

Kaushik, P. and Dhiman, A.K., 2000. *Medicinal Plants and Raw Drugs of India.* Bishen Singh Mahendra Pal Singh, Dehradun.

Khanna, S., Gupta, S.R. and Grover, J.K., 1986. Effect of long term feeding of tulsi on reproductive performance of adult albino rats. *Indian Journal of Experimental Biology*, 24: 302–304.

Khurana, M., 1959. *Indian Journal of Pharmacology*, 21: 331.

Kirtikar, K.R. and Basu, B.D., 1975 (Reprint of 1935 Edition). *Indian Medicinal Plants*, 2nd Edition. vol. I–IV, Revised by E. Blatter, J.F. Caius and K.S. Mahaskar, Bishen Singh Mahendra Pal Singh, Dehradun.

Nadkarni, K.M., 1976 *Indian Material Medica.* Popular Book Depot, Bombay.

Navneet, Prabhat and Shri Krishna, 2004. *A. catechu:* A valuable medicinal plant. *Vedic Path, Gurukul Research Journal*, p. 158–163.

Purohit, S.S., Sharma, A.K. and Kumar, T., 2003. The antiplatelet activity of *Acacia nilotica* is due to blockade of calcium influx through membrane calcium channels. *Pharmacology*, 29: 251–255.

Reddy, B.M., Rao, N.K. and Radhmesh, M., 1993. *International Journal of Pharmacognosy*, 32(4): 553–556.

Sharma, P., Dyal, R. and Ayyar, K.S., 1997. Chemical constituents of *A. catechu* leaves. *Journal of the Indian Chemical Society*, 74: 60.

Subramanian, P.M. and Misra, G.S., 1978. Leucoanthocyanidins of *Vitex negundo*. *Indian J. Chem.*, 16 B(7): 615–616.

Tewari, R.K., Dadhwal, K.S. and Solanki, K.R., 2001. *National Research Center for Agroforestry*, Jhansi. 1607–8317, Issue January to March, Volume, 11, 1.

Thakkar, G.C., 1994. *Introduction of Ayurveda* A.S.I. Publishers. Incorporated, New York.

Yadav, R.N. and Sodhi, S., 2002. A new flavone glycoside 5,7,3,4-tetrahydroxy-3 methoxy flavone 7-O-β-D glactopyranosyal (1 to 4) O-β-glucopyranoside from the stem of *A. catechu* wild. *Journal of Asian Natural Product Research*, 4: 11–15.

Zhu., P.Y., 1998. *Chinese Material Medica*. Hartwood Academic Publishers, Amsterdam, Netherlands, pp. 633.

Medicinal Plants: Conservation, Cultivation and Utilization (2007) *Pages 319–323*
Editors: **A.K. Chopra, D.R. Khanna, G. Prasad, D.S. Malik and R. Bhutiani**
Published by: **DAYA PUBLISHING HOUSE**

Chapter 40

Conservation Practices and Utilization Strategies of Medicinal Plants in Bhandara District of Vidarbha Region

Deepak D. Ramteke[1], Nitin Dongarwar[2], S.B. Zade[3] and C.J. Khune[3]
[1]Department of Botany, M.B. Patel College, Sakoli
[2]P.G. Department of Botany, Nagpur University Nagpur
[3]Department of Zoology, M.B. Patel College, Sakoli

ABSTRACT

We have rich tradition of medicine and health care. Our cultural heritage is enriched with presence of Unani and Siddha system of medicine. Fairly comprehensive information about herbs has been recorded in Charak Samihita and Sushruta Samhita.

The present work has been done in Bhandara district of east Vidarbha region of Maharashtra. The paper includes important medicinal plants, which are endangered and threatened. It also include survey, conservation, cultivation along with their utilization with respect to economic, ethnomedicinal and ethnobotanical properties.

The Bhandara district is a part of east Vidarbha region, Maharashtra State and occupied tropical dry deciduous forest with max-range of annual rain fall is 176.9 mm and minimum rainfall is 146.6 mm as well as max temp. is 21.00°C. and possess vast biodiversity in Medicinal Plant's. It is a tribal area and includes the main tribes like Gond, Halbi, Bhill, Korku, Katkari, Dhiwar, Mana.

Keywords: *Bhandara, Charak Samhita, Sushrut Samhita, Vidharbha, Gond, Korku, Katkari, Dhiwar.*

Introduction

Medicinal plants are the local heritage with global importance. Herbs have always been the principle form of medicine in India. It is estimated that around 70 thousand plant species at one time have been used for medicinal purposes. The Rigveda, Yajurveda, Charak Samhita, Sushrata Samhita, describes properties and uses of various medicinal plants in Ayurvedic system of medicine.

There is a great commercial demand for pharmacopoeial drugs and their products in India. Efforts have been made to introduce many drug plant under conservation and utilization. The present research have undertaken studies on conversation along with utilization of medicinal plants which are economically, ethanobotanically and ethanomedically important. There is need to give priority to conservation of endangered and threatened medicinal plants.

Methodology

The various medicinal plants for this study are collected from different locations of the district. The different medicinal plants or plant parts are brought in laboratory. The plant is morphotaxonomically studied. Information related to its chemical analysis is studied. This is important to study mode of action of chemical constituent on organism. Then study the information regarding the uses of particular plant or its parts to cure various diseases have been collected. Some times decoction of plant is used. In some cases the different plant parts are mixed together and used as drug. The specimens are preserved in herbarium. The visual charts of plants with various information is prepared and stored.

Generally following methods are applied for the study and chemical constituents of the plants like alkaloids, steroids, glycosides, corticosteroids essential oil etc.

The plant was defatted with Petroleum ether, especially in case of seeds and leaf, before applying this treatment alkaloid should be tested for its solubility in Petroleum ether. The drug should be pretreated with acid to convert the alkaloid into their salts. In second stage the drug may be extracted with Polar Solvent like water, ethanol, methanol, aqueous alcohol mixture or with acidified aqueous solution. It also helps in removing pigment, sugars and other organic secondary constituents. The alcohol solution is evaporated to a thick syrup and was subjected to partitions between aqueous acid solution and an organic solvent.

Following ways does further Purification of crude extract:

1. *Direct crystallization from solvent*: It is very simple method of isolation and may not be useful in case of complex mixture.
2. *Steam distillation*: This method was specially employed for extraction of volatile oils and some alkaloids.
3. *Chromatographic techniques*: This method proved to be ideal for separation of vest number of plant alkaloids and other chemical constituents. The different techniques of chromatography were used for separation of alkaloids, starch, hormones etc. from complex mixture.
4 *Gradient pH technique*: The extraction of plants have variation in asicity depending upon their pH value now pH of aqueous solution was increased gradually by 0.5 increment to pH 9 and extraction was carried out to each pH level with organic solvent.

Observations

Medicinal plants have curative properties due to the presence of various complex chemical substances of different compositions, which are found as secondary plant metabolites. These plants metabolites according to their composition are grouped as alkaloids, glycosides, corticosteroids, essential oil etc. The alkaloids from largest group which includes morphine and codein (poppy), strychnine and brucine (nuxvomica), quinine (cinchona), ergotamine (ergot), hyocyamine (belladona), scolaphomine (datura), reserpine (rauwolfia), aconitine (aconitum), and large number of other. Glycosides froms another important group represented by glycyrrihzin (liquorice), barboline (aloe), cannocides (senna) etc. Cortico steroids have been reported from solasodine (solanum sp.), sennocides (senna), diosgenonin (discorea) etc.

Bhandara district is a part of east Vidarbha region of Maharastra and Vacated neat two national reserve's, Nagzira Wildlife Sanctuary and Navegaon Band National Parks which is rich is medicinal plant and give priority to conserve them for upliftment of tribal peoples of the region.

The plants have different habit and habitat. Generally it is either herb, shrub or tree. These plants are naturally occurring in the region and need specially care. So these plants are considered for study. Due to limitation of paper it is not possible to name all the plants here, but some important plant species are listed here with botanical name, Vernacular Name, Chemical Constituent along with parts used as medicine to cure the disease.

Discussion

Harvesting too much, growing and protection too little.

Medicinal plants needs special protection. Conservation practices and management of medicinal plant for the benefit of life including humankind of the biosphere so that it may yield sustainable benefit to the present generation.

1. Conversation of vulnerable species at grassroots level.
2. Adopt sustainable collection and management practices on public land.
3. Agricultural development.
4. Research have focused to improve basic knowledge about conservation practices and dissemination of plant species.
5. Future research should also link management and conservation of medicinal plant with the development of these resources.

In situ Conservation

Medicinal plants diversity should be conserved at the genetic, species and ecosystem level on long-term basis. There are also some endemic species. Conversation of these widely spread population is possible only through setting up a network of representative medicinal plant reserve.

Ex situ conservation

1. Development of ethnomedicinal and ethnobotanical plant garden. All the medicinal plant known to the various ethnic communities of Bhandara District.
2. Gene banks are developed for medicinal plants found in the region with priority to known rare, endangered, threatened and endemic species.
3. Nursery network is most urgent task in order to ensure immediate availability of plants.

Table 40.1: Some important Medicinal Plants under Study

Sl.No.	Botanical Name	Vernacular Name	Chemical Constituent	Part's Used
1.	*Abelmoschus muschatus*	Maskdana	β-sitosterol	Seed, leaves, root
2.	*Acorus calamus*	Buch	Calaminaol	Rhizome
3.	*Adhatoda vasica*	Adhulsa	Vasicine	Root leaves
4.	*Aloebardadensis*	Ghrit Kumari	Barbaloin	leaves
5.	*Andrographis paniculata*	Bhuinimba	Glucosides	Whole plant
6.	*Asperagus recemosus*	Satavari	Saponins	Root
7.	*Atropa belladonna*	Belladonna	Arparoqines	Leaves, Root
8.	*Bacopa monnieri*	Brahmi	Brahmine	Whole plant
9.	*Bixa orellana*	Sinduri	Bixin	Root, Seed
10.	*Biophytum sensitivum*	Lajollu	Insulin	Whol plant
11.	*Boerhavia diffusa*	Punarnava	Tria contonol	Whole plant
12.	*Cannabis sativa*	Ganja	Terahydo canabinal	Leaves, ft. shoot.
13.	*Casia angustifolia*	Senna	Sennosides	Leaves, pods
14.	*Catharanthus roseus*	Sadabahor	Serpentine	Leaves, pods
15.	*Centella asitica*	Manduk parni	Asiaticoside	Whole plant
16.	*Cinnamonum camphera*	Kapur	Cineol	Root, wood
17.	*Colchicum autumnale*	Saffron	Colchicine	Corm, Seeds
18.	*Coleus forskohli*	Patharchur	Diterpenes	Root, leaves
19.	*Clitoria ternatea*	Aparajeeta	taraxinol	Root, leaves, seeds
20.	*Commiphora mukul*	Gugal	gugulsterone	gum
21.	*Curcumma amada*	Amba haldi	Myrcene	Rhizome
22.	*Chlorophytum borivilianum*	Safed Musli	Saponine	Root
23.	*Equisetum debile*	Khadya nag	Eqicetine	Whole plant
24.	*Holarrhena antidysentrica*	Kurchi	Conessine	Fruit, bark
25.	*Phyllanthus niruri*	Bhuinimba	Lignans	Whole plant
26.	*Rauwolfia serpentina*	Strapgandha	Resrpine	Bark, root, leaves
27.	*Santalum album*	Safed Chandan	Santalbic acid	Wood
28.	*Swertia chirayita*	Chirata	Ophelic acid	Seeds
29.	*Withania somnifera*	Ashwaqandha	Withaferin	Leaves, Root

Conclusion

1. The present research work provides valuable information about medicinal, ethanomedicinal, Ethanobotanical as well as economic importace of these plants.
2. Medicinal study of agricultural tracts and forests of particular area will provide information regarding the significant plants and their parts having medicinal value.
3. The study is important to find out various chemical constituents found in various plants or plant part like alkaloids, glycosides, corticosteroides, essentials etc.
4. The research helps to provide self-employment and upliftment to the tribal people of region.

Acknowledgements

We are very thankful to Prof Dr. R. D. Singh Prinicpal M.B.Patel College Sakoli for providing facilities, encouragement and inspiration.

References

Auhanrkar, S.P., 1991. *Medicinal Plants of Bombay Presidency*, Jodhpur.

Choma, R.N., 1932. *The Indigenous Drugs of India*, Calcutta.

Hooker, J.D., 1875–1891. *Flora of British India, Vols.*, 1-11, London.

Kokate, K.C., Purohit, A.P. and Gohkale, S.B., 1990. *Pharmacognosy*.

Kotwal, P.C., 2004. *Biodiversity Conservation in Managed Forests and Protected Area.*

Nadkarni, K.M., 1927. *Indian Plants and Drugs with their Medical Properties and Uses*, Bombay.

Prajapati, N.D., 2004. *A Handbook of Medicinal Plants*, Jodhpur.

Robinson, T., 1968. *The Biochemistry of Alkaloid.*

Trivedi, P.C., 2004. *Biodiversity Assessment and Conservation.*

Medicinal Plants: Conservation, Cultivation and Utilization (2007) *Pages 325–330*
Editors: A.K. Chopra, D.R. Khanna, G. Prasad, D.S. Malik and R. Bhutiani
Published by: DAYA PUBLISHING HOUSE

Chapter 41

Industrial Utilization and Promotion of Medicinal Plants in India

Shikha Singhal[1] and Amit Agarwal[2]
[1]S-69, Shivalik Nagar, BHEL, Haridwar – 249 403 (UA)
[2]Assistant Professor, Department of Computer Science and Information Technology
Graphic Era Institute of Technology, Dehradun – 248 002 (UA)

ABSTRACT

Medicinal plants are nature's wonderful gift to mankind and are India's ancient heritage of traditional systems of medicines such as ayurveda, siddha, yoga and unani. There has been increasing trend in the awareness and utility of medicinal plants in the health care management. A medicinal herb has attained significant role in health system for both human and animals as a potential source of therapeutics aids. Herbal medicines are being utilized by about 80 per cent of the world's population in the developing countries like India for primary health care system. India is rich in biodiversity of medicinal plants. Industrial utilization of herbal medicine requires the knowledge of plant species and its use as herbal medicine. There are over 1.5 million practioners of traditional medicinal system brings medicinal plants in preventive, promotional and creative application. There is 7800 medicinal drug manufacturing units in India, which require about 2000 tones of herbs annually. Two of the largest users of medicinal plants are China and India. Today scientist, doctors and pharmaceuticals companies are looking at countries like India, China etc for their requirement of medicinal plants. India has opportunity to act as a major player in the global herbs based medicines and products by developing its research development capability. Dabur research foundation, Himalayas health care, Zandu pharmaceuticals, and Reliance life sciences, Hamdard etc are few of them. Due to side effects of synthetic products,

* E-mail: [1]aashikha@gmail.com; [2]agarwals69@ieee.org.

herbal products are gaining popularity in the world market. Recently, considerable attention has been paid to utilize eco-friendly and bio-friendly plant based products for the prevention and cure of different human diseases. Governments or entrepreneurs have not exploited the real potential of these plants. Industrial utilization of these medicinal plants will be helpful in enhancing greenery, generating employment and income to the people and conserving biodiversity. India has the knowledge and skills to develop its research and development capabilities. It is the second largest exporter of medicinal plants. Instead of exporting such large amount valuable resource with very low returns it can think about developing its own research and development capabilities and produce finished goods in the form of modern medicines and health care products derived from plants origin and based on the knowledge of alternative system of medicine. Standardization of products is essential to compete in the market. India has to take us the challenge of leading the drug and herbal market while conserving its rich heritage through proper planning and implementation of policies.

Keywords: *Medicinal plants, Herbal medicine, Health care products, Traditional knowledge.*

Introduction

India is rich in biodiversity of medicinal plants. India has 24 per cent of world's area with 8 per cent of global bio-diversity. Only about 10 per cent of the known medicinal plants are restricted to non-forest habitats. Two of the largest users of medicinal plants are China and India. According to WHO, nearly 80 per cent of the population of developing countries like India rely on traditional medicine, mostly plant drugs for their primary health care needs.

Medicinal plants are nature's wonderful gift to mankind and are India's ancient heritage of traditional systems of medicines such as ayurveda, siddha, yoga and unani. India is sitting on a gold mine of well-recorded and well-practiced knowledge of traditional herbal medicine. Due to the side effect of synthetic products herbal products are gaining popularity in the world market. Recently considerable attention has paid to utilize eco-friendly and bio-friendly plant based products for the prevention and cure of different human diseases. India has not yet exploited the real potential of these medicinal plants.

Strategically, India should enter through these plant-based medicines, which are already accepted in Europe, USA and Japan. Simultaneously it should identify those medicinal plants, which are time tested and dispersed all over in India.

The basic requirement to compete the global market include:

1. Well-documented traditional use.
2. Single plant medicines.
3. Medicinal plants free from pesticides having metal etc.
4. Standardization of herbal medicine.
5. Safety and sustainability.

Medicinal Plants in India

The plants used for medicinal purpose are clubbed under the category of medicinal plants. According to WHO, a medicinal plant is any plant which, in one or more and its organs, contain substances that can be used for therapeutic purposes, or which are precursors for chemo-pharmaceutical semi synthesis. India has 20 per cent plant species of medicinal value (Table 41.1).

Table 41.1: Numbers and Plants Used Medicinally Worldwide (Schippmann *et al.*, 2002)

Country	*Plants Species*	*Medicinal Plant Species*	*Percentage*
China	26092	4941	18.9
India	15000	3000	20.0
Indonesia	22500	1000	4.4
Malaysia	15500	1200	7.7
Nepal	6973	700	10.0
Pakistan	4950	300	6.1
Philippines	8931	850	9.5
Sri Lanka	3314	550	16.6
Thailand	11625	1800	15.5
USA	21641	2564	11.8
Vietnam	10500	1800	17.1

But according to Hamilton (2003), India has about 44 per cent of flora, which is used medicinally.

Table 41.2: Numbers and Percentage of Medicinal Plant Worldwide (Hamilton, 2003)

Country	*Total No. of Native Species of Flora*	*No. of Species of Medicinal Plants*	*% of Flora which is Medicinal*
China	27100	11146	41
India	17000	7555	44
Mexico	30000	2237	7
North America	20000	2572	13
World	297000-510000	52885	10-18

India with rich bio-diversity ranks first in percent flora, which contain active medicinal ingredients. 80 per cent of the exports to developed countries are of crude drugs and not finished formulations leading to low revenue for the country. Thus the export of herbal medicine from India is negligible despite the fact that the country has a rich traditional knowledge and heritage of herbal medicine. Table 41.3 shows the list of some medicinal plants being exported from India.

Indigenous System of Medicine

The traditional health care systems such as Ayurveda, Siddha, Yoga and Unani have been recognized as the original health care systems of India. The name ayurveda comes from two Sanskrit words: Ayur meaning "life" and Veda meaning "knowledge". Siddha means achievements of a process of perfection, through the practice of yoga. Arab and Persian coming from Greece evolved the Unani System of medicine in India. Table 41.4 shows the major Indian medicinal plants used in indigenous systems of medicines.

Table 41.3: Medicinal Plants being Exported from India

Botanical Name	*Part of the Plant*
Aconitum species	Root
Acorus calamus	Rhizome
Adhatoda vasica	Whole plant
Berberis aristata	Root
Cassia angustifolia	Leaf and pod
Colchicum luteum	Rhizome and seed
Hedychium spicatum	Rhizome
Heracleum candicans	Rhizome
Inula racemosa	Rhizome
Juglans regia	Bark
Juniperus communis	Fruit
Juniperus macropoda	Fruit
Picrorhiza kurrooa	Root
Plantago ovata	Seed and husk
Podophyllum emodi	Rhizome
Punica granatum	Flower, root and bark
Rauvolfia serpentina	Root
Rheum emodi	Rhizome
Swertia chirayita	Whole plant
Valeriana jatamansi	Rhizome
Zingiber officinale	Rhizome

There are estimated to be around 25000 effective plant based formulation, used in folk medicine and known to rural communities in India. There are 1.5 million practitioners of traditional medicinal system using medicinal plants in preventive, promotion and curative application. The Department of Indian Systems of Medicine and Homeopathy, responsible for the development and protection of indigenous systems of medicine and utilization of the country's heritage and knowledge base, should take the lead in developing suitable strategies and evolving action programmes to ensure high value addition to these valuable resources.

Opportunity for Industrial Utilization and Promotion of Medicinal Plants in India

Industrial utilization of medicinal plants requires the knowledge of plants species and its use as herbal medicine. India is the second largest exporter of medicinal plants in the world. Instead of exporting such large amount valuable resources with very low returns it can think about developing its own research and development capabilities and produce finished goods in the form of modern medicines and health care products derived from plants origin and based on the knowledge of alternative system of medicine. There is 7800 medicinal drug manufacturing units in India, which require about 2000 tones of herbs annually. Today scientists, doctor and pharmaceuticals companies are looking at countries like India, China etc for their requirement of medicinal plants.

Table 41.4: Major Indian Medicinal Plants Used in Indigenous Systems of Medicine

Botanical Name	*Sanskrit Name*
Abies webbiana	Taleespatra
Achyranthes aspera	Apamarga
Acorus calamus	Vacha
Aloe sp.	Kumari
Andrographis paniculata	Bhoonimba (Kalmeg)
Asparagus adscendens	Mushali
Asparagus racemosus	Shatavari
Bauhinia variegata	Kachnar
Berginia ligulata	Pashan bheda
Clerodendrum serratum	Bharangi
Convolvulus pluricaulis	Shankhapushpi
Hedychium spicatum	Shathi
Mesua ferrea	Nagkesar
Nardostachys jatamansi	Jatamansi
Ocimum sp.	Tulsi
Phyllanthus emblica	Amalika (Amla)
Picrorhiza kurrooa	Kutki
Piper longum	Pippali
Pluchea lanceolata	Rasna
Terminalia arjuna	Arjuna
Terminalia chebula	Haritaki (Harad)
Tinospora cordifolia	Guduchi
Tribulus terrestris	Gokshura
Valeriana jatamansi	Tagar
Vitex negundo	Nirgundi
Withania somnifera	Ashwagandha

A significant number of modern pharmaceuticals drugs are thus based on or derived from medicinal plants. The derivatives of medicinal plants are non-narcotic with little or no side effects. Almost 70 per cent modern medicines in India are derived from medicinal plants. It has been observed that plant based medicines take much less time and expenses than synthetic medicines. Therefore plants based medicines would be cheaper.

In terms of volume of medicinal plants exported, India ranks second in the world. There is a scope for India to act as a major player in the International herb based medicines and products by developing its research and developing capability.

Although India has not been able to convert the grey areas of ayurveda as a major contributor to National Economy, it has huge opportunity for the development of the pharmaceutical and phyto-chemical industry. There has been capability building in India in recent years in the research and development sector of medicinal formulations involving plants and its compounds both in private sector (*i.e.* industry oriented) as well as government funded research. Among the industry oriented research and development institutes in India are Dabur Research Foundation, Himalaya Health Care, Zandu Pharmaceutical, Avestha Gengrein Technologies, Reliance, Hamdard etc. Table 41.5 shows the some of the medicinal plants being imported in India by many pharmaceutical industries.

Table 41.5: Medicinal Plants Being Imported in India

Botanical Name	*Native Name*
Cuscuta epithymum	Aftimum vilaiyti
Glycyrrhiza glabra	Mullathi
Lavendula stoechas	Ustukhudus
Operculina turpethum	Turbud
Piminella anisum	Anise fruit
Smilax china	Chobchini
Smilaxornata	Ushba
Thymus vulgaris	Hasha

Conclusion

Governments or entrepreneurs have not exploited the real potential of medicinal plants. About 2 million hectares of forest area in India can produce medicinal plants for export and domestic use to provide health for our millions. Industrial utilization of medicinal plants will be helpful in enhancing greenery, generating employment and income to the people and conserving biodiversity. The prevalence of a variety of climate conditions puts India in a supreme position with respect to richness of medicinal flora. India should form an agro-technology process technology, standardization, and quality control research development of herbal medicine. It is the time to compile and document the available knowledge on our valuable plant resources and to prove their utilization scientifically through detailed phyto-chemical, biological and pharmacological investigations.

Medicinal Plants: Conservation, Cultivation and Utilization (2007) *Pages 331–339*
Editors: **A.K. Chopra, D.R. Khanna, G. Prasad, D.S. Malik and R. Bhutiani**
Published by: **DAYA PUBLISHING HOUSE**

Chapter 42

Biodeterioration of Aonla (*Emblica officinalis*) and Their Products

Anjma Bhanti, Manisha, Divya Goyal and Seema Bhadauria
Department of Botany, Raja Balwant Singh College, Agra – 282 002, India

ABSTRACT

Aonla is one of the most important indigenous fruit of India, it is highly nutritive and rich source of vitamin C, it is known for its medicinal value and fruits are used in many forms like dry, murabba, pickle, candy, confectionaries, embolic powder, Chutney, tablet, juice etc. It is major component of Triphala, an Ayurvedic medicine. Aonla fruits and their products were found infected by mycoflora that cause diseases. In the present investigation, *Emblica* fruits and *Emblica* products screened for the qualitative and quantitative analysis of different moulds associated with them. The analysis of various samples of *Emblica* fruits and their products revealed the presence of a no. of fungal species such as *Aspergillus, Fusarium, Alternaria, Penicillium, Curvularia, Mycelia sterilia, Rhizopus, Cephalosporium, Cladosporium* and *Mucor.*

Introduction

The medicinal and allied plants offer not only a vast and rich field for investigation but also for utilization in the economy of our country.

For the present investigation *Emblica officinalis* Gaertn. Syn. *Phyllanthus emblica* Lin. (Aonla) has been selected on account of its large scale use in manufacturing of indigenous drugs. Aonla belongs to the family Euphorbiaceae, Sub family Phyllanthiodeae. It is known by several other names such as amla, amlika (Hindi) and Emblic (English). Aonla fruit is found to be acrid, cooling, refrigerant, astringent, diuretic, laxative, tonic and useful in burning sensations, vomiting, urinary discharges, leprosy, the dry fruit is used as an appetizer. The fruit is green changing to light yellow colour when mature. The fruit pulp contains moisture 81.2 per cent, protein 0.5 per cent, fat 0.02 per cent, Fe 1.2 mg/100 gm. Nicotinic acid 0.2 μg/100 gm and vitamin C 600 mg/100 gm of fresh pulp and 921 mg/100 ml of juice, it is a rich source of pectin and perhaps the richest for vitamin C. The fruit is rich in tannins having 28 per cent, which gives on hydrolysis gallic acid, ellagic acid and glucose. The Chemicals derived from plants are being used as architect for various synthetic products in field of medicines, cosmetics and other health risks.

Fungal growth on materials which are used as food and feed not only deteriorate their nutritive value but also contaminate them by producing physiologically active secondary metabolites *i.e.*, mycotoxins. Mycotoxins are a diverse of compounds produced by an equally wide range of fungi. Following infection with these fungi, seeds, nuts and fruits regularly become contaminated with mycotoxins, which may directly or indirectly enter the human food chain. Mycotoxin problems that include associated mycoflora with crude herbals under storage, their role in biodeterioration and mycotoxin contamination have drawn worldwide attention for quality maintenance and therapeutic potential of plant drugs (Bilgrami, 1984). WHO has also paid serious attention on mycotoxin contamination in herbal drugs considering it as a global problem. In the present investigation samples of dried fruits of *Emblica*, Triphala, Chawanprash, Hair oil and Aonla syrup were collected from different areas and analysed to assess magnitude of microbial contamination.

Material and Methods

Collection

In all a total number of 100 samples of *Emblica* products were collected. In each case, sample weighing 100-500 g. were collected in sterilized polythene bags, which were sealed over flame soon after collection and kept in refrigerator at 4°C till analyzed. Usually, samples were screened within a week but never later than a fortnight of their collection.

Determination of Mycoflora Associated with *Emblica* Fruits and their Products

Isolation of Mycoflora from Emblica Fruits and their Products

The mycoflora associated with samples was determined by agar plate technique, using Czapek's media (Hesseltine, 1966, Anonymous, 1966), fruits were surface sterilized with 2 per cent sodium hypochlorite solution for 10 min. and subsequently plated on petridishes containing medium. The plate were incubated at 28 ± 2°C for 5 days in an alternating cycle of 12 hours fluorescent light and 12 hours darkness. After incubation, the plates were examined under stereobinocular microscope on 6th day and fungal population was determined. After incubation period, the plates were studied and colonies of different fungi were counted. Finally, population of fungi per gram of sample was determined. The fungi were identified, subcultured and maintained on Czapek's medium for further study.

Identification, Purification and Maintenance of Fungal Cultures

The different fungal isolates were purified using standard techniques and maintained on Czapek's agar medium. The identification of fungal isolates was made following illustrations and description given by Gilman (1957), Barnett (1960), and Subrahmaniam (1971) and also with the isolates maintained in the Laboratory.

Primary Screening of Aflatoxigenic isolates: Orange Yellow Pigmentation Method

In this Method *Aspergillus* differential Medium (ADM) and coconut agar medium (Raper and Fennel, 1965) were used for determine aflatoxigenic nature of isolates of *Asperillus flavus*. For this purpose, conidia from a test culture were transferred to a plate containing ADM and incubated at 28 ± 1°C for 2 days. Mycelial plug (3 mm in diameter) from the ADM plates were transferred to plate containing coconut agar medium. Each mycelial plug from ADM was placed on the center of a plate-containing test medium and incubated for a period of 1 week. Plates were examined visually for colony morphology and orange yellow pigmentation and then with a UV lamp in a dark room for fluorescence. Intensity of yellow pigmentation was expressed by number of '+' signs.

Determination of Aflatoxins in Samples

The aflatoxin contamination in samples was worked out as follows:

Visual Detection

The samples were screened for blue green yellow fluorescence (BGYF test) under longwave UV light. The samples were placed on a glass sheet and observed under long wave UV light in chromatoview cabinet.

Extraction of Aflatoxins

The samples positive to BGYF test were extracted chemically from natural contamination of aflatoxin. In this method, 50g of powdered samples was taken and blended with 250ml of methanol: water (60:40 V/V) for 15 min at high speed in mixer cum blender. The methanolic extract was filtered through whatman no. l filter paper, than 125 ml of filtrate was taken in 500ml separating funnel, and 30ml of saturated NaCl and 50ml of n-Hexane were added. Separating funnel, as shaken vigorously for 5 minute and upper hexane layer was discarded. Further, 40 ml of chloroform was added and shaken again. The layers were allowed to separate. The lower chloroform layer was obtained into a flask containing 5 g of cupric carbonate and was allowed to settle down. Finally, chloroform layer was decanted through Whatman No 1 filter paper passing through the bed of anhydrous sodium sulphate. The chloroform extract was evaporated to dryness and residue was dissolved in 1 ml of chloroform and used in TLC for qualitative estimation of aflatoxins.

Qualitative Estimation of Aflatoxins

Qualitative estimation of aflatoxin was made by thin layer chromatography (TLC) technique for the preparation of TLC plates, uniform and cleaned glass plates 92 × 20 cm were used. Silica gel-G weighing, 36g was thoroughly mixed with 72ml distilled water to form a slurry, which was immediately used for coating six plates uniformly 90.25-0.30mm thickness with the help of an applicator. The plates were dried at room temperature and then activated in oven at 120°C for 1 hour. The plates were cooled before used finally; chloroform extract was spotted on TLC plate along with the aflatoxin standards.

Solvent system comprising Acetone: Chloroform (1: 9 V/V) was also used for developing plates. The plate was developed by standing it in a chromatography tank containing the appropriate solvent to a depth of not more than 0.5 cm the solvent was allowed to run upward for a distance of 15 cm. Thereafter, the plates were air dried and then examined under long wave (360 nm) UV light in a sample, five replicates were used to study. The characteristics blue and green fluorescence at the same Rf value as that of standard aflatoxin was used identification criteria of aflatoxin B_1, B_2, G_1 and G_2.

Results and Discussion

In the present investigation, emblica fruits and emblica products screened for the qualitative and quantitative analysis of different moulds associated with them. The mycoflora found associated with different products. During storage, the fungal organisms thrive on drug plants by utilizing various components including active ingredient. Biodeterioration in alkaloid, Phenol and protein contents of seeds; fruit and root samples of 21 plants by *A. flavus and P. citrinum, A. niger* was studied at optimum temperature (26±2°C) and RH (90 ± 6 per cent). A general trend of decrease (10–40 per cent) in concentration of all important constituents (except phenols) was recorded under fungal infestation within 60 days of storage.

Table 42.1: Mycoflora Associated with Aonla Based Products

Sl.No	Name of Fungi	Dried Aonla	Chawanprash	Hair oil	Triphala	Aonla Syrup
1.	*Alterneria alternata*	+	+	+	–	+
2.	*Aspergillus flavus*	+	+	+	+	+
3.	*Aspergillus fumigatus*	+	+	+	+	+
4.	*Aspergillus parasiticus*	–	–	+	–	+
5.	*Aspergillus niger*	+	+	+	+	+
6.	*Aspergillus nidulans*	+	+	+	+	+
7.	*Aspergillus sulphureus*	+	–	+	+	–
8.	*Cephalosporium acremonium*	+	+	–	+	–
9.	*Curvularia lunata*	+	–	+	+	+
10.	*Cladosporium epiphyllum*	–	–	+	–	+
11.	*Fusarium epiphyllum*	–	+	–	–	–
12.	*Fusarium moniliforme*	+	+	+	–	+
13.	*Fusarium acuminata*	+	+	–	–	+
14.	*Mucor hiemalis*	+	+	–	–	+
15.	*Mycelia sterilia*	–	–	–	–	+
16.	*Penicillium chrysogenum*	+	–	+	+	–
17.	*Penicillium citrinum*	+	–	+	+	–
18.	*Penicillium janthinellum*	–	+	–	–	+
19.	*Penicillium funiculosum*	+	+	–	+	+
20.	*Rhizopus stolonifer*	+	+	+	+	–
	Total no. of Fungi	**15**	**13**	**15**	**11**	**14**

Total no. of sample analyzed = 100.

Mycoflora Associated with Medicinal Products

Among the various fungal species, *A. flavus* was most dominant and frequent species in most of the foodstuffs studied. The total population of *A. flavus* was recorded in range of 20.30 × 10^3–89.50 × 10^3 colonies/10 g in dried Aonla, 2.00 –18.13 × 10^3 colonies/10 g in chawanprash, 8.00–42.25 × 10^3 colonies/10 g Triphala, 1.25 × 10^3–19.83 × 10^3 colonies/g in hair oil and 1.20-27.00 × 10^3 colonies/g in Aonla syrup.

Emblica Dry Fruit

Emblica dry fruits are commonly used in all Ayurvedic medicines. The analysis of 20 samples of this commodity revealed the presence of 15 fungal species representing 9 genera. These include

5 species of *Aspergillus,* 2 species of *Penicilium* and *Fusarium* and one species each of *Curvularia, Mycelia sterillia, Rhizopus, Cephalosporium, Cladosporium and Alternaria* (Table 42.2). Among all *Aspergillus* species *A. flavus* was found to be most frequent and abundant species. The frequency of *A. flavus and A.fumigatus* were 100.00 per cent.

Table 42.2: Mycoflora of Dried *Emblica* Fruit

Sl.No	Name of Fungi	T.P (Mean)	%F	%A
1.	*Alternaria alternata*	1.33	50	0.93
2.	*Aspergillus flavus*	44.83	100	30.71
3.	*Aspergillus fumigatus*	35.66	100	25.08
4.	*Aspergillus niger*	4.33	50	3.04
5.	*Aspergillus nidulans*	2.5	17.2	5
6.	*Aspergillus sulphureus*	2	12.8	0.18
7.	*Cephalosporium acremonium*	0.16	16.6	0.11
8.	*Curvularia lunata*	1	26	0.12
9.	*Fusarium acuminata*	1	14.2	11
10.	*Fusarium moniliforme*	0.16	16.6	0.11
11.	*Mucor hiemalis*	1.33	27	2.3
12.	*Mycelia sterilia*	1.16	16.6	0.82
13.	*Penicillium citrinum*	2.5	19.5	0.15
14.	*Penicillium funiculosum*	1.5	23	0.73
15.	*Rhizopus stolonifer*	4.16	33.3	6.44
TP	Total population × 10^3/10 gms	103.62		
%F	Percentage frequency		522.8	
%A	Percentage abundance			86.72

Mycoflora Associated with Chawanprash

The analysis of 20 samples of chawanprash obtained from different regions revealed presence of 13 fungi. These include 4 species of *Aspergillus,* 2 species *of Fusarium,* 1 species each of *Penicilium, Alternaria, Cladosporium, Cephalosporium, Curvularia, Mucor, Mycelia sterilia* and Rhizopus. *A. flavus* was most frequent and abundant is chawanprash and was recorded from all samples, its percentage frequency is 100 per cent but the percentage abundance is 30.82 per cent.

Mycoflora Associated with Hair Oil

The analysis of 20 samples of hair oil, showed the presence of 13 fungi. Among them, there are, 6 species of *Aspergillus,* 2 species of *Penicilium,* 1 species each of *Curvularia, Cladosporium, Mycelia sterilia, Rhizopus, Fusarium and Alternaria*

Mycoflora Associated and Triphala

11 fungal species was isolated from 20 samples of Triphala. There were 5 species of *Aspergillus,* 3 species of *Penicilium,* and one species of *Curvularia, Cephalosporium, Rhizopus.*

Table 42.3: Mycoflora of Chawanprash

Sl.No	*Name of Fungi*	*T.P (Mean)*	*%F*	*%A*
1.	*Alternaria alternata*	0.8	30	2.11
2.	*Aspergillus flavus*	4	100	30.82
3.	*A. fumigatus*	4	100	13.69
4.	*A. niger*	3.2	100	10.93
5.	*A. nidulans*	1.2	60	5.74
6.	*Cephalosporium acremonium*	2.2	55	3
7.	*Fusarium epiphyllum*	3	100	12.6
8.	*Fusarium moniliforme*	1	60	4.79
9.	*Fusarium accuminata*	2	50	4
10.	*Mucor hiemalis*	0.5	25	1.2
11.	*Mycelia sterilia*	0.2	20	0.68
12.	*Penicillium funiculosum*	1.4	60	4.79
13.	*Rhizopus stolonifer*	1	60	3.42
TP	Total population × 10^3/10 gms	24.5		
% F	Percentage frequency		820	
% A	Percentage abundance			97.77

Table 42.4: Mycoflora of Aonla Hair Oil

Sl.No	*Name of Fungi*	*T.P (Mean)*	*%F*	*%A*
1.	*Alternaria alternata*	3.11	40.1	1.11
2.	*Aspergillus parasiticus*	0.7	20.1	1.25
3.	*Aspergillus flavus*	4.33	66.6	9.73
4.	*Aspergillus fumigatus*	14.16	66.6	31.83
5.	*Aspergillus nidulans*	0.83	33.3	1.87
6.	*Aspergillus niger*	10.5	100	23.59
7.	*Aspergillus sulphureus*	0.66	17.8	1.8
8.	*Cladosporium epiphyllum*	4	50	4.2
9.	*Curvularia lunata*	11.16	34.8	10.7
10.	*Fusarium moniliforme*	8.5	24.8	9.7
11.	*Penicillium chrysogenum*	0.66	16.6	1.49
12.	*Penicillium citrinum*	0.5	15.6	1.12
13.	*Rhizopus stolonifer*	0.33	33.3	0.74
TP	Total population × 10^3/10 gms	97.77		
%F	Percentage frequency		519.6	
% A	Percentage Abundance			99.13

Table 42.5: Mycoflora of Triphala

Sl.No	Name of Fungi	T.P (Mean)	%F	%A
1.	*Aspergillus flavus*	23.6	100	25.7
2.	*Aspergillus fumigatus*	21.6	100	33.52
3.	*Aspergillus nidulans*	5.6	80	6.1
4.	*Aspergillus niger*	17.6	100	19.17
5.	*Aspergillus sulphureus*	8.8	70	9
6.	*Cephalosporium acremonium*	11.2	80	11.6
7.	*Curvularia lunata*	17.8	80	5.86
8.	*Penicillium chrysogenum*	18.5	60	5.9
9.	*Penicillium citrinum*	3.4	80	3.7
10.	*Penicillium funiculosum*	7.6	30	1.2
11.	*Rhizopus stolonifer*	1.4	40	1.52
TP	Total population × 10^3/10 gms	137.1		
%F	Percentage frequency		820	
%A	Percentage abundance			123.27

Table 42.6: Mycoflora of Syrup

Sl.No	Name of Fungi	T.P (Mean)	%F	%A
1	*Alternaria alternata*	1	66.6	2.38
2	*Aspergillus flavus*	27	100	64.28
3	*Aspergillus fumigatus*	3.33	66.6	7.93
4	*Aspergillus nidulans*	1	66.6	2.38
5	*Aspergillus niger*	1	66.6	2.38
6	*Aspergillus parasiticus*	2.3	75	2.45
7	*Cladosporium epiphyllum*	3.1	72	7.86
8	*Curvularia lunata*	2	100	4.76
9	*Fusarium moniliforme*	2.7	34.5	1.2
10	*Fusarium acuminata*	0.45	29	0.36
11	*Mucor hiemalis*	0.33	33.3	0.79
12	*Mycelia sterilia*	1	33.3	2.38
13	*Penicillium funiculosum*	0.65	27	0.65
14	*Rhizopus stolonifer*	0.34	31.7	0.23
TP	Total population ´ 103/10 gms	46.2		
%F	Percentage frequency		802.2	
%A	Percentage Abundance			100.03

Mycoflora Associated with Aonla Syrup

From 20 samples of Aonla syrup, in all 14 fungi are isolated. These include 2 species of Fusarium and one species of *Cladosporium, Curvularia, Mucor, Mycelia sterilia, Rhizopus, and Penicilium*. The percentage abundance of *Aspergillus* species was highest. The frequency of *A. flavus* was 100 per cent in samples.

In all 20 fungal species belonging to 10 genera were counted in 100 samples of different products: Among them the most common fungi were *A. flavus, A. niger, A. fumigatus*, and *Rhizopus stolonifer* which were found associated with all five products.

Table 42.7: Aflatoxin Associated with Aonla Based Products

Sl.No	Types of Aflatoxin	Dried Aonla	Chawanprash	Hair oil	Triphala	Aonla Syrup
1.	B_1	+	+	–	+	–
2.	B_2	–	+	+	+	+
3.	G_1	+	–	–	+	+
4.	G_2	–	–	–	–	–

Occurrence of Alfatoxin in Emblica Based Medicinal Products

4 Aflatoxins namely B_1, B_2 and G_1 were found in samples.

In case of dried Aonla, samples collected were noted to contain aflatoxin B_1 (12 out of 20) samples were found contaminated with aflatoxin. Aflatoxin G_1 could be detected in the dried emblica fruits samples. Among the 20 samples of chawanprash Aflatoxin B_1 was detected in 16 samples, aflatoxin B_2 was recorded in 10 samples. All together 7 samples (out of 20) of Hair oil were found contaminated with aflatoxins B_2. The analysis of 20 samples of Triphala revealed presence alfatoxin B_1 in 7 samples (out of 20) aflatoxin–B_2 was recorded in 5 samples Alftatoxin G_1 was present in 3 samples. In case of Aonla syrup, 20 samples were analyzed and out of them 12 were found contaminated with different aflatoxins (B_2 and G_1).

Conclusion

The analysis of various samples of *Emblica* fruits and their products revealed the presence of a no. of fungal species such as *Aspergillus, Fusarium, Alternaria, Penicilium, Curvularia, Mycelia sterillia, Rhizopus, Cephalosporium, Cladosporium and Mucor*. Being rich source of vitamin C and useful in Ayurvedic preparations, these products were found to be highly infected but only 3 Aflatoxins were recorded *i.e.* B_1, B_2, G_1. So there is a great need of quality assured production of these medicinal products for Good Manufacturing Practices (GMP).

References

Anonymous, 1960. *Herb, IM, Handbook*. Commonwealth Mycological Institute, Ferry lane, Kew, Surrey, England.

Barnett, H.L. and Hunter, B.B., 1972: *Illustrated Genera of Imperfect Fungi*, 3rd edn. Burgess Publishing Company, pp. 241.

Bilgrami, K.S., 1984. Mycotoxins in food. *J. India Bot. Soc.*, 63: 109–120.

Gilman, J.C., 2001. *A Manual of Soil Fungi*. Biotech Books, Delhi, pp. 392.

Hesseltine, C.W., 1952. A survey of the Mucorales. *Trans N.Y. Sci. Ser.*, 2. 14: 210–214.

Subramaniam, C.V., 1975. *Hyphomycetes*. Publ. ICAR, New Delhi, pp. 930.

Raper, K.B. and D.I. Fennel, 1965. *The Genus Aspergillus*. Williams and Wilkins Co., Baltimore.

Medicinal Plants: Conservation, Cultivation and Utilization (2007) *Pages 341–356*
Editors: A.K. Chopra, D.R. Khanna, G. Prasad, D.S. Malik and R. Bhutiani
Published by: DAYA PUBLISHING HOUSE

Chapter 43

Studies on *in vitro* Antimicrobial Activity of Essential Oil of the *Nardostachys jatamansi* and *Zanthoxyllum armatum*

Anupama Gautam[1], Shailu Dalal[2] and G.R.S. Bisht[3]
[1]Department of Botany and Microbiology, Gurukul kangri University, Haridwar
[2]Department of Biotechnology, IIT, Roorkee
[3]Sardar Bhagwan Singh (P.G) Institute of Biomedical Sciences and Research, Balawala, Dehradun

ABSTRACT

Emerging resistance against conventional antibiotics among microbes resulted into shortage of effective chemotherapeutic agents, it was considered worthwhile to look for natural products like essential oils as an alternative to in effective chemotherapeutic agents, pure essential oils have high frequency. Clinical research shows that essential oils have the highest frequency of any natural substance known to man, creating an environment in which disease, bacteria, virus, fungi etc cannot live. In this study essential oils from two medicinal plants namely *Nardostachys jatamansi* and *Zanthoxyllum armatum* were extracted from roots and seeds respectively, their antimicrobial activity were tested against cultures of bacteria and fungi and five essential oils were used to compare the results. The extracts from the medicinal plants showed more activity against the microbes.

Introduction

Essential oils are the subtle, aromatic and volatile liquids extracted from the flowers, seeds, leaves, stems, bark and roots of herbs, bushes, shrubs and trees through distillation. According to ancient Egyptian and Chinese manuscripts, priests and physicians were using essential oils thousands of years before to heal the sick. They are the oldest form of medicine and cosmetic known to man and were considered more valuable than gold. There are 188 references to oils in the Bible.

Aromatherapy is one of the most actively growing forms of alternative medicine combining massage together with counseling and a nice odour. The actual mode of action of essential oil *in vivo* is still far from understanding although there is strong *in vitro* evidence that essential oils can act as an antimicrobial or antioxidant agent or have a pharmacological effect on various tissues. Studies have shown that essential oils have an effect on brain waves and can also alter behavior. (Lis-Balchin, 1997).

The antimicrobial effects of many herbs and spices have been well known for centuries. These properties are attributed to essential oil fraction with inhibition observed against bacteria, yeasts and fungi.

The roots and rhizomes of *Nardostachys jatamansi* DC (Valerianaceae) are used in Indian system of medicine as tranquilizer, nervine tonic, intellect promoting, antihypertensive, antidiarrhoeal and anticolic. The infusion of root is given in hysteria, palpitation and menopause. Recently antidepressant activity of *Nardostachys jatamansi* DC have been investigated (Metkar *et al.*, 2002).

Nardostachys jatamansi DC (Valerianaceae) is critically endangered rhizome bearing medicinal plant, is restricted to specialized habitat since high altitudes of the Himalaya; ranging from 3000 to 5000 m (Airi, *et al.*, 2000). Due to its bactericidal, deodorant, fungicidal, sedative, tonic and anti-inflammatory effects, it has been found to help conditions like insomnia, migraine and stress related conditions etc. It is a good alternative to valerian root (Mishra *et al.*, 1995, Miczak, 1999).

Fennel essential oil is extracted from *Foeniculum vulgare* or *Anethum foeniculum* (Family–Apiaceae). Therapeutic properties of fennel include: aperitif, antiseptic, antispasmodic, carminative, diuretic, insecticide, laxative, stimulant, stomachic, tonic and vermifuge.

Citronella essential oil is obtained from two types of grasses *i.e. Cymbopogon nardus* which is called Ceylon citronella grass, Another species is *Cymbopogon winterians* called Java citronella grass and leaves.

Lemongrass essential oil is extracted from *Cymbopogon citrates* (West Indian Lemongrass).They are found in forests of Karnataka, Maharashtra, Gujarat, Punjab and Uttar Pradesh. Another species is *Cymbopogon flexuosus* (East Indian Lemongrass). Oil is extracted from leaves and flowers It is mainly found in Kerala and forests of Kumaon region of Uttaranchal.

The study regarding the antimycotic activity of the essential oil from Japanese mint promise a good source of natural fungitoxic agents (Pandey, 2003).

In the present investigation essential oils from the roots and rhizome of *Nardostachys jatamansi* DC and seeds of *Zanthoxyllum armatum* were extracted through hydrodistillation apparatus and five other oils *viz.*, Cinnammon, Ajowain, Fennel, Citronella and Lemon grass and tested for their antimicrobial potential.

The literature is scanty regarding the studies on antimicrobial activity in *Nardostachys jatamansi* and *Zanthoxyllum armatum.* It was considered worthwhile to compare these two essential oil with other essential oils with regard to their antimicrobial potential. Uttaranchal state is considered one of the best habitats of these two plants in the country. The work was carried out on the following lines:

1. The procurement of plant materials
2. Isolation of essential oil from root/rhizomes or seeds by steam distillation

3. Preliminary *in vitro* antimicrobial activity of essential oil on some bacterial and fungal species
4. Determination of MIC by disc diffusion method.

Materials and Methods

Plant Materials

The plant materials used for the project are dried seeds of *Zanthoxyllum armatum* (Family Rutaceae) and dried rhizomes of *Nardostachys jatamansi* (Family Valerianaceae) collected from an Ayurvedic shop at Roorkee Pahari Bazar in Uttaranchal State for isolation of their essential oils while following essential oils were used for comparison.

1. Ajowain (*Cuminum cyminum*)
2. Citronella (*Cymbopogon nardus*)
3. Cinnamon (*Cinnamomum zeylanicum*)
4. Fennel (*Anethum foeniculum*)
5. Lemongrass (*Cymbopogon citratus*)

Plant Sample Processing

The dried rhizomes of *Nardostachys jatamansi* (Plate 43.1) and dried seeds of *Zanthoxyllum armatum* (Plate 43.2), were crushed before filling in the Clevenger's apparatus.

Apparatus Used for Isolation

Clevenger's extractor

Isolation of *Nardostachys jatamansi* and *Zanthoxyllum armatum* Essential Oils

Isolation through Clevenger's Extractor

Weighed amount of the dried powdered rhizomes of *Nardostachys jatamansi* or dried powdered seeds of *Zanthoxyllum armatum* are taken in the round bottom flask and distilled water is added to it. The flask is heated with the help of the mantle when vapours of the plant material get collected, in the receiving tube over water (already placed in it).

Media Used for Antimicrobial Assay

For Antibacterial Assay

Nutrient Agar and Nutrient Broth

Constituents	$g\,l^{-1}$
Beef extract	3.0
Sodium chloride	5.0
Peptone	5.0
Agar	15.0
pH	7.5

(For nutrient broth, agar is not added)

Maintenance of Bacterial Cultures

The Bacterial cultures were maintained on nutrient agar slants or in the nutrient broth tubes as and when required and kept at 4°C for further use.

For Antifungal Assay

Sabouraud's Agar Medium

Constituents	gl^{-1}
Peptone	10.0
Dextrose	400
Agar	15.0
pH	5.6

(An antibacteria dye rose bengal was added at the rate of 50 mgl^{-1})

Maintenance of Fungal cultures

The fungal cultures were maintained on potato dextrose agar slants. We have used commercial potato dextrose agar, which comes in powdered form in packet. 39 gms (Hi-media) of PDA was dissolved in 1000 ml of distilled water.

Table 43.1: Cultures Used for Antimicrobial Assay

Numerals	*Bacterial Cultures*
1	*Bacillus cereus*
2	*Salmonella typhi* MTCC 531
3	*Staphylococcus aureus* (AIIMS)
4	*Staphylococcus aureus* (MRSA) KI 2
5	*Staphylococcus aureus* (VRSA) KI 30
6	*Pseudomonas aeruginosa*
7	*Escherichia coli*
8	*Salmonella* sp.
9	*Shigella dysenteriae*
Numerals	*Fungal Cultures*
1	*Aspergillus niger*
2	*Aspergillus flavus*
3	*Aspergillus fumigatus*
4	*Penicillium monotrichales*
5	*Trichoderma viride*
6	*Fusarium graminearum*
7	*Trichoderma* sp.
8	*Candida albicans*
9	*Saccharomyces* cerevisae
10	*A. dermatophyte*

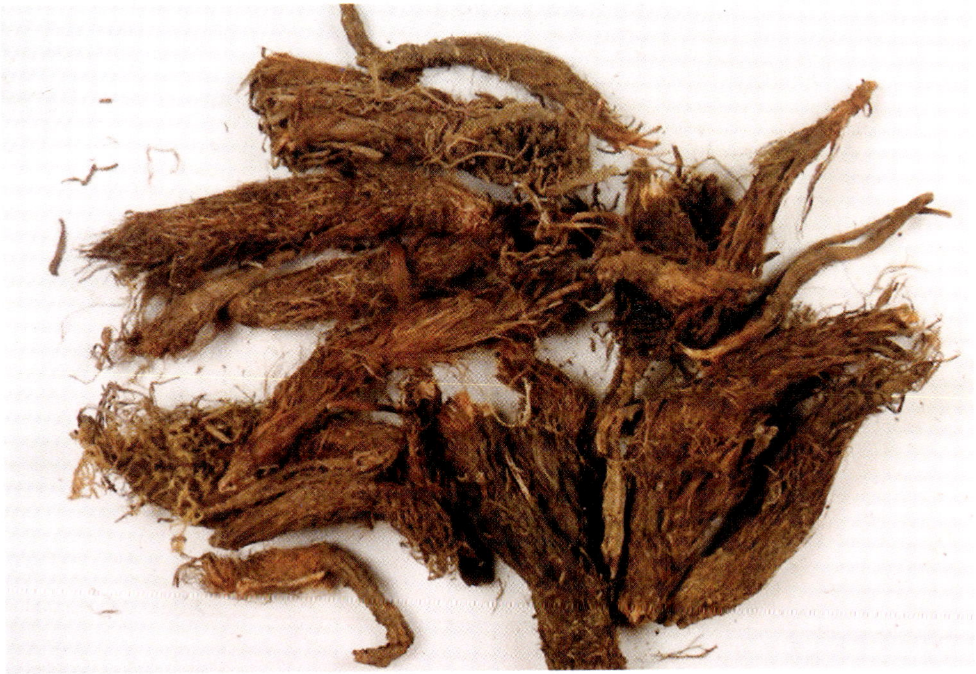

Plate 43.1: Dried Roots and Rhizomes of *Nardostachys jatamansi*

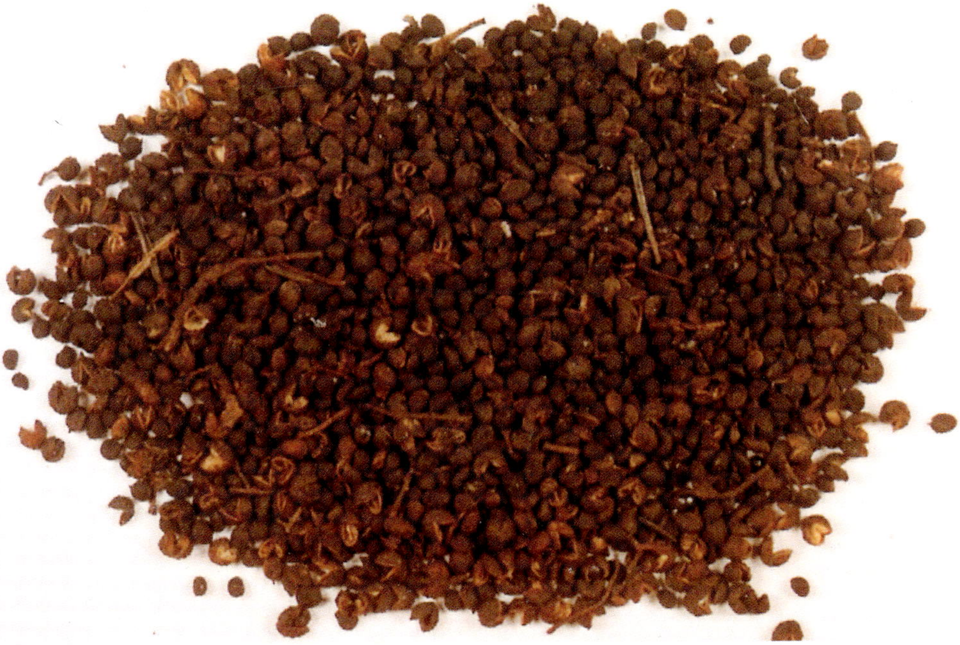

Plate 43.2: Dried Seeds of *Zanthoxyllum armatum*

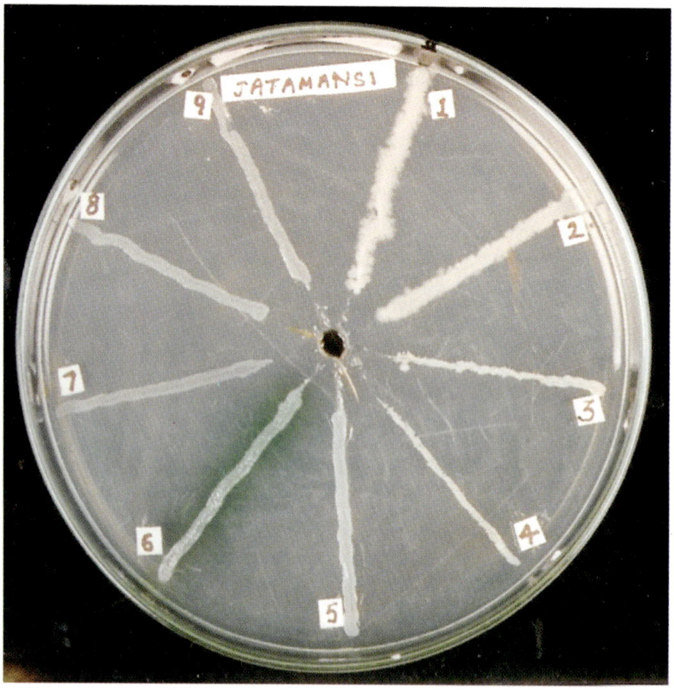

Plate 43.3: Antibacterial Activity of *Nardostachys jatamansi*

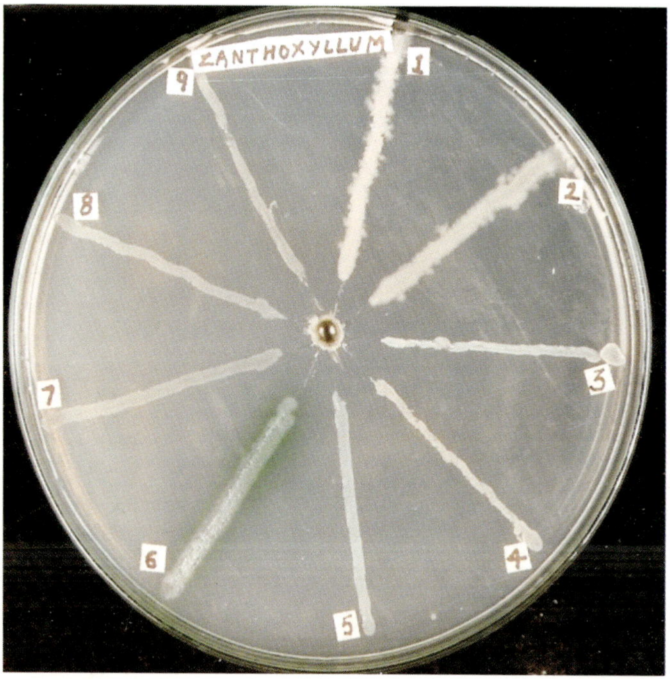

Plate 43.4: Antibacterial Activity of *Zanthoxyllum armatum*

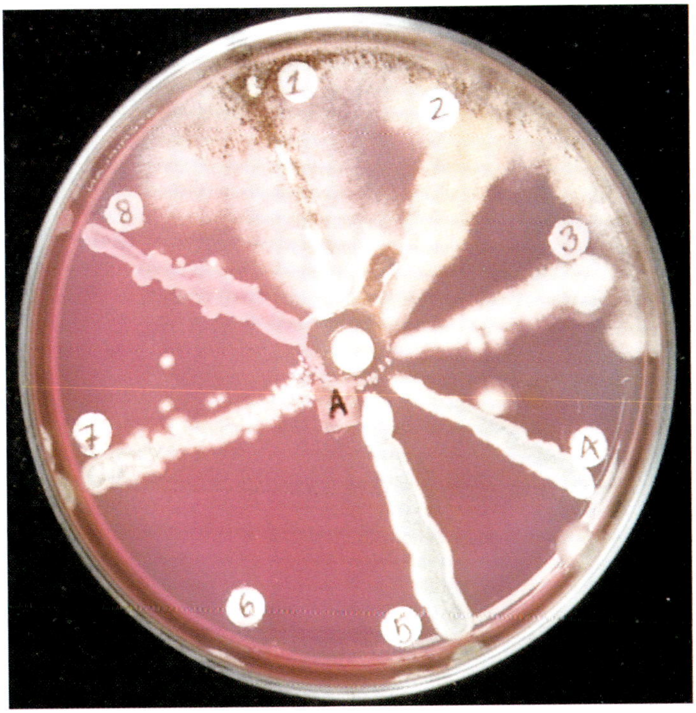

Plate 43.5: Antifungal Activity of *Nardostachys jatamansi*

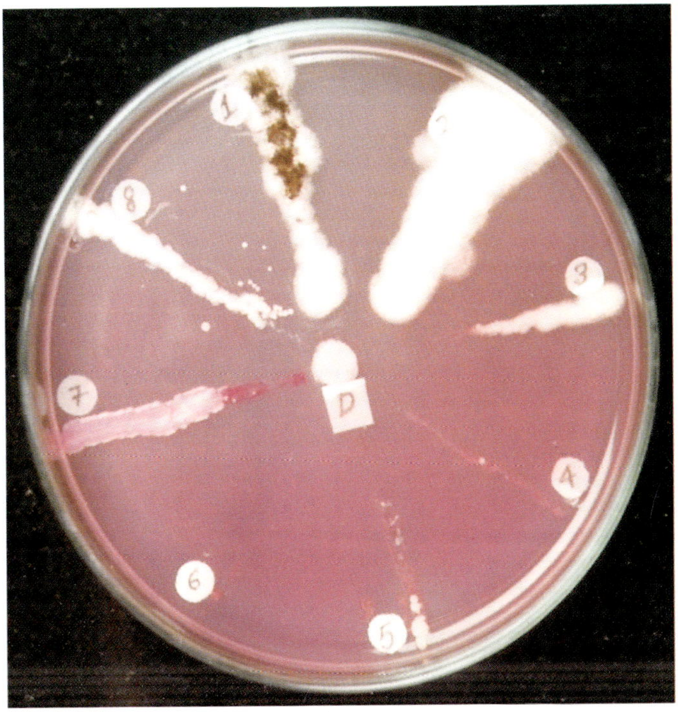

Plate 43.6: Antifungal Activity of *Zanthoxyllum armatum*

Apart from above fungal cultures *Mucor mucedo* has also been used as test organism for determining the MIC values of Cinnamon essential oil.

Assay for Antimicrobial Activity

Assay for Antibacterial Activity

Preparation of Nutrient Agar Plates

About 60 ml to 70 ml of molten nutrient agar medium cooled to 45ºC was added to pre-sterilized Petriplates (150mm) and allowed to solidify. Solidified nutrient agar plates were taken and wells were made with the help of a sterilized cork borer (6 mm diameter).

Determination of Antibacterial Activity

A Petriplate was taken for each essential oil and 20µl oil was poured in the well with the help of a sterilized micropipette. Then nine cultures of bacteria were streaked one by one from center to the periphery of the Petriplate radially of the well with the help of an inoculating loop. The Petriplates were incubated at 37ºC for 24 hours. The inhibition zone diameter (mm) were observed and recorded.

Assay for Antifungal Activity

Preparation of Sabouraud Agar Plates

About 60ml to 70 ml of molten Sabouraud agar medium cooled to 45ºC was added to pre-sterilized Petriplates (150 ml) and allowed to solidify.

Disc Diffusion Method for Antifungal Activity

Whatmann No.1 filter paper was used to cut 6mm size paper discs by a punching machine. These discs were sterilized at 121ºC for 30 minutes at 15 lbs. At the centre of the Petriplate a disc was positioned and then 20µl of each essential oil was soaked on the disc. Then 3-4 days old cultures of fungal strains were streaked one by one over the agar plates radially. The Petriplates were incubated at 27ºC for 3-5 days. The inhibition zone diameter (mm) were observed and recorded.

Determination of Minimum Inhibitory Concentration (MIC) of essential oils of Ajowain, Cinnamon and Zanthoxyllum

Minimum Inhibitory Concentration (MIC) level of any antimicrobial substance is the lowest concentration that inhibit the microbial growth. The MIC value of those microorganisms against a particular fraction is considered which exhibits a maximum activity in preliminary screening process by disc diffusion plate method.

For determining lowest active concentration of respective essential oils, the methodology applied in preliminary screening methods were followed except that different concentrations of essential oils diluted in 2 per cent Dimethylsulfoxide (DMSO) *viz.*, 12.5, 6.25, 3.12, 1.56, 0.78 and 0.19 percent (v/v) for Ajowain and Zanthoxyllum while 6.25, 3.12, 1.56, 0.78, and 0.19 percent for Cinnamon oil.

These concentrations were added to the respective seeded petriplates with different test organisms and incubated as required for optimum growth. The inhibition zone diameters were observed and recorded.

Results and Discussion

Screening for Antimicrobial Activity of Various Essential Oils

The antimicrobial activity is shown in terms of Inhibition Zone Diameter in millimeter in parenthesis along with the microorganism.

Screening for Antibacterial Activity

Analyzing the experimental results from Table 43.2 it is evident that seven essential oils show antibacterial activity.

1. *Jatamansi* essential oil found to be active against *Bacillus cereus, Salmonella typhi* MTCC 531,*Staphylococcus aureus* (AIIMS), *Staphylococcus aureus* KI 2, *Staphylococcus aureus* KI 30, *Pseudomonas aeruginosa, Escherichia coli, Salmonella sp.* and *Shigella dysentriae* with the highest activity against *Staphylococcus aureus* KI 2 (36) and lowest against *Salmonella typhi* (20) (Plate 43.3).

Table 43.2: Preliminary Antibacterial Activity of Different Essential Oils on Various Species of Bacteria by Agar Well Diffusion Method

Sl.No.	*Test Organism*	*Inhibition Zone Diameter (mm)**							
		Jatamansi	*Cinnamon*	*Lemongrass*	*Ajowain*	*Citronella*	*Fennel*	*Zanthoxyllum*	*Gentamycin 10µg*
1.	*Bacillus cereus*	24	30	26	28	18	22	24	24
2.	*Salmonella typhi* MTCC531	20	32	28	28	26	22	24	20
3.	*Staphylococcus aureus* (AIIMS)[1]	26	34	30	30	26	24	24	20
4.	*S. aureus* KI2[2]	36	32	32	32	24	32	28	15
5.	*S. aureus* KI30[2]	28	32	32	32	20	32	26	12
6.	*Pseudomonas aeruginosa*	24	32	38	34	26	34	24	22
7.	*Escherichia coli*	28	26	36	26	30	34	24	20
8.	*Salmonella* sp.	32	38	38	36	26	36	18	20
9.	*Shigella dysenteriae*	26	32	32	34	28	32	24	20

* Average of three wells (20µl/well); [1] Methicillin and Vancomycin sensitive strain;
[2] Methicillin and Vancomycin resistant strains.

2. *Cinnamon* essential oil found to be active against *B. cereus, S. typhi* MTCC 531, *S. aureus* (AIIMS), *S. aureus* KI 2, *S. aureus* KI 30, *P. aeruginosa, E. coli, Salmonella sp.* and *S. dysentriae* with the highest activity against *Salmonella sp.* (38) and lowest against *E. coli* (26).
3. *Lemongrass* essential oil found to be active against *B. cereus, S. typhi* MTCC 531,*S. aureus* (AIIMS), *S. aureus* KI 2, *S aureus* KI 30, *P. aeruginosa, E. coli, Salmonella sp.* and *S. dysentriae* with the highest activity against *P. aeruginosa* and *Salmonella sp.* (38) and lowest against *B. cereus* (26).
4. *Ajowain* essential oil found to be active against *B. cereus, S. typhi* MTCC 531,*S. aureus* (AIIMS), *S. aureus* KI 2, *S. aureus* KI 30, *P. aeruginosa, E. coli, Salmonella sp.* and *S. dysentriae* with the highest activity against *Salmonella sp.* (36) and lowest against *E. coli* (26).
5. *Citronella* essential oil found to be active against *B. cereus, S. typhi* MTCC 531, *S. aureus* (AIIMS), *S. aureus* KI 2, *S. aureus* KI 30, *P. aeruginosa, E. coli, Salmonella sp.* and *S. dysentriae* with the highest activity against *E. coli* (30) and lowest against *B. cereus* (18).
6. *Fennel* essential oil found to be active against *B. cereus, S. typhi* MTCC 531, *S. aureus* (AIIMS), *S. aureus* KI 2, *S. aureus* KI 30, *P. aeruginosa, E. coli, Salmonella sp.* and *S. dysentriae* with the highest activity against *Salmonella sp.* (36) and lowest against *B. cereus* and *S. typhI* MTCC 531 (22).

7. *Zanthoxyllum* essential oil found to be active against *B. cereus, S. typhi* MTCC 531, *S. aureus* (AIIMS), *S. aureus* KI 2, *S. aureus* KI 30, *P. aeruginosa, E. coli, Salmonella sp.* and *S. dysentriae* with the highest activity against *S. aureus* KI 2 (28) and lowest against *Salmonella sp.* (18) (Plate 43.4).

Screening for Antifungal Activity

Analyzing the experimental results from Table 43.3 it is evident that Cinnamon, Ajowain and Zanthoxyllum essential oil show maximum antifungal activity.

Table 43.3: Preliminary Antifungal Activity of Different Essential Oils on Various Species of Fungi by Disc Diffusion Method

Sl.No.	Test Organism	Inhibition Zone Diameter (mm)*						
		Jatamansi	Cinnamon	Lemongrass	Ajowain	Citronella	Fennel	Zanthoxyllum
1.	*Aspergillus niger*	12	>40	12	NI	12	12	18
2.	*A. flavus*	12	36	10	NI	10	12	20
3.	*A. fumigatus*	14	>40	12	NI	20	14	40
4.	*Penicillium monotrichales*	14	>40	14	20	16	12	>40
5.	*Trichoderma viride*	14	>40	16	>40	14	14	>40
6.	*Fusarium graminearum*	–	–	–	–	–	–	–
7.	*Trichoderma sp.*	16	40	16	10	18	14	25
8.	*Candida albicans*	16	18	12	10	16	14	18

*: Average of triplicate discs; –: No growth; NI: No Inhibition

1. *Jatamansi* essential oil found to be active against *Aspergillus niger, Aspergillus flavus, Aspergillus fumigatus, Penicillium monotrichales, Trichoderma viride, Trichoderma sp.* and *Candida albicans* with the highest activity against *Trichoderma sp.* and *Candida albicans* (16) and lowest against *Aspergillus niger* and *Aspergillus flavus* (12) (Plate 43.5).
2. *Cinnamon* essential oil found to be active against *A. niger, A. flavus, A. fumigatus, P. monotrichales, T. viride, Trichoderma sp.* and *C. albicans* with the highest activity against *A. niger, A. fumigatus, P. monotrichales* and *T.* viride (>40) and lowest against *C. albicans* (18).
3. *Lemongrass* essential oil found to be active against *A. niger, A. flavus, A. fumigatus, P. monotrichales, T. viride, Trichoderma sp.* and *C. albicans* with the highest activity against *T. viride* and *Trichoderma sp.*(16) and lowest against *A. flavus* (10).
4. *Ajowain* essential oil found to be active against *P. monotrichales, T. viride, Trichoderma sp.* and *C. albicans* with the highest activity against *T. viride* (>40) and lowest against *Trichoderma sp.* and *C. albicans* (10).
5. *Citronella* essential oil found to be active against *A. niger, A. flavus, A. fumigatus, P. monotrichales, T. viride, Trichoderma sp.* and *C. albicans* with the highest activity against *A. fumigatus* (20) and lowest against *A. flavus* (10).
6. *Fennel* essential oil found to be active against *A. niger, A. flavus, A. fumigatus, P. monotrichales, T. viride, Trichoderma sp.* and *C. albicans* with the highest activity against *A. fumigatus, T. viride, Trichoderma sp.* and *C. albicans* (14) and lowest against *A. niger, A. flavus* and *P. monotrichales* (12).

7. *Zanthoxyllum* essential oil found to be active against *A. niger, A. flavus, A. fumigatus, P. monotrichales, T. viride, Trichoderma sp.* and *C. albicans* with the highest activity against *P. monotrichales* and *T. viride*, (>40) and lowest against *A. niger*, and *C. albicans* (18) (Plate 43.6).

Antifungal Susceptibility Test Against Three Antibiotics

The three antibiotics Amphotericin-B, Nystatin, Fluconazole were taken as control and show antifungal activity as shown in Table 43.4.

Table 43.4: Antifungal Susceptibility Test of Different Fungi Against Three Antibiotics

Sl.No.	*Test Organism*	*Inhibition Zone Diameter (mm)**		
		Amphotericin B	*Nystatin*	*Fluconazole*
1.	*Aspergillus niger*	16	18	NI
2.	*A. flavus*	NI	NI	NI
3.	*A. fumigatus*	NI	14	10
4.	*Penicillium monotrichales*	NI	ND	ND
5.	*Trichoderma viride*	NI	ND	ND
6.	*Fusarium graminearum*	NG	NI	NI
7.	*Trichoderma sp.*	14	ND	ND
8.	*Candida albicans*	16	12	NI
9.	*Saccharomyces cerevisae*	ND	14	NI

*: Average of three discs; NI: No Inhibition; ND: Not determined; NG: No growth.

1. Amphotericin-B shows antifungal activity against *Aspergillus niger, Trichoderma sp.* and *Candida albicans* with highest activity against *Aspergillus niger* and *Candida albicans* (16) and lowest against *Trichoderma sp.* (14).
2. Nystatin shows antifungal activity against *A. niger, A. fumigatus, C. albicans* and *Saccharomyces cerevisae* with highest activity against *A. niger* (18) and lowest against *C.albicans* (12)
3. Fluconazole shows low antifungal activity against *Aspergillus fumigatus* (10) among all antifungal antibiotic tested.

It is noteworthy to mention here that the antifungal antibiotics *viz.*, Amphotericin-B, Nystatin and Fluconazole has shown lower *in vitro* antifungal activity against some fungal species than tested different essential oils.

Determination of Minimum Inhibitory Concentration (MIC) of Three essential Oils Namely Ajowain, Cinnamon and Zanthoxyllum

MIC tests lack reliability because their outcome depends too heavily on variable experimental conditions such as medium composition, pH, temperature and inoculum size etc. (Koneman, 1997).

MIC of Zanthoxyllum Essential Oil

Different MIC are observed in terms of inhibition zone diameter (mm) which is shown in Tables 43.5 and 43.9.

Zanthoxyllum essential oil against *Aspergillus flavus* has MIC value at 6.25 per cent concentration, against *Penicillium monotrichales* has MIC value at 3.12 per cent concentration, against *Trichoderma viride* has MIC value at 1.56 per cent concentration while against *Fusarium graminearum* it has MIC value at 0.78 per cent concentration.

The above results indicate that the MIC levels of Zanthoxyllum essential oil are different for different fungal species.

Table 43.5: Determination of Minimum Inhibitory Concentration (MIC) of Essential Oil of *Zanthoxyllum armatum* against Some Fungal Species

Sl.No.	% Concentration (v/v)	Inhibition Zone Diameter (mm)*			
		Aspergillus flavus	*Penicillium monotrichales*	*Trichoderma viride*	*Fusarium graminearum*
1.	12.5	20	25	28	30
2.	6.25	10	16	16	20
3.	3.12	–	12	10	18
4.	1.56	–	–	08	16
5.	0.78	–	–	–	10
6.	0.39	–	–	–	–
7.	Cycloheximide (50 μg/ml)	11	20	20	25

*: Average of triplicate discs; –: No Inhibition.

MIC of Ajowain Essential Oil

Different MIC are observed in terms of inhibition zone diameter (mm), which is shown in Table 43.6 and 43.9.

Table 43.6: Determination of Minimum Inhibitory concentration (MIC) of Essential Oil of Ajowain Against Some Fungal Species

Sl.No.	% Concentration (v/v)	Inhibition Zone Diameter (mm)*		
		Aspergillus flavus	*Trichoderma viride*	A Dermatophyte
1.	12.50	18	25	20
2.	6.25	10	18	15
3.	3.125	08	14	10
4.	1.56	–	12	–
5.	0.78	–	–	–
6.	0.39	–	–	–
7.	Cycloheximide (50 μg/ml) (as control)	11	18	10

*: Average of triplicate discs; –: No Inhibition.

Ajowain essential oil against *A. flavus* has MIC value at 3.125 per cent concentration, against *T. viride* has MIC value at 1.56 per cent concentration and with a dermatophyte it has MIC value at 3.125 per cent concentration.

The above results indicate that the MIC levels of Ajowain essential oil are same for two fungal species *i.e.* for *A. flavus* and a dermatophyte.

MIC of Cinnamon Essential Oil

Different MIC are observed in terms of inhibition zone diameter (mm), which is shown in Table 43.8 and 43.9.

Table 43.7: Determination of MIC Values of Essential Oil of Cinnamon Against Some Fungal Species

Sl.No.	*% Concentration (v/v)*	*Inhibition Zone Diameter (mm)**				
		Aspergillus niger	*Penicillium monotrichales*	*Trichoderma viride*	*A. dermatophyte*	*Mucor mucedo*
1.	6.25	22	32	40	15	36
2.	3.12	15	20	35	10	22
3.	1.56	08	16	24	–	12
4.	0.78	–	10	15	–	–
5.	0.39	–	08	10	–	–
6.	0.19	–	–	–	–	–
7.	Cyclohexiemide (50 μg/ml)	10	20	18	14	12

*: Average of triplicate discs; –: No Inhibition.

Cinnamon essential oil against *A. niger* has MIC value at 1.56 per cent concentration, against *P. monotrichales* has MIC value at 0.39 per cent concentration, against *T. viride* has MIC value at 0.39 per cent concentration, against a dermatophyte has MIC value at 3.12 per cent concentration, while against *Mucor mucedo* it has MIC value at 1.56 per cent concentration.

The above results indicate that the MIC levels of Cinnamon essential oil are same for some fungal species.

Determination of MIC Values of Three Essential Oils Against *Staphylococcus aureus* (AIIMS)

Different MIC are observed in terms of inhibition zone diameter (mm), which is shown in Table 43.8.

Table 43.8: Determination of MIC Values of Three Essential Oils Against– *Staphylococcus aureus* (AIIMS)

Sl.No.	*% Concentration (v/v)*	*Inhibition Zone Diameter (mm)**		
		Ajowain	*Cinnamon*	*Zanthoxyllum*
1.	6.25	26	28	26
2.	3.12	22	22	22
3.	1.56	20	20	20
4.	0.78	18	18	16
5.	0.39	14	16	–
6.	0.19	–	–	–
7.	Gentamycin 10 μg/disc	20	18	20

*: Average of triplicate discs; –: No Inhibition.

Above results indicate that MIC of Ajowain and Cinnamon essential oils are same against *Staphylococcus aureus* (AIIMS).

1. *Ajowain* essential oil against *Staphylococcus aureus* (AIIMS) has MIC value at 0.39 per cent concentration.
2. *Cinnamon* essential oil against *Staphylococcus aureus* (AIIMS) has MIC value at 0.39 per cent concentration.
3. *Zanthoxyllum* essential oil against *Staphylococcus aureus* (AIIMS) has MIC value at 0.78 per cent concentration.

Minimum Inhibitory Concentration (MIC) of three essential oils for different organisms

Different MIC are observed in terms of inhibition zone diameter (mm), which is shown in Table 43.9 and Figure 43.1.

Table 43.9: Minimum Inhibitory Concentration (MIC) of Three Essential Oils for Different Organisms

Sl.No.	Organism	% Concentration (v/v) of Essential Oil*		
		Ajowain	Cinnamon	Zanthoxyllum
1.	*Staphylococcus aureus*	0.39	0. 39	0.78
2.	*Aspergillus flavus*	3.125	–	6.25
3.	*Penicillium monotrichales*	–	0.39	3.12
4.	*Trichoderma viride*	1.56	0.39	1.56
5.	*Fusarium graminearum*	–	–	–
6.	*Aspergillus niger*	–	1.56	–
7.	*Mucor mucedo*	–	1.56	–
8.	*A dermatophyte*	3.125	3.12	–

*: Average of triplicate discs; –: No Inhibition.

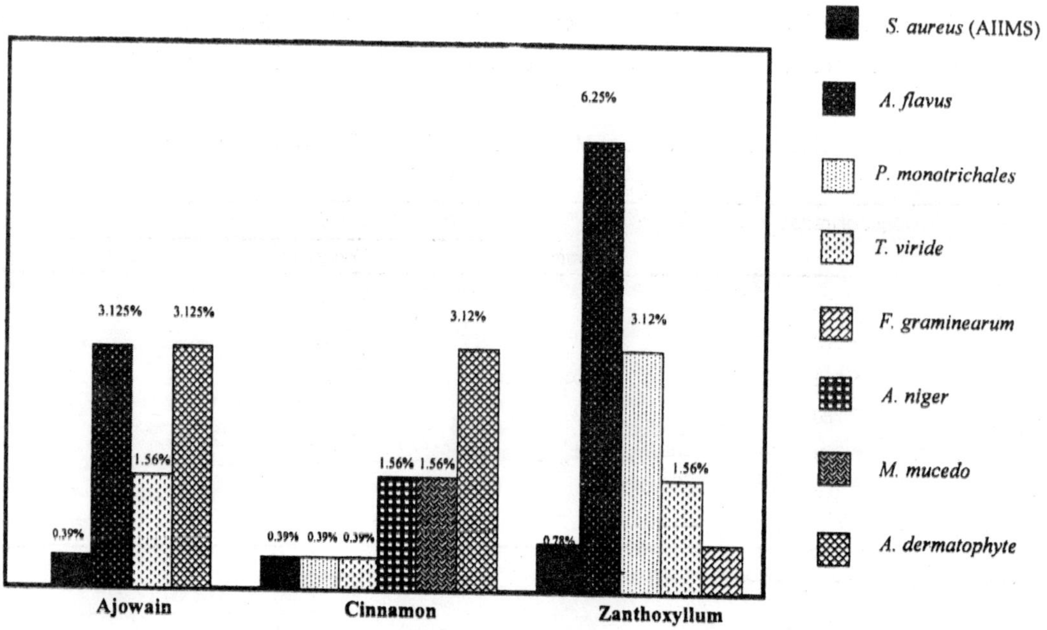

Figure 43.1: MIC Values (%, v/v) of Three Essential Oils Against Different Organisms

1. *Ajowain* essential oil against *Staphylococcus aureus* (AIIMS) has MIC value at 0.39 per cent concentration, against *Aspergillus flavus* and against a dermatophyte it has MIC value at 3.125 per cent concentration while against *Trichoderma viride* it has MIC value at 1.56 per cent concentration.
2. *Cinnamon* essential oil against *S. aureus* (AIIMS), *Penicillium monotrichales* and *T. viride* has MIC value at 0.39 per cent concentration, against *Aspergillus niger* and *Mucor mucedo* it has MIC value at 1.56 per cent concentration while against a dermatophyte it has MIC value at 3.12 per cent concentration.
3. *Zanthoxyllum* essential oil against *S. aureus* (AIIMS) and *Fusarium graminearum* has MIC value at 0.78 per cent concentration, against *A. flavus* has MIC value at 6.25 per cent concentration, against *P. monotrichales* has MIC value at 3.12 per cent concentration and against *T. viride* it has MIC value at 1.56 per cent concentration.

Most of the previous work on antimicrobial activity of essential oils has been reported on Cinnamon and other spices yielding herbs but the literature is scanty to report the MIC values of Jatamansi and Zanthoxyllum. In the present investigation Jatamansi yielded low antimicrobial activity as compared to other essential oils. Zanthoxyllum has comparable antimicrobial activity to Cinnamon and Ajowain.

There are reports of use of Zanthoxyllum essential oil (seeds) for source of aroma compounds.

References

Airi, S., Rawal, R.S., Dhar, U. and Purohit, A.N., 2000. Assessment of availability and habitat preference of jatamansi, a critically endangered medicinal plant of Western Himalaya. *Curr. Sci.*, 47(10): 1467–1471.

Annon., 2000. Convention on international trade in endangered species of wild flora and fauna. In: *Tenth Meeting of the Plants Committee*. Shapherdstonon (USA), 11th–15th December, p. 1–14.

Annon., 2003. Young living essential oils transport nutrients to body cells. *http://www.therapure.com/ yleo/eowhatr.htm*: 1–4.

Attar-ur-rehman, M.,Chaudhary, I., Farooq, A., Ahmed, A., Iqbal, M.Z., Demirci, B., Demirci, F. and Susnu Can Baser, K., 1999. Antifungal activities and essential oil constituents of some spices from Pakistan. In: *Third International Electronic Conference on Synthetic Organic Chemistry*, ECSOC–3 www.reprints.netc/ecsoc–3.htm.

Brizzo, J., Nunoz, L., Chirife, J., Herszage, L. and Aquino, M., 1989. Antimicrobial activity of clove oil disposed in a concentrated sugar solution. *J.Appl. Bact.*, 66(1): 69–75.

Das, D.K., Kulkarni, Meshram, S.U. and Shanmare, A.S., 2000. Assessment of antifungal activity of some essential terpenic oils *in vitro* against isolates of oral Candidiasis from immunosuppressive patients. In: *43rd AnnualConference of AMI CCS Haryana Agricultural Univ. Hissar*, December 11–13.

Das, P., 2000. Studies on the antimicrobial activity of *Valeriana wallichii* DC. Mem.Valer., 15t. 4 and *Zanthoxyllum armatum* Roxb. *M.Sc. Dissertation*, C.C.S. Univ., Meerut, p. 1 –67.

Faraz, R.S., Daw-zy., Howodi, F.M., El-Baroty-GSA, 1989. Antimicrobial activity of some essential spice oils. *Journal of Food Protection*, 52(9): 665–667.

Girgune, J.B., Jain, N.K. and Garg, B.D., 1978. Antimicrobial activity of some essential oils. *Curr. Sci.*, 47(13): 454–455.

Islam, S.N., Monira Ahsani, Ferdous, A.J. and Faroque, A.B.M., 1990. *In vitro* antibacterial activities of commonly used spices. *B.J. Bot.*, 19(1): 99–101.

Jirovertz, L., Buchbauer, G., Shafi, M.P. and Saidutty, A., 1998. Analysis of aroma compounds of the essential oil of seeds of spice plant *Zanthoxyllum rhetsa* from Southern India. *Chem. Abstr.*, 124 294093f.

Koneman, E.W., Allen, S.D., Janda, W.M., Schreckenberger, P.C. and Winn, W.C., 1997. Tests for determining inhibitory activity of antibiotics. In: *Diagnostic Microbiology*, 5th edn. pp. 822–823, Lippincot, Philadelphia, New York.

Lis-Balchin, M., 1997. Essential oils and aromatherapy: Their modern role in healing. *J. Royal Soc. Health*, 117(5): 324–329.

Mallavarapu, G.R., Ramesh, S., Chandrasekhara, R.S., Rao, BRR., Kaul, P.N. and Bhattacharya, A.K., 1995. Investigation of the essential oil of Cinnamon leaf grown at Banglore and Hyderabad. *Flavour and Fragrance Journal*, 10(4): 239–242.

Medici, Dde., Pieretti, S., Salvatore, G., Nicoletti, M. and Rasoanaivo, P., 1992. Chemical analysis of essential oils of Malagasy medicinal plants by gas chromatography and NMR spectroscopy. *Flavour and Fragrance Journal*, 7(5): 275–281.

Miczak, M.A., 1999. Single oil look. *Spikenard–Suite 101.com.*

Mishra, D., Chaturvedi, R.V. and Tripathi, S.C., 1995. The fungitoxic effect of the essential oil of the herb *Nardostachys jatamansi* DC. *Trop. Agri.*, 72(1): 48–52.

Nath, S.C., Pathak, M.G. and Akhil Baruah, 1996. Benzyl benzoate, the major component of the leaf and stem bark oil of *Cinnamomum zeylanicum* blume. *Journal of Essential Oil Research*, 8(3): 327–328.

Pandey, A.K., 2003. Composition and *in vitro* antifungal activity of the essential oil of menthol mint (*Mentha arvensis*) growing in Central India. *Indian Drugs*, 40(2): 726–728.

Prasad, Y.R., Alankararao-GSJC and Baby, P., 1983. Antimicrobial studies on essential oil of *Hemidesmus indicus* R.Br. *Indian Perfumer*, 27(3–4): 197–199.

Rana, R., Gupta, M.K. and Kanwar, S.S., 1998. Antimicrobial activity of *Eupatorium adenophorum* on beneficial soil bacteria. *Ind. J. Microbiol.*, 38(1): 49–50.

Rath, C.C., Mahapatra, S., Dash, S.K. and Mishra, R.K., 2002. Antimicrobial susceptibility of ten essential oils against 15 bacterial and fungal pathogens isolated from a variety of wounds. In: *43rd Annual Conference of Association of Microbiologist of India*, CCS Haryana Agricultural University, Hissar, December 11–13.

Tiwari, R. and Dixit, V., 1994. Fungitoxic activity of vapours of some higher plants against predominant storage fungi. *Nat. Acad. Sci. Lett.*, 17(3–4): 55–57.

Yadav, P. and Dubey, D.K., 1994. Screening of some essential oils against ring worm fungi. *Ind. J. Pharma. Sci.*, 56(6): 227–230.

Medicinal Plants: Conservation, Cultivation and Utilization (2007) *Pages 357–367*
Editors: A.K. Chopra, D.R. Khanna, G. Prasad, D.S. Malik and R. Bhutiani
Published by: DAYA PUBLISHING HOUSE

Chapter 44

Clinical Evaluation of the Effect of *Centella asiatica* on Cerebral Higher Functions

Uttam Kumar Sharma[1], Ajay Kumar Sharma[2] and C.M. Sharma[3]

[1]Reader, Department of Kayachikitsa, State Ayurvedic College, Gurukul Kangri, Hardwar

[2]Professor and Head, P.G. Department of Kayachikitsa, National Institute of *Ayurveda*, Jaipur

[3]Associate Professor, P.G. Department of Neurology, SMS Medical College, Jaipur

Introduction

The psychological aspect of *Ayurveda* is probably the most important part of the system and the least understood. *Ayurveda* has a group of certain drugs highly appreciated for their effect to promote various faculties of human body. In this respect *Rasayana* is one of the important branches of *Astanga Ayurveda*, which deals with promotion of physical and mental health. All *Rasayana* drugs are supposed to improve mental faculties, in addition to their beneficial effects on the body. However, the *Medhya Rasayana* has specific effect on mental functions.

Rasayana drugs used with the objective of promotion of intellect, memory and other mental capabilities, are called *Medhya Rasayana*. These drugs are supposed to provide nutrition and other essential elements to the cells and tissues of the brain and possess tranquilizing effect, which in turn increases the functional capacity of brain and promote mental health.

Medha encompasses the processes like *grahana*, *dharana* and *smarana* which are similar to encoding, storage and retrieval respectively. Thus *Medha* can be appropriately correlated with the process of memory and other higher functions of the brain.

In *Ayurvedic* literature the term *'Medha'* seems to represent higher functions of brain, as it involves (i) Dhee which incorporates thinking, reasoning, analysing, learning, understanding etc. (ii) *Dhriti* which encompasses power of retention, regulation and self control and (iii) *Smriti*, which includes reproduction, auto suggestion, remembering past experiences etc. Thus it appears logical to correlate the term *'Medha'* with cerebral higher functions.

The present study has been conducted with the objective to evaluate clinically the *Medhya* effect of *Manukaparni* (*Centella asiatica*) in 100 cases with minor disturbances of cerebral higher functions on scientific parameters.

Materials and Methods

For clinical studies 100 clinically diagnosed patients of minor disturbances of cerebral higher functions were selected and registered for the present trial on the basis of specially designed proforma for the purpose. As already stated, these 100 patients were randomly divided in to following two groups of 50 patients each:-

1. Group A (*Mandukaparni* group): These patients were treated with *Mandukaparni* syrup in the dose of 20ml b.d. for three months.
2. Group B (Placebo/Control group): These patients were treated with placebo "Glucose powder" in the dose of 250 mg b.d. in capsule form for three months.

The subjects were selected on the basis of complaints and features of minor disturbances of cerebral higher functions in the form of poor memory, disturbances of concentration and orientation, poor intellectual performance, poor retention power, disturbed sleep pattern, and anxiety leading to disturbed mental functions etc.

Patients having major mental or neurological disorders like psychosis, psychoneurosis, dementia, epilepsy, hysteria, delirium etc. were excluded.

Method of Preparation of *Mandukaparni* Syrup

The drug *Mandukaparni* (with its panchanga) was taken in dry form and its *kwatha* (decoction) was made. For making *kwatha* the crude drug was boiled in eight times of water till 1/4 part was left behind. Then it was filtered and collected in an open vessel and the sugar was added in it in double quantity of the filtered *kwatha*. The mixture was heated and stirred till sugar dissolves. After that the liquid was kept open till it comes to the normal temperature. Then sodium benzoate, as a preservative was added in this mixture in the proportion of 0.1 percent. This syrup was stored in air tight containers and then bottled for convenient dispensing.

Calculations of the ingredients of the syrup revealed that each 10ml. of syrup contained 2.21 gm *Mandukaparni* and each 10ml. of *Mandukaparani* syrup contained 4.5ml. liquid extract of *Mandukaparani*. Detailed calculations for the purpose are given below:

Quantity of crude dry drug: 60 kg.

Quantity of *kwatha* obtained: 120 Ltr.

Quantity of syrup formed: 266 Ltr.

$$\text{Quantity of } Mandukaparni \text{ in 10 ml syrup (in gm)} = \frac{\text{Quantity of Crude drug (gm)}}{\text{No. of doses (each of 10 ml) in total quantity of syrup}}$$

$$= \frac{60,000}{266,00}$$

$$= 2.21 \text{ gm}$$

$$\text{Quantity of liquid extract of } \textit{Mandukaparni} \text{ in 10 ml syrup} = \frac{\text{Quantity of } \textit{kwatha} \text{ (liquid extract) ml}}{\text{No. of doses (each of 10 ml) in total quantity of syrup}}$$

$$= \frac{120,000}{266,00}$$

$$= 4.5 \text{ ml.}$$

Criteria of Assessment

The follow up studies of the patients were made at the interval of one month. During the trial and follow up studies the parameters of assessment were as described below:-

Subjective Improvement

It was assessed in terms of increase in the growing feeling of well being with physical and mental fitness, if any produced after the treatment. In addition all the patients were assessed in terms of various *Rasayana* and *Medhya Rasayana* effects produced in their body on the basis of the characteristics described in *Charaka Samhita* (Ch. Sh 1/99-101).

Clinical Improvement

All the patients were assessed in terms of improvement in following six types of cerebral higher functions on the basis of various tests:

1. Attention
2. Memory
3. Calculation
4. Abstract thought
5. Spatial appreciation
6. Visual and body perception

Scoring for Cerebral Higher Function Tests

The complete clinical test for each higher function was divided in to three major groups. Each group was given maximum 10 marks. The scoring was done on the basis of the performance of the patient out of 10 marks. The better performance was marked towards increasing number and worst performance towards decreasing number. Thus collectively, each function was assessed in terms of maximum 30 marks.

Other Tests

Mini Mental Scale Test

Mini mental state test is a scale used in neurology for the gross assessment of cerebral higher functions. It was used to assess the improvement in terms of score achieved by the patient out of 30.

Mental Fatigue Rate

Mental fatigue rate was assessed by asking the patient to cut a particular digit in the sheet prescribed. Same process was adopted during follow ups and after treatment. It was decided to assess mental fatigue rate on the following two parameters -

1. The time consumed, before and after the treatment
2. Number of mistakes done, before and after the treatment.

Anxiety Level

For assessment of Anxiety level, Sinha Anxiety Scale (Sinha W.A. Self Analysis Form) constructed and standardized by D. Sinha, Prof. and Head, Department of Psychology, University of Allahabad, U.P., India was used. It is a self–administered evaluating scale. The scale contains 100 questions to which patient has to answer in 'Yes' or 'No' after reading them carefully. The positive score gives directly the percentage of anxiety level. Statistical difference before and after the therapy was worked out.

Laboratory Profile

1. Hematological changes in terms of TLC, DLC, E.S.R. and Hbgm per cent.
2. Lipid profile in terms of Total Lipids, L.D.L., V.L.D.L., H.D.L., Serum Cholesterol, S. Tryglycerides.

Observations made and results obtained after clinical trial were computed statistically to draw various conclusions.

Observations and Results

It was observed that most of the patients treated with the trial drug *Mandukaparni*, reported a growing feeling of well being, more mental and physical fitness and considerable improvement in their psychological make up after the therapy, which supports the *Medhya* effect of *Mandukaparni*.

Medhya prabhava of *Mandukaparni* was also worked out in terms of Dhee, *Dhriti*, *Smriti*, *Prabha*, *Varna*, *Swara*, *Dehabala*, *Indriyabala* and *Arogya*. All the subjects of group A (*Mandukaparni*) showed statistically highly significant improvement in these factors except in *Varna* and *Swara* where less significant improvement was noticed after the course of the therapy. On the other hand the subjects of group B (Placebo) witnessed a trend of slight clinical improvement in all factors but it was statistically insignificant. Probably the improvement was noticed in these subjects due to the psychological effect of placebo therapy.

The assessment of *Medhya Prabhava* of *Mandukaparni* in comparison to control group was observed in all the subjects in terms of cerebral higher functions namely 1. Attention, 2. Memory, 3. Calculation, 4. Abstract thought, 5. Spatial appreciation and 6. Visual and body perception. It was observed that there was statistically significant improvement in the level of all the six cerebral higher functions in group A treated with *Mandukaparni* as in comparison to the group B treated with placebo. It was noticed that in two cerebral higher functions. Attention and Perception improvement in their level after the therapy in group A (*Mandukaparni*) was statistically less significant.

The gross improvement in cerebral higher functions was also observed in all the subjects with applying the Mini Mental State Test. The observations made before and after the treatment show that the subjects treated with *Mandukaparni* (group A) scored much higher as in comparison to their initial scoring rate. These results were found statistically highly significant. On the other hand the subjects of group B (placebo) although showed slight improvement in Mini Mental State Test, but it was found statistically insignificant. Since, it was observed that there was highly significant improvement in Mini Mental State Test Scoring in group A (*Mandukaparni*) after the therapy, it suggests collectively marked improvement in cerebral higher functions produced by *Mandukaparni* which is possible only due to *Medhya* effects of *Mandukaparni*.

Improvement in mental functions was also observed in all the subjects in terms of two parameters namely 1. Anxiety level and 2. Mental fatigue rate. It was observed that there was significant reduction in the level of anxiety in group A (*Mandukaparni*) in comparison to group B (placebo), which suggests the marked tranquilizing and psychotropic effect produced by the *Mandukaparni*. The improvement observed in the level of anxiety in group B (placebo) was found to be statistically insignificant.

Mental fatigue rate was worked out with the help of a self administered scale. It was observed on two factors–(i) Time consumed to complete a specific task and (ii) mistakes committed during completion of the task. Statistical datas show that the time consumed for completion of a specific task was reduced insignificantly in group B (placebo), whereas it was markedly reduced in the subjects of group A (*Mandukaparni*). Similarly the subjects of group B (placebo) showed insignificant reduction in number of mistakes committed for completion of a task, while in the subjects of group A (*Mandukaparni*), there was highly significant reduction in the number of mistakes committed after the therapy.

The *Mandukaparni* has been found effective in improving the feeling of well being and in improving the quality of sleep in the subjects after the therapy. Out of 50 patients of group A (*Mandukaparni*) 30 (60 per cent) patients were reported to have developed growing feeling of well being, whereas the number of patients noticed in this respect was very small 8 (16 per cent) in group B (placebo). The quality of sleep was improved in 33 (66 per cent) patients in group A (*Mandukaparni*) in comparison to subjects of group B (placebo), in which 16 (32 per cent) patients were reported to have improved their sleep pattern towards better side after the therapy, showing better *Medhya Prabhava* of the drug *Mandukaparni*.

It was observed that there were significant changes in the pattern of lipid profile in the subjects of group A treated with *Mandukaparni*. The level of S. Cholesterol decreased significantly. There was a trend of decrease in *S. Triglycerides* which was insignificant statistically. Similarly Higher Density Lipoprotein have shown statistically significant increase in it's level while Low Density Lipoprotein and Very Low Density Lipoprotein registered significant decline after the therapy with *Mandukaparni*. These observations confirm the Cardio-protective effects of drug *Mandukaparni* which is probably due to its *Rasayana* effects.

Table 44.1: Showing the Response of *Mandukaparni* (Group A) in Comparison to Placebo (Group B) in Respect of its *Rasayana* Effects (Subjective Improvement)

Rasayana Effects		*Dhee*	*Dhriti*	*Smriti*	*Prabha*	*Varna*	*Swara*	*Dehabala*	*Indriya Bala*	*Agrogya*
Percent	Group A	56.94	96.92	72.37	73.33	31.03	40.7	58.97	77.46	80.86
Improvement		P<0.001	P<0.001	P<0.001	P<0.001	P<0.010	P<0.010	P<0.001	P<0.001	P<0.001
	Group B	16.87	13.65	15.38	18.39	14.61	13.65	13.95	15.56	16.85
		P<0.10	P<0.10	P<0.10	P<0.10	P<0.10	P<0.10	P<0.10	P<0.10	P<0.10

Studies show statistically significant decrease in the level of ESR after the therapy with *Mandukaparni*. Similarly there was significant improvement in Hb gm per cent after *Mandukaparni* therapy which is possible because of its *Rasayana Prabhava*. It is observed that *Mandukaparni* helps in producing good quality *Rasa, Rakta* etc. *dhatus* which is the *Rasayana Prabhava* of *Mandukaparni*. No significant changes were observed on hematological parameters in the subjects treated with placebo.

Table 44.2: Showing the Response of *Mandukaparni* (Group A) in Comparison to Placebo (Group B) in Respect of Cerebral Higher Functions (Clinical Improvement)

Cerebral Higher Functions		*Attention*	*Memory*	*Calculation*	*Abstract Thought*	*Spatial*	*Perception*
Percent Improvement	Group A	9.16	27.4	20.42	16.21	18.72	3.28
		P<0.01	P<0.001	P<0.001	P<0.001	P<0.001	P<0.01
	Group B	3.17	3.54	3.73	3.04	3.35	1.87
		P<0.10	P<0.10	P<0.10	P<0.10	P<0.10	P<0.10

Table 44.3: Showing the Level of Improvement in Certain Mental Faculties in Subjects of Group A (*Mandukaparni*) and Group B (Placebo)

Tests for Mental Faculties		*Mini Mental State Test*	*Anxiety Level*	*Mental Fatigue Rate (P)*	*Mental Fatigue Rate (E)*
Percent Improvement	group A	19.62	33.08	22.46	68.29
		P<0.001	P<0.001	P<0.001	P<0.001
	group B	3:26	7.57	5.16	19.11
		P<0.10	P<0.10	P<0.10	P<0.10

Table 44.4: Showing the Comparison of the Pattern of Changes in Lipid Profile Amongst the Subjects of Group A (*Mandukaparni*) and Group B (*Placebo*)

Biochemical Parameters of Lipid Profile		*S. Cholesterol*	*S. Triglyceride*	*HDL*	*LDL*	*VLDL*
Percent improvement	Group A	6.1	5.48	6.52	12.24	5.48
		P<0.025	P<0.20	P<0.025	P<0.01	P<0.20
	Group B	4.8	9.64	3.11	8.09	9.64
		P<0.40	P<0.10	P<0.10	P<0.20	P<0.10

Table 44.5: Showing the Comparison of the Pattern of Haematological Changes in the Subjects of Group A (*Mandukaparni*) and Group B (*Placebo*)

Haematological Parameters		*ESR*	*Hb*	*TLC*	*P*	*L*	*E*	*B*	*M*
Percent Improvement	Group A	32.61	6.31	3.45	19.48	26.54	66.67	0	2.27
		P<0.001	P<0.001	P<0.40	P<0.010	P<0.010	P<0.40		P<0.50
	Group B	7.87	1.56	1.68	7.33	11.13	66.67	0	5.17
		P<0.20	P<0.50	P<0.40	P<0.10	P<0.05	P<0.10		P<0.50

Table 44.6: Showing the Comparison of the Pattern of Physiological Changes in the Subjects of Group A (*Mandukaparni*) and Group B (*Placebo*)

Physiological Parameters		*Body weight*	*Systolic B.P.*	*Diastolic B.P.*	*Pulse Rate*	*Respiration*
Percent Improvement	Group A	1.88	0.79	0.52	0.97	3.43
		P<0.05	P<0.025	P<0.40	P<0.10	P<0.025
	Group B	1.41	0.68	0.05	0.71	1.94
		P<0.20	P<0.10	P<0.50	P<0.10	P<0.10

Table 44.7: Showing the Response of *Mandukaparni* (Group A)/Placebo (Group B) on Feeling of Well Being After the Therapy

Sl.No.	*Group*	*Feeling of Well Being After the Therapy*		
		Present (++)	*Present (+)*	*Unchanged*
1.	A (50) *Mandukaparni*	9 (18 per cent)	21 (42 per cent)	20 (40 per cent)
2.	B (50) Placebo	0	8 (16 per cent)	42 (84 per cent)

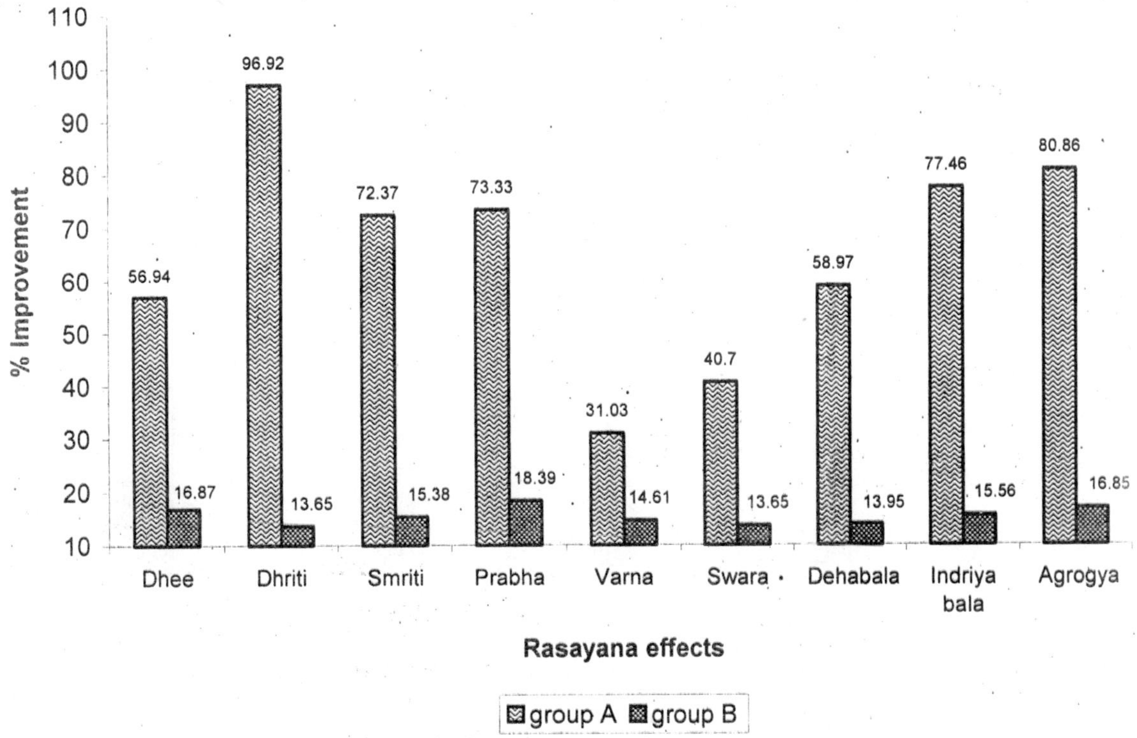

Figure 44.1: Showing the Response of *Mandukaparni* (Group A) in Comparison to Placebo (Group B) in Respect of its Rasayana Effects (Subjective Improvement)

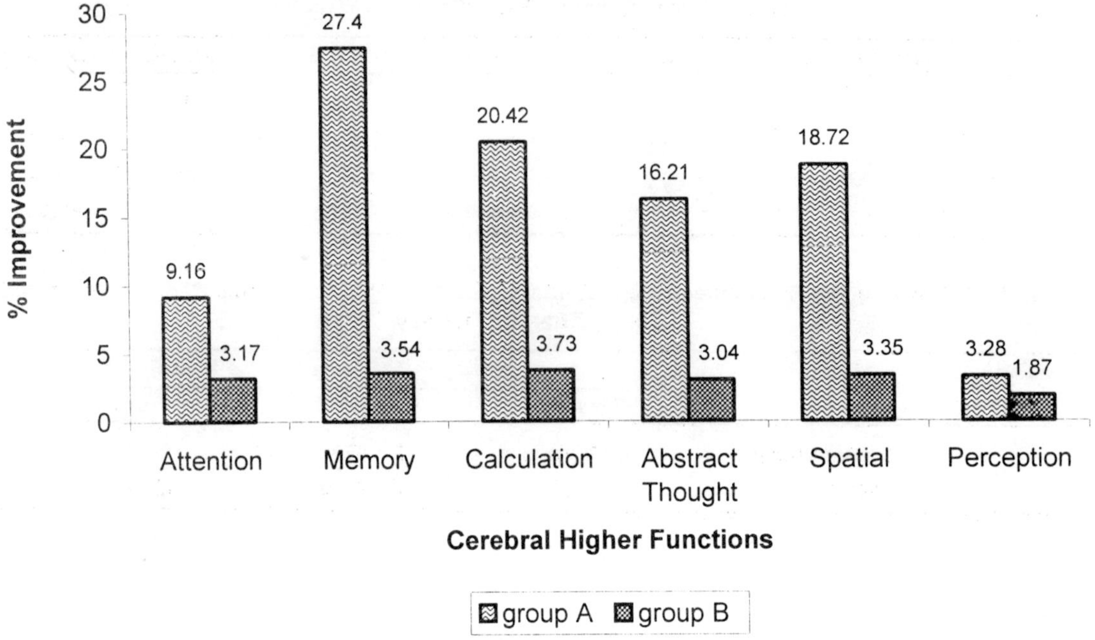

Figure 44.2: Showing the Response of *Mandukaparni* (Group A) in Comparison to Placebo (Group B) in Respect Cerebral Higher Functions (Clinical Improvement)

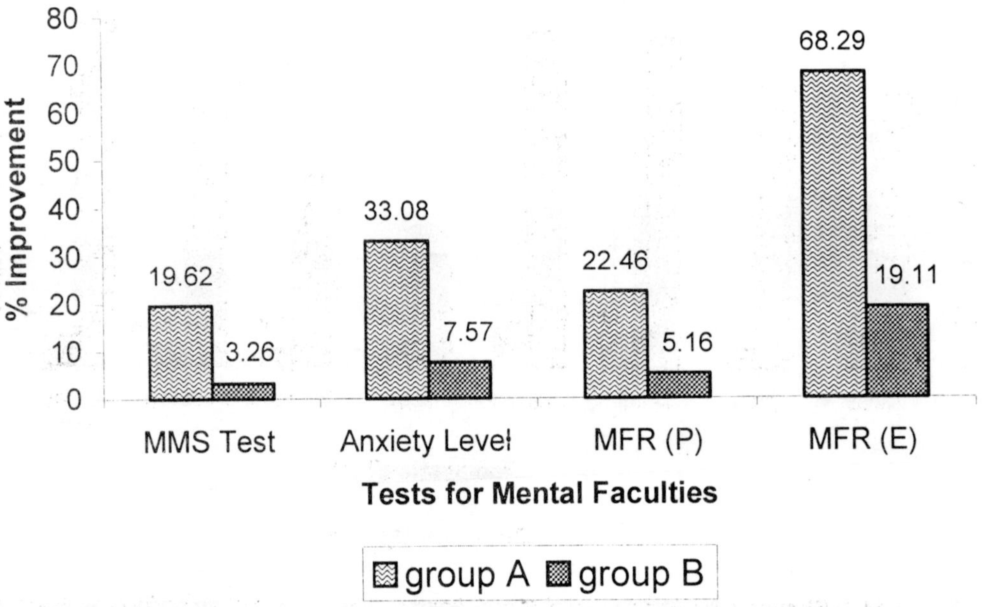

Figure 44.3: Showing the Level of Improvement in Certain Mental Faculties in Subjects of Group A (*Mandukaparni*) and Group B (Placebo)

While reviewing the pattern of physiological changes in subjects of *Mandukaparni* treated group it is evident that there was considerable gain in body weight in subjects of group A after the course of therapy which is possible due to its *Rasayana Prabhava*. No significant changes were observed in other parameters, that in the subjects of group B *i.e.* placebo treated group no significant changes were observed in any of the physiological parameters after the therapy.

Table 44.8: Showing the Response of *Mandukaparni* (Group A)/Placebo (Group B) on Quality of Sleep After the Therapy

Sl.No.	Group	Quality of Sleep		
		Unchanged	Better	Worse
1.	A (50) *Mandukaparni*	17 (34 per cent)	33 (66 per cent)	–
2.	B (50) Placebo	30 (60 per cent)	16 (32 per cent)	4 (8 per cent)

Discussion

Mandukaparni (Centella asiatica) possesses various effects on central nervous system such as stimulatory nervine tonic, rejuvenant, sedative, tranquilizer and intelligence promoting properties. It is reported to have the capacity to produce improvement in learning and memory. It has cognitive enhancing effects which involves antioxidant mechanism. *Mandukaparni* (Centella asiatica) has potent anxiolytic effect. It has been reported that long term treatment with *Mandukaparni* decreases locomotor activity and enhances mental performance. *Mandukaparni* is known to possess good wound healing activity by induction of antioxidant levels at initial stage of healing. It has been reported that *Mandukaparni* increases learning ability significantly, enhances concentration ability and promotes overall mental growth.

Probable Modes of Action of *Mandukaparni* (*Centella asiatica*)

Like other *Medhya Rasayana* Drugs *Mandukaparni* is likely to act at various levels:

1. In *Ayurveda Mandukaparni* (*Centella asiatica*) is described as "*Medhya Rasayana* or "Brain Tonic" with the ability to promote mental functions along with providing general rejuvenating effects.
2. *Medhya Rasayana Prabhava*: At one or all the following levels *viz.* at the level of Guna (properties), at the level of Panchabhautic composition, at the level of Rasa, at the level of Agni, at the level of Srotasa.

   Mandukaparni may act:

   (*a*) at the level of *Poshaka Rasa i.e.* by improving the quality of *Rasa dhatu* produced in the body.

   (*b*) at the level of *Agni i.e.* by improving the digestion, metabolism and assimilation of food in the body.

   (*c*) at the level of *Srotasa i.e.* by improving the circulation in micro circulatory channels in the body leading to better bio availability of the nutrients to the tissues and improved tissue perfusion which may in turn help in promotion of nutritional status of nervous system and brain.

   Mandukaparni has *sheeta veerya,* tiikta-madhura rasa and *snigdha-laghu guna* which may produce *kaphaja prabhava* (anabolic response) and similar effects in the subjects. It is expected that due to its properties, *Mandukaparni* may produce improvement in the physique and exert soothing effect over the mind (*Manasa*) and ultimately improving *Dhee, Dhriti, Smriti*.

3. Tranquilizing action: *Mandukaparni* may have anxiolytic (anti anxiety) activity by virtue of its comprehensive *Rasayana* and adaptogenic effects, producing non specifically increased resistant against stressful conditions.
4. Regulating Neurotransmitters
   (*a*) Electrophysiological-mechanism of action:

   Mandukaparni is likely to increase the CNS a wave activity and simultaneously may decrease the CNS β wave activity. Increase in a wave activity in the EEG has been shown to be associated with a state of relaxation of the body and mind and thereby decreased fluctuation of attention/minute and increased concentration ability, leading to improved learning powers and overall positive mental health. High β wave activity, on the other hand, causes distractibility, low concentration powers and is not conducive to learning.

   (*b*) Biochemical mechanism of action: *Mandukaparni* may regulate the altered levels of brain biogenic amines [glutamate, gama aminobutyric acid (GABA)] and thereby improve the process of learning.
5. Antioxidant action: One of the contributing factors to the decline of cognitive function is the damaging effect of free radicals exposure. The mechanism of action of *Mandukaparni* and other *Medhya Rasayana* drugs could be through chelation of free radicals (ferrous ions) and also as a chain breaker. It has been reported by scientific studies that *Mandukaparni* (*Centella asiatica*) is a potent antioxidant drug.
6. By improving the nutritional status of brain cells: It has been reported that *Medhya Rasayana* drugs like *Mandukaparni* (*Centella asiatica*) and *Brahmi* (*Bacopa* monnieri) possess properties similar to nootropic aagents which are supposed to improve oxygen supply and glucose utilization of the brain cells with undue alteration in blood circulation or any psychostimulation, producing positive effects on the cerebral higher function like, memory, intelligence, and learning etc. Similarly *Medhya Rasayana* drugs do not produce undue psychostimulation or sedation and produce positive effect on *Medha* along with improved physiological status of the body.

Conclusion

It can be concluded from the current research project that *Mandukaparni* (*Centella asiatica*) is a potent psychoprotective, anxiolytic, mood elevating, rejuvenating, intellect and mental health promoting and immunomodulator drug with specific properties of enhancing Cerbral Higher Functions due to its *Medhya* effects.

References

Ahuja, Neeraj , 2001. *A Short Textbook of Psychiatry*.

Ajay Kumar Sharma, 2002. *The Panchakarma Treatment of Ayurveda including Keraliya Panchakarma*. Sri Satguru Publications, Delhi.

Arthur C. Guyton, 1986. *Text book of Medical Physiology*. Igaku-shoin/Saunders, W.B. Saunders Company.

Ashtanga Hridaya, 1990. Hindi translation by Lal Chandra Vaidya. Motilal Banarasidas Publishers Pvt. Ltd., Delhi.

Bal Krishna Amarji Pathak, *Manas Vigyana*, Nagpur, 1983. Sri Baidyanath *Ayurveda* Bhavan Ltd..

Bhaishjya Ratnavali, 1997. Translation by Ambika Datt Shastri. Chaukhambha Sanskrit Sansthan, Varanasi.

Bhava Mishra, 1993. Bhava Prakasha (Poorvardha). Chaukhambha Sanskrit Sansthan, Varanasi.

Dwarkanath, C., 1996. *Introduction to Kayachikitsa*. Chaukhambha Orientalia, Varanasi.

Dwarkanath, C, 1998. *The Fundamental Principles of Ayurveda*, Part 1, 2, 3. Krishnadas Academy, Varanasi.

Dwivedi, B.K., 1997. *Ayurvedeeya Bhoot Vidya Vivechana* (Hindi). Krishnadas Academy, Varanasi

Chakrapani Datta, 1981. *Charaka Samhita* (*Ayurveda* Deepika Commentary), edited by Jadavji Trikamji Acharya. Munshiram Manoharlal Publishers Pvt. Ltd., New Delhi.

Charaka Samhita, 1994.

C.C.R.A.S., 1997. *Journal of Research in Ayurveda and Siddha*, Jan-June.

Nadkarni, K.M., 1996. *Indian Materia Medica*, Vol. 1. Popular Prakashan, Bombay.

Sharma, Priyavrat, 1994. *Ayurveda Darshanam (Philosophy of Ayurveda)*. Chaukhambha Vishvabharati, Varanasi.

Sharma, Priyavrat, 1998. *Charaka Samhita: Critical Notes*. Chaukhambha Orientalia, Varanasi

Sharma, Priyavrat, 1998. *Dravya-guna Vijnana*, Vol. 2. Chaukhambha Bharti Academy, Varanasi.

Singh, Ram Harsh, 1986. *Ayurvedeeya Manas Vigyana*. .

Singh, Ram Harsh, 1998. *The Holistic Principles of Ayurvedic Medicine*. Chaukhambha Sanskrit Pratishthan, Delhi.

Sushruta Samhita, 1993. Hindi translation by Ambika Datta Shastri. Chaukhambha Sanskrit Sansthan, Varanasi.

Tripathi, Brahmananda . Chaukhambha Surbharti Publication (Hindi Translation), Varanasi.

Udupa, K.N. and R.H. Singh, 1993. *Clinical and Experimental Studies on Rasayana Drugs and Panchakarma Therapy*. Central Council for Research in *Ayurveda* and Siddha, New Delhi.

Vinayak Jayan and Thakar, 1985. *Ayurvedeeya Maulik Siddhanta*. *Ayurveda* Mudranalaya, Gujarat *Ayurveda* University, Jamnagar.

Medicinal Plants: Conservation, Cultivation and Utilization (2007) *Pages 369–374*
Editors: A.K. Chopra, D.R. Khanna, G. Prasad, D.S. Malik and R. Bhutiani
Published by: DAYA PUBLISHING HOUSE

Chapter 45

Green Tea and Benefits

Shailu Dalal[1] and Anupama Gautam[2]
[1]Department of Biotechnology, IIT, Roorkee
[2]Department of Botany and Microbiology, GKV, Hardwar

ABSTRACT

Green tea is one of the best health drinks with innumerable benefits. These includes green tea being anticancerous, good against rheumatoid arthritis, a boon for high cholesterol levels, against infection, cardiovascular disease and also impaired immune function. In this study a survey was made and green tea was given in doses at intervals thereby its effect was evaluated against two important aspects of weight loss and cholesterol levels and encouraging results were obtained. Graphs were plotted against the data and hence green tea proved to be very effective.

Introduction

Why Drink Tea?

Tea is the second most popular beverage in the world next to water. Green, oolong and Black teas all come from the leaves of *Camellia sinensis* plant. Tea has a natural occuring compound called as flavonoids, these have strong antioxidant properties. Of these teas green tea has the highest amount of flavonoids or antioxidants. Tea contains two to three times less caffiene than coffee.

Green Tea

Green tea was first brewed in China where it was known as MIRACLE MEDICINE. The Chinese have known about the medicinal benefits of green tea since ancient times, using it to treat everything from headaches to depression. In her book, Green tea: The natural secret for a healtheir life, Nadine Taylor states that green tea has been used as a medicine in China for at least 4000 years. Today research shows us how true that ancient claim was. Green tea, with its medicinal properties, is a boon for the health conscious and a wonder even to modern science.

What Makes Green Tea so Special?

The secret of green tea lies in the fact that it is rich in Catechin polyphenols, particularly epigallocatechin gallate (ECGC). Catechins give green tea its astringent flavor, ECGC is a powerful antioxidant besides inhibiting the growth of cancer cells, it kills cancer cells without inhibiting the normal tissues. It has also been effective in lowering LDL cholestrol levels, and inhibiting the abnormal formation of blood clots. Green tea lies way apart because of the process it is prepared. Green tea leaves are steamed, which prevents the ECGC compound from being oxidised. By contrast, oolong and black tea leaves are made from fermented leaves which results in the ECGC being converted into other compounds that are not nearly as effective in preventing and fighting various diseases.

Caffeine Content

Caffeine is a natural component of tea, which is present in green tea much in smaller amounts as in black tea or coffee. Caffeine in small amounts can be an excellent energy enhancer, but it is best to limit its intake, as excessive consumption of caffeine may be unhealthy.

Table 45.1: Comparison Chart of Caffeine Content

Standard Beverage Serving	*Average Milligrams Caffeine*
Coffee(brewed)	80-120
Coffee(instant)	30-60
Coffee(decaffeinated)	1-5
Soft drinks	40-60
Black tea	40-90
Green tea	20-30
Cocoa	5-10

Health Benefits of Green Tea

Health benefits of green tea are many

Inhibits Cancer

The latest news about green tea comes from a study done at the Karolinsska Institute in Stockholm. The team of researchers headed by Dr. Yihai Cao found that green tea can block Angiogenesis,the development of new blood vessels that tumors need in order to grow. Studies from Case Western University, Cleveland, shows that the risk of stomach cancer goes down as consumption of green tea goes up.

Prevents High-Blood Pressure and Heart Disease

Scientific studies show that daily consumption of green tea can prevent high blood pressure. 3 to 4 cups of Green tea a day can substantially reduce an individuals risk of heart disease and stroke. Substances in green tea known as Catechins can increase the antioxidant capacity of human plasma, which could help reduce cardiovascular disease risk.

Boon for Dieters

Green Tea can actually help burn Fat. Study at the University of Geneva, in Switzerland, researchers found that men who were given a Green tea extract burned more calories, since Green tea helped to excrete more fat.

Strengthens Immune System

Our body needs to be strong enough to fight common diseases like the flu and other infections. Green Tea helps to strengthen a weak immune system, guarding us from illness and infections that take a long time to heal.

Lowers the Blood Sugar Level

The extract of Green tea has the ability to actually lower blood sugar. It is believed that both the EGCG and polysaccharides in Green tea are factors in lowering blood sugar.

Oral Hygiene and Dental Care

Fluoride in Green tea protects tooth enamel and EGCG reduces the development of bacteria growing in the plaque. Green tea can also kill other oral bacteria, which cause bad breath. It also stimulates the production of saliva and reduces the harmful acids that are formed in the mouth.

Prevents Ageing

Oxygen is very important to us, but it can also be a very harmful agent in form of active or free radical oxygen. One way to slow the ageing process is to prevent the accumulation of active oxygen in our body. This can be done by antioxidants, which are strongly present in Green tea.

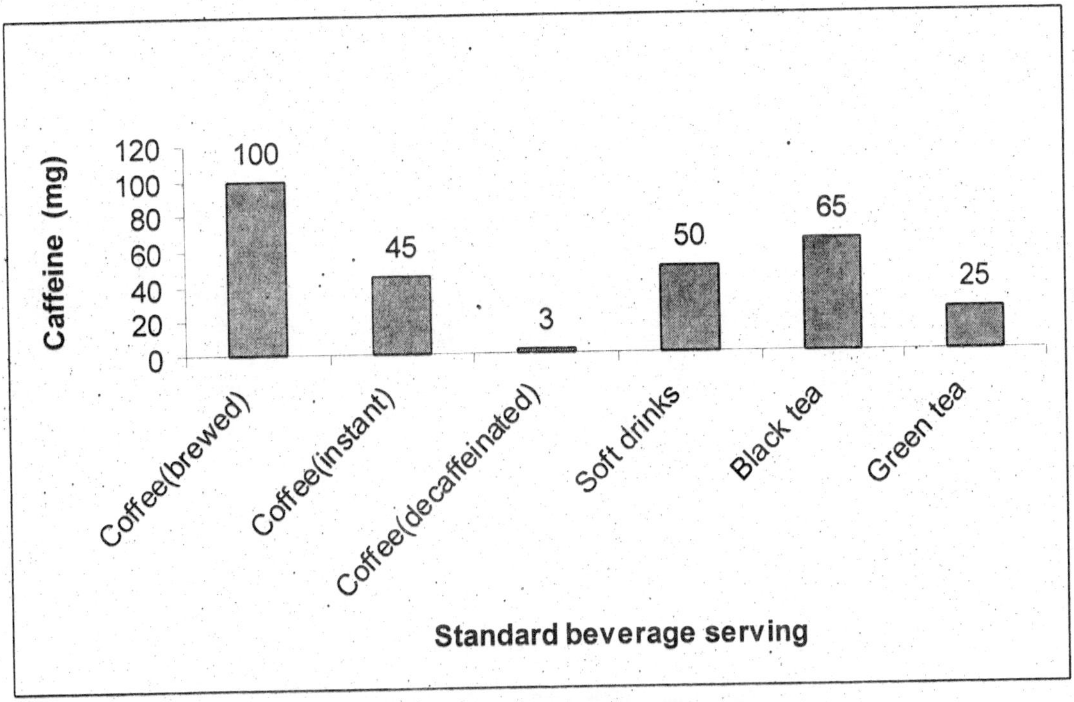

Figure 45.1: Comparison Chart of Caffeine Content

Table 45.2: Correlation Between Age, Height, Initial Weight and Final Weight

	Age (Year)	*Height (cm)*	*Initial Weight (kg)*	*Weight After 3 Months*
Age (Year)	1			
Height (cm)	-0.02942	1		
Initial Weight (kg)	-0.31678	0.812828	1	
Weight After 3 Months	-0.34052	0.763301	0.990017	1

Prevents Arthritis

Antioxidants in green tea may prevent and reduce the severity of rheumatoid arthritis.

Improves Digestion

Recent research speaks about the benefits of green tea as a very good appetizer. Green tea, after meals help to digest even high cholesterol food taken in heavy quantity.

Out of the above health benefits, two benefits were tested on few people.

1. Reduction of excessive fats
2. Control of high blood cholesterol

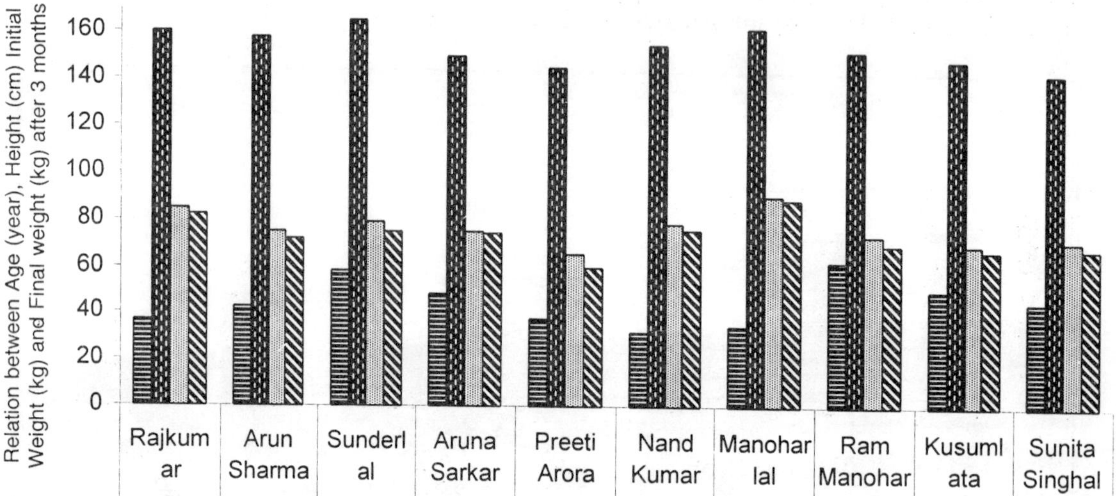

	Rajkumar	Arun Sharma	Sunderlal	Aruna Sarkar	Preeti Arora	Nand Kumar	Manoharlal	Ram Manohar	Kusumlata	Sunita Singhal
Series1	37	43	58	48	38	32	35	62	50	45
Series2	160	158	165	150	145	155	162	152	148	143
Series3	85	75	79	75	65	78	90	73	69	71
Series4	82	72	75	74	60	76	89	69	67	68

Patient's name

Figure 45.2: Effect of Green Tea on Weight

Results

Results showing in Tables 45.3 and 45.4.

Green tea was given three times a day after each meal in a combination with lemon. During the period patients were kept on a diet check. Their weights were observed at regular intervals and final weight was taken after 3 months.

Table 45.3: Effect of Green Tea on Weight

Sl.No.	Patient's Name	Age (in Years)	Height (in cms)	Initial Weight (in Kgs)	Final Weight (Kg) After 3 Months
1.	Rajkumar	37	160	85	82
2.	Arun Sharma	43	158	75	72
3.	Sunderlal	58	165	79	75
4.	Aruna Sarkar	48	150	75	74
5.	Preeti Arora	38	145	65	60
6.	Nand Kumar	32	155	78	76
7.	Manoharlal	35	162	90	89
9.	Ram Manohar	62	152	73	69
10.	Kusumlata	50	148	69	67
11.	Sunita Singhal	45	143	71	68

Table 45.4: Effect of Green Tea on Controling High-cholestrol Level

Sl.No.	Patient's name	Age	Weight (in kgs)	Initial Cholesterol level	Final Cholesterol Level
1.	Vandana Sharma	48	80	148	145
2.	Kamal Kishore	49	78	145	140
3.	Dinesh Kumar	53	89	159	154
4.	Uma Joshi	58	91	160	155
5.	A.K. Asthana	60	94	153	150
6.	Nirmala Devi	45	88	149	145
7.	Sanjeev	56	78	160	154
8.	Anil Batola	40	85	158	155
9.	Gurpreet Singh	48	90	161	159
10.	Rita Sharma	49	82	160	157

Table 45.5: t-Test Means Between Initial and Final Weight (kg)

	Initial Weight	*Final Weight*
Mean	76	73.2
Variance	55.11111	66.4
Observations	10	10
Pearson Correlation	0.990017	
Hypothesized Mean Difference	0	
df	9	
t Stat	6.725382	
P(T<=t) one-tail	4.3E-05	
t Critical one-tail	1.833113	
P(T<=t) two-tail	8.6E-05	
t Critical two-tail	2.262157	

References

American Journal of Clinical Nutrition 1999, November.

Journal of the college of the physicians and surgeons of Columbia university (P and S Journal: Fall 1997, Vol. 17, No. 3).

www.Kalyanitea.com.

Medicinal Plants: Conservation, Cultivation and Utilization (2007)
Editors: A.K. Chopra, D.R. Khanna, G. Prasad, D.S. Malik and R. Bhutiani
Published by: DAYA PUBLISHING HOUSE

Pages 375–376

Chapter 46

Medicinal Plant Conservation

Rekha Sharma
Assistant Professor, Government P.G. College, Mhow

ABSTRACT

Medicinal plants continue to be an important therapeutic aid for alleviating ailments of humankind. The importance of plant based medicine waxed and waned during the last 200 years. Advancements made in synthetic chemistry along with the discovery of antibiotics and cortico-steroids and their artificial synthetics caused rapid decline of plant-based medicines particularly in the developed nations during the century. The developing nations depend on the other hand mostly on plants for their medicine. In recent times, however, due to the increasing realization of the health hazards and toxicity associated with the indiscriminate use of synthetic drugs and antibiotics, there has been a renewal of interest in the use of plants and plants based drugs throughout the world. According to WHO, the resurgence of public interest in traditional medicine is on the increase because of a sweeping green wave and a large number of plant drugs are now sold in the 'health food shops' all over the world including the developed world (Pushpangadan and Narayanan Nair, 1997). The preventive and promotive aspects of the Eastern traditional systems of medicine particularly that of India and China are finding increased popularity and acceptance through out the world and scope for developing plant based drugs assumes greater significance at a time when modern medicine has failed to provide cure for the dreadful diseases like cancer, AIDS, arthritis, liver diseases and other diseases of unknown etiology.

Introduction

"The quest for good health and immortality has been a continuous human endeavor since the beginning of civilization throughout the world. Plants have been used as a source of medicine by men from ancient times. Initially, these formed the bulk of folk or ethnomedicine, practised in India and some other parts of the world. Later, a considerable part of this indigenous knowledge was formulated, documented and eventually passed into the organised systems of medicine, such as Ayurveda, Unani, Sidha or some other systems outside India. Subsequently, with the advance in techniques of phytochemistry and pharmacology, a number of active principles of medicinal plants were isolated and introduced as valuable drugs in modern medicine.

The resurgence of public interest in plant based medicine coupled with the rapid expansion of pharmaceutical industries have necessitated an increased demand for medicinal plants leading to over-exploitation that threaten the survival of many rare species. Confronted by such unprecedented genetic loss, disappearance of species and ecosystems conservation of our national heritage assumes paramount urgency. According to a recent study carried out by scientists of Tropical Botanic Garden and Research Institute (TBGRI), over-exploitation and unsustainable harvesting of medicinal plant resources are posing great danger to the survival of several invaluable plant species in the wild. Habitat degradation due to increased human activities (human settlements, agriculture and other developmental projects), illegal trades in rare and exquisite plant species and loss of regeneration potential of the degraded forests have further accelerated the current rate of genetic erosion and species extinction. TBGRI team has listed 19 critically endangered medicinal plants in Kerala, the southern most state in the Indian Union. Considering the rapid loss of medicinal plants various measures has been initiated in India for conserving and sustainably utilizing the medicinal plant genetic resources.

Medicinal Plants: Conservation, Cultivation and Utilization (2007) *Pages 377–382*
Editors: A.K. Chopra, D.R. Khanna, G. Prasad, D.S. Malik and R. Bhutiani
Published by: DAYA PUBLISHING HOUSE

Chapter 47

Antibacterial Activity of Polar Fraction of *Callistemon lanceolatus* and *Callistemon viminalis*

Harish Chandra*[1], Arun Pratap Singh[1], Jatin Kumar Srivastava[2], Gyanendra Awasthi[3] and Ajay Singh[4]

[1]Department of Microbiology, [3]Department of Biochemistry, [4]Department of Chemistry
Dolphin (P.G.) Institute of Biomedical and Natural Science, V.P.O. Manduwala, Near to Suddhowala, Chakrata Road, Dehradun – 248 007 (U.A.)
[2]Department of Environmental Sciences
Institute of Biosciences and Biotechnology Chatrapati Shahu Ji Maharaj University, Kalyanpur, Kanpur, India

ABSTRACT

Callistemon lanceolatus a small evergreen tree with alternate linear–lanceolate leaves having crimson flower in spike (like the brush of bottle). Commonly medium sized tree, cultivated as an ornamental plants in the garden. *Callistemon viminalis* is exotic tree very commonly cultivated in the Indian garden. The farmer produces very large quantities of nectar and is much sought after in flowers by bees. Callistemon belong to family *Myrtaceae*. The family *Myrtaceae* consists of 100 to 150 genera and 3000 to 3500 sp distributed in tropical and sub-tropical regions confined mostly to Australia. In the present study antibacterial activity of methanolic and Acetone extract of *Callistemon lanceolatus* and *Callistemon viminalis* were investigated against six bacterial strains *i.e. Staphylococcus aureus, Escherchia coli, Klebsiella pneumoniae, Micrococcus luteus, Bacillus cereus*

* Corresponding Author: Phone 91+135+26945 45, 47,49 Ext. 124, Telefax: 2694547; E-mail: hreesh5@rediffmail.com.

and Bacillus pumilus. It was found that both plant extract shows significant activity against *Micrococcus luteus, Bacillus cereus* and *Bacillus pumilus* and no activity shown against *E. coli, Klebsiella pneumoniae* and *Staphylococcus aureus.* Different concentration of acetone and methanolic extract were tested against these bacteria against which they had shown activity and it was found that at 30 per cent concentration of methanolic extract of *C. lanceolatus* shown good activity (*i.e.* zone of inhibition) against *B. cereus* (*i.e.* 30 mm) in comparison to acetone extract *i.e.* 28 mm. In case of *C. viminalis* at 30 per cent concentration acetone extract has good activity against *M. luteus* (*i.e.* 26 mm) in comparison to methanolic extract *i.e.* 24 mm.

Keywords: Callistemon viminalis, Callistemon lanceolatus, Bacillus pumilus Micrococcus luteus and Bacillus cereus.

Introduction

Callistemon lanceolatus a small evergreen tree with alternate linear–lanceolate leaves having crimson flower in spike (like the brush of bottle). Commonly medium sized tree, cultivated as an ornamental plants in the garden *Callistemon viminalis* is exotic tree very commonly cultivated in the Indian garden. The farmer produces very large quantities of nectar and is much sought after in flowers by bees. Callistemon belong to *Myrtaceae.* The family *Myrtaceae* consists of 100 to 150 genera and 3000 to 3500 sp distributed in tropical and sub-tropical regions confined mostly to Australia. *Callistemon lanceolotus* leaves after extraction with a combination of organic solvents have afforded 3-methyltetradec-2-en-7-ol and the rare C-methylated flavones: 5-hydroxy-7,4'-dimethoxy-6,8-dimethylflavone and 5-hydroxy-7,4'-dimethoxy-6-methylflavone. Structures have been established by spectroscopic methods. Isolation of C-methylated flavones from *C. lanceolatus* supported the view that they are characteristic to Myrtaceae. (Huq *et al.*, 1997)

Analysis of leaf essential oils in *Callistemon viminalis* (Sol. ex Gaertner) G.Don ex Loudon was used to determine the validity of infraspecific taxa recognised in the taxon. The leaf essential oils obtained, in 0.08-0.63 per cent yield, have been found to be qualitatively similar over the wide geographic distribution of the species (from 12 degree 28' S to 29 degree 43' S) but to differ quantitatively over this range. All oils contained alpha-pinene, beta-pinene, myrcene and 1,8-cineole as their major compounds and traces of the beta-triketones, leptospermone and flavesone. Overall the essential oils that contained the most 1,8-cineole (60-82 per cent) came from the more southern latitudes (29 degree 14' S to 20 degree 16' S) while those oils with less 1,8-cineole (0.5-47 per cent) came from the more northerly latitudes (12 degree 53' S to 25 degree 18' S). There was overlap in the region 25 degree S to 22 degree S, although the majority of samples from this region contained high 1,8-cineole values. Partial least squares analysis allowed the latitude to be calibrated by the leaf oil concentrations. These data would lend only equivocal support for the establishment of two intraspecific taxa of *C. viminalis* (Brophy *et al.*, 1997). The leaves of *Callistemon viminalis,* on hydrodistillation, gave 0.45 per cent of an oil on a fresh weight basis. GC and GC-MS analysis of the oil resulted in the identification of 42 constituents, representing 99.5 per cent of the oil. 1,8-Cineole (61.7 per cent), alpha-pinene (24.2 per cent) and menthyl acetate (5.3 per cent) were the major components (Srivastava *et al.*, 2003). Bhore *et al.* (1995) investigated one of the attempt to test the efficacy of four natural plant extracts and two commercially available plant products against the test fungi *Aspergillus flavus* and *Curvularia lunata* causing collar rot of groundnut and leaf spot of sunflower respectively. Fifteen plant extracts were tested by spore germination. The extracts from *Allium sativum. Callistemon lanceolatus, Emblica officinalis* and *Punica granatum* and commercially available plant products *viz.,* Indiara and Neemark were selected and used for seed germination test, seed treatment and foliar sprays against the test fungi. The crude extract of *Callistemon lanceolatus* against *Aspergillus flavus* and acetone extract of the same against *Curvularia-lunata* and 1 per cent Indiara were found effective in inhibition of spore germination, suppressing collar rot and minimizing the leaf spot of the test fungi.

Material and Methodology

Collection of Plant Material

Plant material *Callistemon viminalis* (Seed), were bought from the local nursery, Panditwari, Dehradun. Leaves of *Callistemon lanceolatus* were collected from the local area of Dehradun.

Processing of Plant Material

Plant material collected from the local market and local areas were hand sorted and shed dried in the room. Leaves collected from the local areas were washed under the tap water and finally rinse with Distilled water and shed dried. Dried plant material of these plant were powdered with the help of Mortar pestle.

Extraction

100 gm of powdered material were exracted in methanol and Acetone in a wide mouth flask separately by using blendor. After homogenizing kept flask unaltered until the particle get settled. When the particle of plant material get settled. Filter the extract with the hilp of filter paper (Whatmann filter paper no 42). Repeat this process until the extract become colorless. (See Flow Chart)

Flow Chart of Extraction

100 gm seed/plant material

↓

Powdered with mortar pestle

↓

Add 250 ml of Methanol/Acetone

↓

Homogenise with Blendor

↓

Kept Unaltered to settle down the particles

↓

Filter it through Whatmann filter paper No 42

↓

Repeat procedure 4-5 times till solvent become colorless

↓

Collect filterate in separate Flask

↓

Concentrate by using Rotary evaporator

After extraction process was completed filterate which was obtained by the extraction were concentrated in Rotary Evaporator (Butchi Type) till all the solvent evaporate. If it is not possible then extract were taken out in preweighed beaker (100 ml) and then the evaporate under water bath with porcelain particle or glass bead to avoid bumping of solvent and temperature should be maintained under boiling temperature of the solvent.

Bacterial Strains

A total six bacterial strains were used for this study *i.e. Staphylococcus aureus, Escherchia coli, Klebsiella pneumoniae, Micrococcus luteus, Bacillus cereus and Bacillus pumilus.*

Maintenance of Bacterial Strain

All the seven bacterial strain maintain in the laboratory on the surface of Nutrient Agar Slant and preserved in the refrigerator at 4°C and taken out and bring it at room temperature whenever required for the study.

Antimicrobial Activity Test

Preparation of Inoculum

The ideal inoculum after overnight incubation gives the even semi confluent growth. Too heavy inoculum may reduce the size of inhibition zone by many antimicrobial agents from plant source. Using a straight wire touch 5-10 well isolated colonies of particular microorganism against which antimicrobial activity to be tested. Inoculate on the nutrient broth. Medium. Incubate at 35-37°C for 4–6 hour. The density of the inoculums is adjusted to 10^8 cfu/ml by comparing with that of 0.5 Mc Farland Standard.

Agar Well Diffusion

0.1 ml of the original cultures (about10^6-10^7 cells) were added into sterile duplicate sets of petri dishes and 25 ml of the molten (45° C) Mueller Hinton Agar (HiMedia, Ltd) were poured into petri dishes. The methanol or Acetone extract (0.1ml) were placed in wells (8mm diameter) cut in the agar media and plates were incubated at 37° C in the case of bacteria and at 30°C in the case of yeasts (Kivanç *et al.*, 1986). The resulting inhibition zones obtained with bacteria were recorded after 24 hour.

Result and Discussion

The result of methanolic and acetone extract of *C. lanceolatus* and *C.viminalis* are shown in Tables 47.1–47.4. It was found that both plant extract shows significant activity against *M. luteus, B. cereus* and *B. pumilus* and no activity shown against *E. coli, K. pneumoniae* and *S. aureus*. Different concentration of acetone and methanolic extract were tested against these bacteria which had shown activity and it was found that at 30 per cent concentration of methanolic extract of *C. lanceolatus* shown good activity (*i.e.* zone of inhibition) against *B. cereus* (*i.e.* 30 mm) in comparison to acetone extract *i.e.* 28 mm. In case of *C. viminalis* at 30 per cent concentration acetone extract has good activity against *M. luteus* (*i.e.* 26 mm) in comparision to methanolic extract *i.e.* 24 mm. In recent years multiple drug/chemical resistance in both human and plant pathogenic microorganism have been developed due to indiscriminate used of commercial antimicrobial drugs/chemical commonly used in the treatment of infectious disease (Davis, 1994). This Situation forced the scientist to the searching of new antimicrobial substance from various sources like medicinal plants (Clark, 1996; Cordell, 2000). Antimicrbial activity of Callistemon spp. have been also reported by other researchers Pandey (1995) reported complete inhibition of the growth of fungal pathogens of sugarcane due to essential oil of *C. lanceolatus* whereas, (Pandey *et al.*, 1982) observed fungistatic effect of essential oil of *C. lanceolatus* against *Fussarium oxysporium* sp. *udum*.

Table 47.1: Antibacterial Activity of Methanolic Extract of Leaves of *C. lanceolatus* at Different Concentration

Plant Part	*Concentration in Percentage (%)*	*Zone of Inhibition in mm*		
		Bacillus pumilus	*Bacillus cereus*	*Micrococus luteus*
Leaves	5	20.5 ± 0.7	19.5 ± 1.4	16.0 ± 0.7
	10	23.0 ±1.4	21.5 ± 0.7	20.2 ± 0.3
	15	23.2 ± 0.3	24.0 ± 1.4	22.0 ± 2.8
	20	24.0 ± 2.8	25.5 ± 2.1	24.0 ± 1.4
	25	24.5 ± 1.4	28.2 ± 0.3	24.0 ± 0.7
	30	26.0 ± 1.4	30.5 ± 0.7	26.0 ± 2.8

Table 47.2: Antibacterial Activity of Acetone Extract of Leaves of *C. lanceolatus* at Different at Different Concentration

Plant Part	*Concentration in Percentage (%)*	*Zone of Inhibition in mm*		
		Bacillus pumilus	*Bacillus cereus*	*Micrococus luteus*
Leaves	5	14.0 ± 1.4	18.0 ± 0.7	18.0 ± 1.4
	10	16.2 ± 0.3	20.5 ± 0.7	20.0 ± 0.3
	15	16.5 ± 1.4	24.2 ± 0.3	20.5 ± 0.7
	20	18.0 ± 1.4	24.5 ± 1.4	22.0 ± 0.7
	25	18.0 ± 0.7	26.0 ± 2.8	22.0 ± 0.7
	30	20.0 ± 2.1	28.0 ± 0.3	24.0 ± 2.1

Table 47.3: Antibacterial Activity of Methanolic Extract of Seeds of *C. viminalis* at Different at Different Concentration

Plant Part	*Concentration in Percentage (%)*	*Zone of Inhibition in mm*		
		Bacillus pumilus	*Bacillus cereus*	*Micrococus luteus*
Seed	5	18.2 ± 0.3	18.0 ± 1.4	16.0 ± 0.3
	10	20.0 ± 0.0	20.0 ± 0.3	18.5 ± 0.3
	15	22.0 ± 2.8	21.0 ± 1.4	20.0 ± 1.4
	20	22.0 ± 0.3	23.0 ± 1.4	23.0 ± 0.3
	25	24.0 ± 1.4	23.5± 2.1	24.0 ± 1.4
	30	25.0 ± 0.3	24.0 ± 0.7	24.5± 0.3

Table 47.4: Antibacterial Activity of Acetone Extract of Seed of *C. viminalis* at Different Concentration

Plant Part	*Concentration in Percentage (%)*	*Zone of Inhibition in mm*		
		Bacillus pumilus	*Bacillus cereus*	*Micrococus luteus*
Seed	5	14.5 ± 2.8	14.0 ± 1.4	14.0 ± 0.7
	10	16.0 ± 1.4	16.5 ± 2.1	18.2 ± 1.4
	15	18.0 ± 1.4	20.5 ± 0.7	20.0 ± 0.7
	20	19.0 ± 0.3	22.0 ± 0.3	22.5 ± 1.4
	25	20.2 ± 0.7	22.5 ± 1.4	24.0 ± 2.8
	30	20.5 ± 1.4	24.0 ± 0.3	26.0 ± 1.4

References

Bhore, S.T., Thakare, C.S. and Kadam, V.C., 1995. Efficacy of some plant extracts and commercial plant products against test fungi. *Journal of Maharastra Agriculture Universities*, 20(2): 251–254.

Brophy, J.A., Forster, P.I., Goldsack, R.J., Hibert, D.B. and Punruckvong, A ., 1997. Variation in *Callistemon viminalis* (Myrtaceae): New evidence from leaf essential oils. *Australian-Systematic-Botany*, 10(1): 1–13.

Clark, A.M., 1996. Natural product as resource for new drugs. *Pharmaceutical Research*, 13: 1133–1141.

Cordell, G.A., 2000. Biodiversity and drug discovery: A symbiotic relationship. *Phytochemistry*, 55: 463–480.

Davis, S.G. and Savoboda, K.P., 1989. Antibacterial activity of summer savory (*Satureja hortensis* L), essential oil and its constituent. *Journal of Horticultural Science*, 64: 205–210.

Huq, F. and Misra, L.N., 1997. An alkenol and C-methylated flavones from *Callistemon lanceolatus* leaves. *Planta-Medica*, 63(4): 369–370.

Pandey, D.K., Chandra, H. and Tripathi, N.N., 1982. Volatile fungi toxic activity of some higher plants with special reference to that of *Callistemon lanceolatus*. *Phytopathologische-Zeitschrift*, 105: 175–182.

Pandey, A.K., 1995. Fungitoxicity of essential oil of *Callistemon lanceolatus* DC. against some sugarcane pathogens. In: *Proceedings of the National Academy of Sciences India, Section B: Biological Sciences*, 65 73–80.

Srivastava, S.K., Ahmad, A., Syamsunder, K.V., Aggarwal, K.K. and Khanuja, S.P.S., 2003. Essential oil composition of *Callistemon viminalis* leaves from India. *Flavour and Fragrance Journal*, 18(5): 361–363.

Kivançc, M. and Akgül, A., 1986. Antibacterial activities of essentialoils from Turkish spices and citrus. *Flavour and Fragrance Journal*, p. 175–179.

Medicinal Plants: Conservation, Cultivation and Utilization (2007) *Pages 383–386*
Editors: A.K. Chopra, D.R. Khanna, G. Prasad, D.S. Malik and R. Bhutiani
Published by: DAYA PUBLISHING HOUSE

Chapter 48

Optimization of Procedure for Dyeing of Cotton and Wool Fibres with Bark of *Juglans regia* as Natural Dyes

S.C. Sati[1]*, J.S. Jagwan[2] and Manisha Dobhal[2]

[1]**Department of Chemistry, H.N.B. Garhwal University Campus, Srinagar, Garhwal**

[2]**Department of Chemistry, H.N.B. Garhwal University Campus, Badhshaithaul Tehri, Garhwal**

Introduction

Vegetable dyes and their uses were known in ancient time more than 2000 years ago. It was found that the discovery of synthetic dyes reduce the use of natural dyes and consequently the export of same was affected in large extent. However due to non toxic nature, eco-friendly behaviour and properties to impart variety of colours, once again natural dyes is getting the more attention of chemists and dyers. The *Juglans regia* (Ankhrot) belong to family *Juglandaceae* is large tree. Flowers green, male and female on the same tree, appearing with the leaves.

The bark of *Juglans regia* (ankhrot) were known to contain substances that could be used for colouring the fabrics, cloths, utensils, and house hold implements. The colouring matter presents in the bark of *Juglans regia* is a mixture of Lignins, Tannins, Anthocyanins and Xanthones. The bark are credited with astringent properties. The fresh bark powder and seed coat of the plant are used as biopesticide in agriculture.

The present article deals with optimization of procedure for dyeing of cotton and wool with bark extract of *Juglans regia* and also the study of dyed sample toward light and washing rastness studies.

* Corresponding Author.

Material and Methods

The bark or the plant were collected from the jungle of Sainti Ghat, Chamoli Garhwal, Uttaranchal. India, during August 2005, and dried in shade. All the chemicals used as mordant were of L.R/A.R and BDH fine chemicals. The white wool and cotton samples were freed from traces of protein, gums and oil impurities by washing it with detergent or soap for a required period, followed by kneading, squeezing and rinsing with lot of water till it was free from traces of detergent. It was then dried in shade and ironed before dyeing and mordanting, the cotton and wool samples was soaked for an hour. The optical density was recorded by using digital spectrophotometer.

The optimum concentration of dye material and the time for extraction of the dye and dyeing of cotton and wool were found out by taking different concentration of dye material (3-18 per cent) in different beakers containing 100 ml water for an hour and measuring the optical density of dye liquor at 345 nm (Table 48.1).

Table 48.1 Optimum Concentration of Dye Material

Conc. of Dye Material g/100 ml of Water	*Optical Density*	*Percentage Rating*
3 gm	0.091	55
6 gm	0.097	58
9 gm	0.123	62
*12 gm	*0.127	*69
15 gm	0.119	62
18 gm	0.102	65

Wavelength 345 nm

* Selected sample.

The optical time for extraction of dye was found out by extracting the optimum concentration of dye material at 80°C for 15, 30, 45 and 60 minutes and the optical density of the liquor was measured (Table 48.2).

Table 48.2: Optimum Time for Extraction of Dye and Dyeing

Time for Extraction of Dye (min.)	*Conc. of Dye Material (gm)*	*Optical Density rating*	*Per cent*	*Dyeing Time/Per Cent*
30	12	0.152	0.78	0.82
*60	12	*0.159	*0.82	*0.89
90	12	0.158	0.80	0.88
120	12	0.155	0.79	0.72
150	12	0.152	0.72	0.72

Wavelength 345 nm

* Selected sample.

In order to find the optimum time for dyeing one gram of cotton and wool fibres was added to four beakers and dyed for 15, 30, 45 and 60 minutes. The samples were stirred occasionally to obtain an even dyeing. The dyed samples were taken out from beakers and dried in shade. The evenness of dye, depth of shade and overall appearance are evaluated by a panel of judges. The highest percentage rating was calculated by judgment Table 48.2.

Number of shades were obtained by mordanting the cotton and wool with different concentration of mordants such as chrome, alum, copper sulphate, ferrous sulphate, stannous chloride etc. and also using the pre-mordanting (mordanting before dyeing). Post-mordanting (mordanting after dyeing) and simultaneous mordanting (dyeing and mordanting together in same pot).

Analysis of Samples Toward Light and Washing Fastness

The dyed samples of cotton and wool to be tested for the light fastness were cut into specimens of 3 × 6 cm, numbered and mounted on a cardboard frame. The blue wool and cotton sample (five of each) standard having a light fastness rating from low to high (1 low–5 high cotton, 1 low–5 high wool) were stapled on cardboard strip. A strip of thick black chart paper was pinned in such a manner that half of it lies on the specimen and the standards thereby leaving the samples half exposed and half covered.

A strip of thick black paper was put inside the fluorescent lamp. The specimens and standards were checked at regular intervals. The samples were compared with blue wool and cotton standards and rated. The different methods of mordanting produce good range of colours having various shades ranging from dark brown to brownish black, black to Greenish, brown to black. The pre-mordanting method gave the best results/colours with Stannous Chloride and Ferrous Sulphate. A variety of shades was also obtained with post and simultaneous mordanting process.

The washing fastness of sample was done by making the specimens of 5 × 7 cm size and placed between two layers of the fabric of the same size. These layers were seen from all sides to form a complex specimen. The soap or detergent solution was prepared by dissolving 6 gram of soap or detergent in 1000ml of water. Each composite sample was tréated with soap solution in Launderometer for 20–30 minutes at a temperature of 60°C. The samples were then removed and rinsed thoroughly under running tap water, dried and ironed.

The rating of washing fastness was done on the basis of the staining of the fabrics. Washing brought a considerable change in the colour of dyed sample Chrome, Alum and Stannous chloride mordanted samples showed very poor fastness. Cotton was stained with $SnCl_2$ whereas wool was noticeably stained with Alum.

Ferrous Sulphate mordanted samples has fair washing fastness while Copper Sulphate and Chrome mordanted samples have poor to fair washing fastness. Chrome and $SnCl_2$ showed slight stain on wool.

Results and Discussion

From the data of Tables 48.1 and 48.2 it is evident that 12 gm of bark powder was optimum to give the maximum optical density of dye liquor while 60 minutes of extraction time and dyeing time was found to be optimum. Best shades of colours were obtained by using 15 gm of Alum, 5 gm of Chrome, 8 gram of $CuSO_4$, 8 gram of $SnCl_2$ and $FeSO_4$ respectively per 100 gm of wool and cotton.

In present study it was observed that cotton samples was noticeable stained with Stannous Chloride using post mordanting technique, while wool was noticeably stained with Alum using same procedure. The washing fastness of both sample of cotton and wool was found fairly good.

Some efforts was also made to mordant the samples with naturally occurring mordants work on natural mordants of plants origin and eco-friendly behaviour in progress.

The whole study points out that the dye extracted form bark of *Juglans regia* can be use to obtained array of colours either alone or in combination with mordants (natural/synthetic) with different fabrics. Dye can be used for commercial purposes by industries or local tribals of Garhwal and Kumaon presently associated with this ancient method of natural dyeing in this synthetic era of carcinogenic and harmful dyes.

Medicinal Plants: Conservation, Cultivation and Utilization (2007) *Pages 387–388*
Editors: A.K. Chopra, D.R. Khanna, G. Prasad, D.S. Malik and R. Bhutiani
Published by: DAYA PUBLISHING HOUSE

Chapter 49

Optimization of Procedure for Dyeing of Wool, Cotton and Silk Fibres

S.C. Sati[1], Manisha Dobhal[2] and J.S. Jagwan[2]
[1]Department of Chemistry, H.N.B. Garhwal University Campus, Srinagar, Garhwal
[2]Department of Chemistry, H.N.B. Garhwal University Campus, Badshahithaul, Tehri, Garhwal

The heritage of medicinal and dye yielding plants use in India has an ancient history and India is famous for its rich bio-diversity throughout the world. Colour has played an important role in adding beauty to the world. Vegetable dyes and their use were known in ancient times more than 2000 years ago. The colouring matters (Secondary Metabolites) present in the plants is a mixture of Anthocyanins, Flavonoids, Xanthones and Lignins (*e.g.* Gallic acid and its dimer).

The present work was carried out to gather information from the tribal community of Garhwal about their traditional knowledge on natural dyes, mordants and dyeing processes. It was found that discovery of synthetic dyes reduce the use of natural dye and consequently the export of the same was affected in a great extent. However, due non-toxic, eco-friendly and properties to impart variety of colours (shades) once again natural dye is getting more attention of chemist and dyers.

Some local dye yielding plants namely *Juglans regia* (Akhrot), *Rhododenderon arboretum* (Burans), *Pinus roxburghii* (Chir), *Symplocos racemosus* (Lodh), *Bombex cieba* (Semal), *Butea monosperma* (Dhak), *Erythrina suberosa* (Madar), *Myrica esculenta* (Kaphal), *Berberis asiatica* (Kingor), *Rheum* species (Archa and Dolu) and few *Polygomlm* species were collected for extraction and processing for natural dyes; Wide ranges of colours were obtained on dyeing with wool, cotton and silk using both the natural and synthetic mordant. Parts of few plant species. *Hemicvia annua, Myrica esculenta, Symplocos racemosa, Juglans regia.* Tea leaves citrus fruits and ash were used as a natural mordant. The best results were obtained with simultaneous mordanting (dyeing mordanting together) in most of the plants extract.

The colourtastness properties were determined by measuring the optical density with the help of digital spectrophotometer. These results could help the best uses of the local plant resources for dyeing besides the medicinal and other properties of the plants.

Table 49.1: Optimun Time for Extraction of Dye and Dyeing

Time for Extraclia of Dye/min	*Conc. of Dye Material*	*Optical Diversity*	*% Rating*	*Dyeing Time/ Per Cent Rating*
30	12	0.152	0.78	0.82
60	12	0.159	0.82	89
90	12	0.158	0.80	88
120	12	0.155	–79	–72
150	12	0.152	–72	–70

The bark of *juglans regia* (ankhrot) were known to contain subston us that could be used for colouring the fabrics, cloths, utensils, and house hold implements. The colouring matter presents in the bark of *Juglans regia* is a mixture of liguins Tannins.

Medicinal Plants: Conservation, Cultivation and Utilization (2007) *Pages 389–391*
Editors: A.K. Chopra, D.R. Khanna, G. Prasad, D.S. Malik and R. Bhutiani
Published by: DAYA PUBLISHING HOUSE

Chapter 50

Medicinal Plant: Utilization and Conservation

Sudha Dubey
Holkar Science College, Indore

ABSTRACT

Today's healthcare systems rely largely on plant material. Much of the world's population depends on traditional medicine to meet daily health requirements, especially within developing countries. Use of plant-based remedies is also widespread in many industrial use. Countries and numerous pharmaceuticals are based on or derived from plant compounds. Similarly, cosmetics and other household products may contain plants of medicinal or therapeutic value.

Since the vast majority of plants that are used to create many of these remedies are collected from the wild, some management of medicinal plant resources is critical, especially where traditional medicine prevails. Within traditional systems, reliance on natural medicinal resources can be attributed to cultural preferences, as well as to the high cost, and inaccessibility of western medicine. On the global level, where demand often exists for medicinal plants originating in distant lands, management is equally important if supplies are to meet the need of a variety of medical systems and a growing number of industries.

Medicinal plants originate from almost every part of the globe. They range from small perennial herbs adapted to high elevation mountain areas, to the enormous baobab, one of Africa's most, renowned trees. Plants are harvested for local use on virtually every continent. For international markets certain regions are important centres of production. These include the Himalayan region with Nepal. India and Pakistan being the source of medicinal plants integral to Ayurvedic and other traditional medicine systems, and Europe and America serving as a source for expanding herbal medicine and botanicals industries popular in the west.

As demand for medicinal plants rises, harvest rates also increase. There are numerous documented cases of over exploitation and even local extirpation in response in intensive harvest.

Trade volumes are large, and of significant value. The result is that the natural resource base is becoming degraded in certain areas, and an increasing number of species are becoming threatened.

Introduction

Maintaining medicinal plant harvest and trade within sustainable levels present a major challenge today and for the foreseeable future. A combined effort by those concerned with the conservation of medicinal plant species and/or the healthcare systems dependent on them will be crucial to ensuring the long-term viability of both. In virtually all corners of the globe, different sectors are working at cross-purpose, with some intent upon exploitation, others devoted to preservation, and most unaware of the interests and motivators of other stakeholders. Cultural differences also impede collaboration and cooperation, and make solutions even more difficult to find.

In India, more than 70 per cent of the rural people use medicinal plants for treating various diseases. The number of plant species in common use exceeds 400 and the specific curative values of many of them are well known. The Himalayan range, Northeastern region and the Western, Central and Southern mountain ranges are the natural habitats of many of these medicinal species.

Although herbs have been in use for medicinal purposes for centuries, their commercial exploitation has seen a rapid increase only in recent years. Consequently, there is a tendency to over-exploit their natural resource base. In addition, medicinal herbs are lost or reduced in numbers because of deforestation. Hence many medicinal plants that have served human popluations for generations are in an endangered state.

Forest areas inhabited by tribal people are a rich source of medicinal plants. They have been conserving these species for a long time and are very knowledgeable about them. They will be able to provide valuable information about their uses, climatic requirements, conservation and sustainable harvesting.

Those who know about the properties of medicinal species are locally known as *Vaidus* or *Bhagats*. They are very popular among the rural population because of their house visits to treat the patients. Their source of medicinal herbs is usually nearby forests. They collect the plant parts leaves, root, bark, stem, flower and seed-from forests.

In spite of continuous harvesting of plant parts for medicinal purposes, these species have survived. A question that may be asked is whether this species conservation happens naturally or do the tribal people have a sustainable management strategy. Probably a combination of both helped in their survival. In the case of some species at least, the germplasm was carefully conserved and passed on to the next generation.

The tribal communities that used medicinal plants usually harvested or extracted the minimum required quantity from forests. A small quantity of root, stem or bark may be kept at home, but the general practice is to harvest them freshly when the need arises. Dry flowers and seeds may be harvested and stored because they are available only during certain seasons of the year.

It is not a practice to plant these species on cropland. However, those growing in the farm or homestead through natural dispersion may be retained if they do not interfere with farm operations. In future, it may become necessary to introduce the practice of cultivating them on farms as the numbers of medicinal plants growing in nature are being reduced drastically.

Knowledge on production and use of medicinal plants is passed on from generation to generation verbally. In the absence of appropriate documentation, there is always a possibility of this valuable information being lost. The chances of this happening are greater nowadays as youngsters tend to move out of their traditional occupations and elders have no one to pass on the knowledge. A systematic documentation effort that takes into confidence the established practitioners will help preserve the knowledge. Research to understand the scientific basis of herbal medicines will also add credibility.

Medicinal Plants: Conservation, Cultivation and Utilization (2007) *Pages 393–401*
Editors: A.K. Chopra, D.R. Khanna, G. Prasad, D.S. Malik and R. Bhutiani
Published by: DAYA PUBLISHING HOUSE

Chapter 51

Demographic Dispersion of Weed Flora of Rice, Maize and Wheat in Doon Valley of Uttaranchal

Arun Gupta[1], S.P. Joshi[1], Pramod Uniyal[2] and Asha Dobhal[2]
[1]Ecology Research Laboratory, Department of Botany, D.A.V. (PG) College, Dehra Dun – 248 007, Uttaranchal
[2]Government (PG) College, Rishikesh, Uttaranchal

ABSTRACT

Vegetational analysis of the weed flora of rice, maize and wheat crops or Doon valley was studied using quadrat method from 124 sites (37 in rice, 30 in maize and 57 in wheat among 57 weed species of rice, 77 of maize and 71 of wheats, *Fimbristylis miliacea, Echinochloa colonum* and *Anagallis arvensis* were the dominant in respective crop. Rice, maize and wheat crops had weed density of 358, 369 and 402 m^{-2} respectively. Weed dry weight was more in maize (153.38 gm^{-2}) followed by rice (8135 gm^{-2}) and wheat (53.94 gm^{-2}) crops.

Keywords: *Phytosociology, Weeds, Community structure and Cereal crops.*

Introduction

Weed flora on arable land can change over time because of farmer's choice of crop, fertilizer and soil have pronounced effect on the development of weed flora (Andersson and Milberg, 1998). Information on weed flora and their population in cereal crops of Doon valley is limited. Present study therefore was undertaken.

Materials and Methods

The study was conducted in 124 sites (57 in wheat, 37 in rice and 30 in maize) from 30 villages of Dehra Dun District (Uttaranchal). The villages were selected randomly from each block. Unweeded and no herbicides sprayed sites under irrigated and unirrigated conditions were selected from each village. At each site 10 quadrats (each 50 × 50 cm) were laid down during flowering stage of each crop. Frequency, density and abundance of weeds were calculated by using following formulae:

$$\text{Frequency (\%)} = \frac{\text{Number of quadrats in which species occurred}}{\text{Total number of quadrats studied}} \times 100$$

$$\text{Density} = \frac{\text{Total number of individual species}}{\text{Total number of quadrat studied}}$$

$$\text{Abundance} = \frac{\text{Total number of individual of species}}{\text{Number of quadrats of occurrence}}$$

Individuals of each species were counted from each quadrat. Culms and branches of grasses and herbs respectively were counted as individual. The dry weight of each weed species was recorded from such site for calculating the relative dominance.

The constancy, relative frequency, relative density, relative dominance and total density of weeds were calculated with following expressions:

$$\text{Constancy (\%)} = \frac{\text{Number of sites in which species occurred}}{\text{Total number of sites studied}} \times 100$$

$$\text{Relative frequency (RF)} = \frac{\text{Number of quadrats in which species occurred}}{\text{Total sum of quadrats in which all the species occurred}} \times 100$$

$$\text{Relative density (RD)} = \frac{\text{Number of individual of species}}{\text{Sum of number of individual of all the species}} \times 100$$

$$\text{Relative abdominance (RA)} = \frac{\text{Dry weight of weed species}}{\text{Total dry matter production by all the weed species}} \times 100$$

The RF + RD + RA combined into index and importance value index (IVI) of each species was calculated (Curtis and McIntosh, 1950) on pooled basis in each crop.

Results and Discussion

Pooled constancy, frequency, density, abundance and relative dominance on dry weight basis and IVI values weed species are presented in Tables 51.1–51.3 for rice, wheat and maize crops, respectively.

Table 51.1: Phytosociological Parameters of Weed Species in Rice

Weed Species	Constancy (%)	Frequency (%)	Density (m^{-2})	Dry Weight ($g\ m^{-2}$)	Abundance (m^{-2})	IVI
Fimbristylis miliacea	83.78	59.77	52.21	8.77	87.35	31.81
Echinochloa colonum	86.49	59.77	21.47	14.04	35.92	29.68
Echinochloa crus-galli	54.05	33.91	12.05	16.64	35.53	27.40
Cyperus iria	70.27	52.87	20.07	8.86	37.96	22.20
Lindernia crustacea	81.08	59.20	21.56	3.89	36.43	17.21
Ageratum conyzoides	64.86	41.38	11.77	5.73	28.44	14.79
Fimbristylis schoenoides	27.03	24.71	28.46	2.06	115.16	13.15
Cyperus difformis	59.46	44.25	20.44	1.74	46.18	12.66
Cyperus pumilus	51.35	35.63	19.52	1.50	54.77	11.17
Bacopa hamiltoniaina	48.65	35.63	19.98	1.15	56.06	10.86
Lindernia anagallis	62.16	43.10	17.31	0.68	40.16	10.36
Cyperus compressus	56.76	37.93	11.29	0.94	29.76	8.43
Bacopa procumbens	40.54	31.61	12.25	0.93	38.76	8.00
Fricaulon cinereum	24.32	15.52	15.79	1.13	101.78	7.48
Cyperus alulatus	27.03	17.82	9.22	1.31	51.74	6.11
Monochoria vaginalis	10.81	6.90	9.36	1.20	135.67	4.83
Eragrostis unioloides	43.24	20.11	5.70	0.80	28.34	4.77
Murdannia nudiflora	43.24	28.16	3.24	0.60	11.51	4.70
Eleocharis atropurpurea	29.73	19.54	6.69	0.53	34.24	4.64
Cynodon dactylon	54.05	27.01	3.66	0.45	13.53	4.51
Caesulia axillaris	13.51	11.49	4.21	1.65	36.60	4.43
Phyllanthus fraternus	45.95	20.69	2.46	0.52	11.89	3.57
Eleusine indica	29.73	16.09	2.00	0.75	12.43	3.22
Lindernia ciliata	29.73	17.82	3.10	0.22	1742	3.08
Mazus pumilus	32.43	16.09	3.40	0.24	21.14	2.99
Oldenlandia corymbosa	27.03	16.09	1.98	0.23	12.29	2.58
Cyperus aristatus	10.81	8.05	4.30	0.13	53.43	2.24
Ammannia multiflora	29.73	13.79	1.82	0.17	13.17	2.20
Ischaemum rugosum	10.81	4.60	0.67	1.19	14.50	2.15
Eragrostis tenella	18.92	8.051	1.77	0.39	22.00	1.85
Leptochloa panicea	18.92	9.20	1.45	0.19	15.75	1.64
Eclipta alba	21.62	9.77	0.57	0.17	5.88	1.43
Alternathera sessilis	24.32	9.20	0.67	0.17	7.25	1.40
Panicum psilopodium	16.22	5.17	0.67	0.45	12.89	1.30
Digitaria abludens	13.51	4.60	0.69	0.41	15.00	1.19
Commelina benghalensis	21.62	6.32	0.32	0.28	5.09	1.13

Contd...

Table 51.1–Contd...

Weed Species	Constancy (%)	Frequency (%)	Density (m^{-2})	Dry Weight (g m^{-2})	Abundance (m^{-2})	IVI
Oldenlandia diffusa	5.41	4.02	0.97	0.27	24.00	1.04
Eragrostis japonica	13.51	4.60	0.69	0.28	15.00	1.03
Galinsoga parviflora	5.41	4.02	1.10	0.06	27.43	0.82
Corchorus aestuans	13.51	4.02	0.16	0.23	4.00	0.76
Paspalum dilatatum	13.51	4.60	0.32	0.11	7.00	0.73
Scirpus squarrosus	2.70	2.30	1.45	0.03	63.00	0.68
Physalis minima	5.41	3.45	0.16	0.13	4.67	0.58
Justicia simplex	10.81	4:02	0.18	0.03	4.57	0.54
Eupatorium adenophorum	5.41	3.45	0.23	0.06	6.67	0.52
Torenia cordifolia	10.81	3.45	0.30	0.04	8.67	0.51
Blainvelleaa acmella	5.41	1.15	0.05	0.16	4.00	0.34
Euphorbia hirta	5.41	1.15	0.05	0.05	4.00	0.20
Dactyloctenium aegypticum.	5.41	1.15	0.05	0.05	4.00	0.20
Alternanthera philoxeroides	5.41	1.15	0.05	0.03	4.00	0.17
Biophytum reinwardtii	2.70	1.15	0.05	0.00	4.00	0.15
Cyporus rotundus	2.70	0.57	0.09	0.03	16.00	0.12
Momordica dioica	2.70	0.57	0.07	0.02	4.00	0.12
Setaria glauca	2.70	0.57	0.07	0.02	12.00	0.11
Oxalis corniculata	2.70	0.57	0.02	0.00	4.00	0.08
Xanthium strumarium	2.70	0.57	0.02	0.00	4.00	0.08
Ipomea pos-tigridis	2.70	0.57	0.02	0.00	4.00	0.07
Total		**918.94**	**358.14**	**81.75**		**300.01**

Weed Constancy and Frequency

Based on frequency and constancy, weed species were grouped into four categories in rice. Group 1 which comprised or *Fimbristylis miliacea, Echinochloa colonum, Cyperus iria* and *Lindernia crustacea* had constancy >70 per cent and frequency > 50 per cent. Group 2 comprised of *Echinochloa crus-galli, Cyperus difformis, Cyperus pumilus, Lindernia anagallis* and *Cyperus compressus,* had constancy 50–70 per cent and frequency 30–50 per cent. Group 3 consisted of *Bacopa hamiltoniana, Bacopa procumbens, Eragrostis, unioloides, Murdannia nudiflora, Phyllanthus fraternus* and *Cynodon dactylon* had constancy 30–50 per cent and frequency between 20–30 per cent. Rests of the species were grouped as infrequent species.

In maize, a total of 77 weed species belonged to Poaceae (16), Cyperaceae (8) and other broad-level weeds (53) was recorded. *Commelina benghalensis* was the most widely distributed with constancy 93.3 per cent followed by *E. colonum* (73.3 per cent) and *Ageratum conyzoides* (70 per cent). Species which infected more than 50 per cent in maize were *Digataria abudents* (63.3 per cent), *Eleusine indica* (56.7 per cent), *P. fraternus* (56.7 per cent), *Brachiaria ramose, Cyperus iria* and *Cyperus alulatus* all (53 per cent). *Galinsoga parviflora, Mollugo pentaphylla, Kyllinga triceps, Lindernia crustacea, M. nudiflora, Cyperus*

Table 51.2: Phytosociological Parameters of Weed Species in Maize

Weed Species	Constancy (%)	Frequency (%)	Density (m^{-2})	Dry Weight (g m^{-2})	Abundance (m^{-2})	IVI
Echinochloa colonum	73.33	61.27	41.94	41.40	68.46	44.46
Commelina benghalensis	93.33	83.10	26.23	18.11	31.56	27.19
Eleusine indica	56.67	48.59	13.49	12.74	27.77	16.79
Cyperus iria	53.33	42.25	29.94	6.59	70.87	16.61
Oxalis latifolia	16.67	16.20	22.99	8.62	141.91	13.45
Ageratum conyzoides	70.00	47.18	21.32	4.27	45.19	13.25
Galinsoga parviflora	30.00	25.35	25.94	4.19	102.33	12.28
Brachiaria ramosa	53.33	38.03	13.52	7.22	35.56	12.16
Cyperus alulatus	53.33	43.66	18.34	4.16	42.00	12.02
Mollugo pentaphylla	46.67	30.28	17.61	6.20	58.14	11.82
Digitaria abludens	63.33	35.21	11.41	7.02	32.40	11.17
Kyllinga triceps	33.33	26.76	20.68	4.29	77.26	11.07
Lindernia crustacea	46.67	42.25	21.66	1.08	51.27	10.78
Murdannia nudiflora	46.67	37.32	18.37	2.31	49.21	10.20
Cyperus rotundus	36.67	30.99	6.82	3.37	22.00	7.13
Cynodon dactylon	40.00	30.28	6.34	3.21	20.93	6.82
Phyllanthus fraternus	56.67	37.32	4.45	1.31	11.92	5.77
Cyparus compressus	33.33	16.90	10.20	0.83	60.33	4.98
Physalis minima	43.33	25.35	2.48	1.44	9.78	4.14
Corchorus aestuans	43.33	23.94	2.51	1.25	10.47	3.89
Dactyloctenium aegypticum	20.00	14.08	2.23	1.54	15.80	3.02
Galinsoga ciliata	16.67	14.08	3.46	0.75	24.60	2.83
Eragrostis tenella	23.33	15.49	2.76	0.49	17.82	2.61
Lindernia ciliata	33.33	16.20	1.63	0.13	10.09	2.14
Euphorbial hirta	26.67	13.38	1.38	0.38	10.32	1.96
Nicandra physalodes	23.33	13.38	0.90	0.35	6.74	1.81
Polygonum nepalense	16.67	11.27	1.27	0.04	11.25	1.50
Lindernia anagallis	23.33	9.15	1.61	0.21	17.54	1.48
Euphorbia geniculata	13.33	7.04	0.59	0.94	8.40	1.47
Setaria palmifolia	10.00	4.93	0.87	1.10	17.71	1.44
Dopatrium junceum	6.67	4.93	1.46	0.82	29.71	1.43
Setaria intermedia	20.00	9.15	1.24	0.16	13.54	1.35
Setaria glauca	16.67	6.34	0.85	0.68	13.33	1.30
Justicia simplex	10.00	9.15	0.96	0.09	10.46	1.23
Cucumis melo var. *agrestis*	20.00	7.04	0.31	0.55	4.40	1.15
Parthenium hysterophorus	16.67	7.04	0.56	0.31	8.00	1.05
Acalypha ciliata	10.00	7.75	0.82	0.09	10.55	1.05
Fimbristylis miliacea	10.00	4.93	11.63	0.17	33.14	1.04
Amaranthus spinosus	16.67	7.04	0.54	0.27	7.60	1.02

Table 51.2–Contd...

Weed Species	Constancy (%)	Frequency (%)	Density (m^{-2})	Dry Weight ($g\ m^{-2}$)	Abundance (m^{-2})	IVI
Cyperus diffonnis	3.33	3.52	2.03	0.09	57.60	0.96
Xanthium strumarium	10.00	3.52	0.45	0.74	12.80	0.95
Malus pumilus	16.67	7.04	0.68	0.03	9.60	0.90
Sorghum halepense	10.00	4.23	0.31	0.41	7.33	0.78
Digitaria bicornis	6.67	3.52	0.65	0.35	18.40	0.75
Pulolzia zeylanica	10.00	4.93	0.28	0.19	5.71	0.69
Leucas cephalotes	6.67	4.23	0.25	0.29	6.00	0.67
Momordica dioica	10.00	3.52	0.17	0.39	4.80	0.65
Ipomea pes-tigridis	10.00	2.82	0.11	0.35	4.00	0.54
Urtica dioica	10.00	3.52	0.14	0.20	4.00	0.52
Scirpus supinus	3.33	0.70	0.20	0.51	28.00	0.45
Paspalum dilatatum	3.33	1.41	0.42	0.25	30.00	0.42
Siegesbeckia orientalis	6.67	3.52	0.20	0.02	5.60	0.42
Cleome viscosa	6.67	2.82	0.28	0.05	10.00	0.39
Brachiaria reptans	6.67	2.11	0.20	0.12	9.33	0.34
Triumfettta rhomboidea	6.67	2.82	0.11	0.03	4.00	0.33
Panicum psilopodium	6.67	1.41	0.23	0.19	16.00	0.32
Eragrostis unioloides	6.67	2.11	0.14	0.04	6.67	0.28
Eclipta alba	6.67	2.11	0.14	0.05	6.67	0.28
Bacopa procumbens	6.67	1.41	0.11	0.07	8.00	0.22
Scirpus squarrosus	6.67	1.41	0.23	0.01	16.00	0.21
Melochia chorchorifolia	6.67	1.41	0.06	0.07	4.00	0.20
Boerhaavia diffusa	3.33	1.41	0.06	0.03	4.00	0.17
Alysicarpus vaginalis	6.67	1.41	0.06	0.02	4.00	0.16
Anagallis arvensis	6.67	1.41	0.06	0.00	4.00	0.15
Medicago polymorphoa	3.33	1.41	0.06	0.01	4.00	0.15
Geranium collinum	3.33	1.41	0.06	0.00	4.00	0.15
Oplismenus burmanrni	3.33	0.70	0.08	0.01	12.00	0.11
Alternanthera sessilis	3.33	0.70	0.06	0.02	8.00	0.10
Anaphalis adnata	3.33	0.70	0.03	0.03	4.00	0.10
Ipomea hederacea	3.33	0.70	0.03	0.02	4.00	0.10
Alternanthera philoxeroides	3.33	0.70	0.03	0.02	4.00	0.09
Fimbristylis schoenoides	3.33	0.70	0.03	0.00	4.00	0.08
Murraya koenigii	3.33	0.70	0.03	0.00	4.00	0.08
Eupatorium adenophorum	3.33	0.70	0.03	0.01	4.00	0.08
Bldens biternata	3.33	0.70	0.03	0.01	4.00	0.08
Rumex nepalensis	3.33	0.70	0.03	0.01	4.00	0.08
Vicia sativa	3.33	0.70	0.03	0.00	4.00	0.08
Total		1003.40	369.35	153.38		299.89

Table 51.3: Phytosociological Parameters of Weed Species in Wheat

Weed Species	*Constancy (%)*	*Frequency (%)*	*Density (m^{-2})*	*Dry Weight (g m^{-2})*	*Abundance (m^{-2})*	*IVI*
Anagallis arvensis	78.95	64.77	92.88	4.173	143.40	37.72
Chenopodium album	85.96	75.00	33.08	7.172	44.08	29.51
Medicago polymorpha	7018	51.89	2332	5.595	44.92	21.69
Phalaris minor	63.16	50.00	1848	5.876	36.92	20.81
Poa annua	33.33	26.89	4580	2.172	170.24	18.28
Soliva anthemifolia	36.84	28.41	30.56	2.172	107.64	14.65
Vicia hirsuta	71.93	50.00	14.12	2.802	28.20	14.03
Vicia sativa	66.67	47.35	7.96	3.319	16.80	13.18
Medicago lupulina	54.39	37.88	14,56	1.791	38.40	10.98
Polygonum plebejum	66.67	50.00	11.64	0.886	23.24	9.86
Lathyrus aphaca	47.37	34.85	8.64	1.927	24.84	9.44
Avena sativa	42.11	20.83	5.76	2.392	27.64	8.08
Trifolium tomentosum	28.07	18.94	11.00	1.627	58.16	7.77
Gnaphalium luteo-album	21.05	12.88	11.64	0.930	90.48	5.98
Ranunculus arvensis	36.84	23.86	4.68	0.937	19.68	5.44
Melilotus indica	33.33	19.70	4.84	1.050	24.52	5.25
Areneria serpyllifolia	40.35	30.68	5.36	0.307	17.52	5.17
Ranunculus muricatus	15.79	11.36	6.28	0.808	55.32	4.27
Vicia tetrasperma	36.84	21.21	3.76	0.502	17.72	4.12
Cynodon-dactylon	45.61	21.97	2.32	0.328	10.48	3.53
Capsella bursa-pastoris	31.58	19.32	3.52	0.310	18.12	3.50
Coronopus didymus	28.07	14.77	2.12	0.469	14.24	2.97
Alopecurus geniculatus	10.53	8.33	4.56	0.478	54.92	2.91
Cyperus rotundus	36.84	18.18	2.20	0.219	12.16	2.90
Rumex dentatus	21.05	9.47	2.24	0.716	23.52	2.90
Veronica persica	19.30	12.12	3.88	0.343	31.88	2.89
Stellaria media	19.30	9.85	3.24	0.481	32.92	2.75
Fumana indica	35.09	16.29	1.56	0.328	9.48	2.74
Spergula arvensis	19.30	10.23	4.68	0.142	45.76	2.51
Silene conoidea	26.32	13.26	0.96	0.405	7.20	2.40
Antirrhinum orontium	19.30	11.36	2.24	0.322	19.60	2.37
Veronica biloba	7.02	3.79	4.96	0.381	131.20	2.34
Brassica juncea	14.04	6.82	1.00	0.380	14.44	1.68
Polypogon monospeliensis	19.30	8.71	0.92	0.080	10.44	1.31
Lathyrus sphaericus	7.02	4.92	0.64	0.246	12.60	1.14
Galinsoga parviflora	7.02	5.68	0.68	0.08.5	12.00	0.94
Tridax procumbens	8.77	4.55	0.80	0.093	18.00	0.86
Cnicus arvensis	3.51	2.27	0.28	0.252	12.00	0.78

rotundus, C. dactylon, Cyperus compressus, Physalis minima and *Lindernia ciliata* showed limited constancy. The value of frequencies was reduced significantly in comparison of constancy almost in all the weed species except *Cyperus difformis* and *E. indica*, which reflected more homogenous distribution.

Weed constancy in wheat revealed that *Chenopdium album* had the highest constancy (86.0 per cent). *Anagallis arvensis, Medicago polymorpha, Phalaris minor, Vicia hirsute, V. sativa, Medicago lupulina, Polygonum plebejum* occurred in 50 per cent or more sites. *Poa annua, Solvia anthemifolia, Lathyrus aphaca, Avena sativa, Ranunculu arvensis, Melilotus alba, Vicia tetrasperma, C. dactylon, Capsella bursa-pastoris, C. rotundus* and *Fumaria indica* were prevalent in 30–50 per cent fields. Rest of the species had constancy less than 30 per cent.

Weed Density and Abundance

The 53 per cent of the total weed density in rice was constituted by the sedges. *F. miliacea* had maximum density (52.2 m^{-2} followed by *F. schoenoides* (28.5 m^{-2}). *C. iria, L. crustacea, E. colonum* and *C. pumilus* had the density of 20 m^{-2} or more. *Monoclzoria vaginalis, F. schoenoides* and *Eriocaulon cinereum* had abundance value more than 100 m^{-2}.

In maize crop, 50 per cent of the weed density was formed by broad leaved weeds. Table 51.2 indicates maximum density of *E. colonum* (41.9 m^{-2}). *C. iria* (29.9 m^{-2}) and *C. benglzolensis* (26.2 m^{-2}) were the other weed species, which had higher density. *Oxalis lafifolia, G. parviflora, L. crustacea* had a high abundance value indicating that these weeds had high infestation in some of the quadrats.

A. arvensis recorded the maximum density (92.9 m^{-2}) followed by *P. annua* (45.8 m^{-2}), *C. album* (33.1 m^{-2}) and *S. anthemifolia* (30.6 m^{-2}). *M. polymorpha, P. minor, V. hisuta, M. lupulina, P. pelebejuln, T. tomentosum* and *Gnapllalium luteo-album* had density of 10–30 individuals m^{-2}. In wheat, only those species reached high degree of abundance value, which were short stature and flourished in the understorey niche of the crop.

Weed Dominance

The dry matter accumulation by weeds in wheat, rice and maize was 53.94 g m^{-2}, 81.75 g m^{-2} and 153 g m^{-2} respectively. In general, more dry weight of weeds in maize crops than rice may be attributed to good amount of rainfall occurred coupled with wider more inter and intra row spacing. Angiras and Singh (1988) also reported similar results.

Phytosociology

F. miliacea was the most dominant weed in rice crop with IVI value of 31.81 followed by *E. colonum* (29.68) and *E. crus-galli* (27.40). The co-dominance was shared by the sedges species, namely *C. iria* (22.20), *F. schoenoides* (13.15), *C. difformis* (12.66) and *C. pumilus* (11.17). Among broad-leaved weeds, *L. crustacea* (17.21), *A. collyzoides* (14.79), *B. hamiltoniana* (10.86), *L. anagallis* (10.36) were important from IVI point of view.

Eighteen per cent (14) 05 total weeds was belonged to dominant group in maize with IVI > 10. Of which 50 per cent were broad leaved (7), and 5, 19 per cent (4) were of grass family [*E. colonum* (44.46), *E. indica* (16.79), *B. ramosa* (12.16), *D. abludens* (11.17)]. The sedges consisted of three species namely *C. iria, C. alulatus* and *K. triceps* with IVI values of 16.61, 12.02 and 11.07 respectively. Among other broad-leaved weeds, *C. benghalensis* (27.19), *O. larifolia* (13.45), *A. collyzoides* (13.25), *G. parviflora* (12.28), *M. penraphylla* (11.82), *L. crustacea* (10.78) and *M. nudiflora* (10.70) were the dominant weeds or this area. *C. rotundus, C. dactylon* and *P. fraternus* had the IVI values ranged from 5.77 to 7.13. Rest of weed species had IVI values less than 5.

A. arvensis was the most dominant weed in wheat (IVI 37.72) followed by *C. albun* (29.51). The grassy weeds were represented by *P. minor* (20.81) and *P. annua* (18.28). Among other broad-leaf weeds *M. polymorpha* (21.69), *V. hirsuta* (14.03), *V. sativa* (13.18), *M. lupulina* (10.98) and *S. anthemifolia* were the dominant weeds of this area. *A. sativa* was the only monocotyledon which had IVI value between 5–10, while rest of species were dicotyledons.

Tripathi and Vaishya (1997), also reported dominance of *F. dichotoma, C. iria, E. colonum* and *P. niruri* in kharif season and *A. arvensis* in wheat.

References

Andersson, T.N. and P. Milberg, 1998. Weed flora arid relative importance of site, crop, crop rotation and nitrogen. *Weed Science,* 46: 30–38.

Angiras, N.N. and C.M. Singh, 1988. Influence of weed control methods in plant population, fertility levels and cropping system on weed management in maize. *Indian J. Weed Sci.,* 20(3): 67–72.

Curtis, J.T. and R.P. McIntosh, 1950. The interrelationship of certain analytic and synthetic phytosociological characters. *Ecology,* 31: 434–455.

Tripathi, J.S. and R.D. Vaishya, 1997. Weed infestation in different cropping systems of Eastern Uttar Pradesh. *Indian J. Weed Sci.,* 29(1 and 2): 50–52.

Medicinal Plants: Conservation, Cultivation and Utilization (2007) *Pages 403–407*
Editors: A.K. Chopra, D.R. Khanna, G. Prasad, D.S. Malik and R. Bhutiani
Published by: DAYA PUBLISHING HOUSE

Chapter 52

A Survey of Wound Healing Plants Used by the Tribal People of Khargone District of Madhya Pradesh

S.K. Mahajan[1]*, Virendra Mandloi[2] and Amit Raghuwanshi[3]
[1]Post Graduate Department of Botany, Government College, Khargone – 451 001 (M.P.)
[2]Kunda Nagar (Near Canal), Khargone – 451 001 (M.P.)
[3]Paharsinghpura, Haweli Path, Khargone – 451 001 (M.P.)

ABSTRACT

The present article deals with the styptic plants used by the tribal people of West Nimar district of Madhya Pradesh. The study revealed 19 taxa belonging to 18 genera and 14 families of flowering plants. The local names, Latin names and their synonyms, if any and plant part used are discussed in each case. An emphasis has been given to protect and cultivate these plants so that tribal people may be benefited which would also save our valuable Indian flora.

Keywords: Styptic plants, Medicinal plants and Ethnobotany.

Introduction

A review of past literature on Ethnobotany indicates that sufficient research work has been done in various part of India in general and Madhya Pradesh in particular (Jain, 1963; Jain and Tarafdar,

* Present address: 31, Jain Mandi Path, Khargone – 451 001 (M.P.).

1968; Maheshwari *et al.*, 1981). In M.P. such type of work has been done only in Mandla, Balaghat, Jabalpur, Sidhi and Sagar districts. A little work has also be done in Southern part of M.P. (Mahajan, 1990, 2002 a and b). The present communication deals with the styptic plants used by the tribals of West Nimar district, M.P.

Materials and Methods

The present work was done during 2002–03 and for this field work was done in tribal villages such as Sirwel, Pipaljhopa and Bhagwanpura. Old tribal persons and tribal medicine men were, contacted to gather the information regarding the plants and plant parts used in healing wounds and various types of bleeding from the body. Standard literature was followed for identification of these plants (Chopra *et al.*, 1956; Cooke, 1957; Kirtikar and Basu, 1935 and Solanki, 1984). The herbarium sheets are deposited in the Post-Graduate Department of Botany, Government College, Khargone for future record. Following is the list of plants which are collected and arranged in the alphabetical order.

Enumeration of Plants

***Acacia arabica* W.**

Local name: Babul

Family: Mimosaceae

Use: bark juice is used.

***Catechu* W.**

Local name: Khair

Family: Mimosaceae,

Use: Katha is extracted from its wood which is used in wound healing and bleeding gums.

***Ageratum conizoides* L.**

Local name: Sahdevi

Family: Asteraceae.

Use: Stem and leaves are used.

***Alocasia indica* S.**

Local name: Manaka

Family: Araceae

Use: Acrid juice extracted from rosted leaf stalk is styptic.

***Borassus flabellifer* L.**

Local name: Tad

Family: Palmae

Use: The light brown downy bloom on the base of the leaves is a styptic for superficial wounds.

Bryphyllum pinnata **K.**

Local name: Patharchatta

Family: Crassulaceae

Use: Leaves are slightly toasted and applied on unhealthy wounds and fresh cut, ulcers, bites of venomous insects etc. Fresh juice is also styptic.

Ceiba pentandra **G.**

Local name: Katan

Family: Bombacaceae

Use: Gum from the trunk is useful in menorrhagia.

Coccinia indica **L.**

Local name: Kanduri

Family: Cucurbitaceae

Use: Leaf and fruit juices are used in wound healing.

Cocos nucifera **L.**

Local name: Nariyal

Family: Palmae

Use: Ash of stem bark is antiseptic and dentifrice.

Curcuma longa **L.**

Local name: Haldi

Family: Zingiberaceae

Use: The rhizome powder when mixed with quicklime or alum is excellent dressing for wounds.

Cynodon dactylon **P.**

Local name: Kali ghas

Family: Graminae.

Use: Juice of entire plant or paste of the plant is used to check bleeding from the nose, cuts and wounds. Its infusion is also orally used with milk.

Diospyros peregrina. **G.**

Local name: Tendu

Family: Ebenaceae

Use: Seed paste is used for abscesses.

Dolichos biflorus **L.**

Local name: Kulthi

Family: Papilionaceae

Use: Decoction of its seeds is useful in menstrual disroders.

***Eclipta alba* H.**

Local name: Bhringraja

Family: Asteraceae

Use: Decoction of its leaves is used in uterine haemorrhages.

***Glycyrrhiza glabra* L.**

Local name: Mulaithi

Family: Fabaceae

Use: Its stem extract when mixed with ghee is useful for healing wounds.

***Gossypium herbaceum* L.**

Local name: Kapas

Family: Malvaceae

Use: Cotton ash is applied to ulcers, sores and wounds.

***Linum usitatissimum* L.**

Local name: Alsi

Family: Liliaceae

Use: Ash of its bark is styptic.

***Mangifera indica* L.**

Local name: Amb

Family: Anacardiaceae

Use: Its bark juice is used for haemorrages from lungs, intestines, uterus and in cases of diarrhoea and bleeding piles. The bark juice is used in two ways: (*a*) Juice of fresh bark is mixed with white of an egg or some mucilage and a little opium is added, (*b*) Mixture of 10 g fresh bark juice + 120 g water is given every hour or two in a teaspoonful quantity.

***Tridex procumbens* L.**

Local name: Kulhara

Family: Asteraceae

Use: Its leaves are crushed and applied on cuts and wounds. It cures deep cuts very quickly.

Results and Discussion

The study revealed in all 19 taxa belonging to 18 genera and 14 families of angiosperms. These plants are used in healing of cuts and wounds, bleeding piles, uterine heamorrhage, blood dysentery, heamorrhages from lungs and intestine and also for dressing purposes. Important taxa which are used as styptic plants by the tribal people are *Acacia arabica, Cocos nucifera, Curcuma longa, Gossypium herbaceum, Tridex procumbens* and others. These useful plants need protection and more cultivation in the present context, so that the tribal people may be benefited and our valuable Indian flora may also survive.

Acknowledgements

Authors are thankful to the Principal and Head, Department of Botany, Government P.G. College, Khargone for encouragement and facilities.

References

Chopra, R.N., S.L. Nayar and I.C. Chopra, 1956. *Glossary of Indian Medicinal Plants*, C.S.I.R., New Delhi.

Cooke, T., 1957. *Flora of the Presidency of Bombay*. Vols. I–II.

Jain, S.K., 1963. Plants used by tribals of Madhya Pradesh, *Bull. Reg. Res. Lab.*, Jammu-Tawi, 1: 126–128.

Jain, S.K. and C.R. Tarafdar, 1968. Native plant remedies for snakebite among adivasis of Central India. *Ind. Med. J.*, 57(12): 307–309.

Kirtikar, K.R. and B.D. Basu, 1935. *Indian Medicinal Plants*, Kolkata.

Mahajan, S.K., 1990. A preliminary ethnobotanical survey in the Sirwel hills of Western M.P., In: *Natl. Seminar on Ethnobotany of Tribes of M.P.* organised by S.G.S. Govt. P.G. College, Sidhi, M.P. and Sponsored by MAPCOST, Bhopal, Abst. No. 14.

Mahajan, S.K. and P. Patel, 2002a. Antiseptic plants of Khargone and its neighbourhood areas of Madhya Pradesh. In: *12th Annual Conference of IAAT and National Seminar on Plant Taxonomy in National* Development, organised by Department of Botany, Goa University. Plant Diversity, Human Welfare and Conservation, (Eds.) M.K. Janarthanan and D. Narsimhan, p. 227–229.

Mahajan, S.K. and P. Patel, 2002b. A preliminary survey of anthelmintic plants used by the tribes of West Nimar district of Madhya Pradesh. *Ibid*, p. 289–292.

Maheshwari, J.K., K.K. Singh and S. Saha, 1981. The ethnobotany of Tharus of Kheri district. *U.P. Economic Botany Information Service*, N.B.R.I., Lucknow.

Solanki, C.M., 1984. Flora of Indore. *Ph.D. Thesis*, Devi Ahilya Vishwavidyalaya, Indore.

Medicinal Plants: Conservation, Cultivation and Utilization (2007) *Pages 409–413*
Editors: A.K. Chopra, D.R. Khanna, G. Prasad, D.S. Malik and R. Bhutiani
Published by: DAYA PUBLISHING HOUSE

Chapter 53

Angiospermic Diversity, Conservation and Documentation of Some Interesting and Rare Angiospermis of West Nimar District of M.P.

S.K. Mahajan[1]*, C.L. Dulkar[1], M.M. Keshare[1] and Chetna Sawale[2]
[1]**Botany Department, Government P.G. College, Khargone – 451 001 (M.P.)**
[2]**Research Student, 7, Kunda Nagar, Khargone – 451 001 (M.P.)**

ABSTRACT

In the present article 19 interesting and rare plant species belonging to 19 genera and 15 families have been reported from Khargone district of M.P.

Keywords: Vegetation, Flowering plants, Exploration.

Introduction

Biogeographically, Khargone district (21°22′ to 22°13′ N Lat., 75°19′ to 76°14′ Long. and 300. m above MSL) is a part of Central India. Its total area is 647789 Hectares, out of which 75308 Hectares is occupied by the forest. On account of large geographical area, variable climate and habitat conditions, it is rich in all aspects of diversity. But urbanization, industrialization and habitat destruction have threatened the biodiversity of this tract and now it has become a challenge. Keeping in view of the above fact the present investigation has been undertaken.

* Present address: 31, Jain Mandi Path, Khargone – 451 001 (M.P.).

A review of literature indicates that some research work on the vegetation of Khargone district has been done in the past. Shastri (1977) is the pioneer worker who for the first time published the flora of the Khargone. Afterwards Mahajan (1984) made a survey about climbers and parasites and also published an additional list of the flora of Khargone in 1987. Earlier to this Mahajan and Paliwal studied the biological spectrum of Sirwel hills of Khargone in 1985 and wall vegetation of Khargone district in 2002. Some research papers have also appeared on ethnobotanical studies of Khargone district (Mahajan, 1990 and Mahajan and Patel, 2004).

Materials and Methods

During plant collection work with post-graduate students of botany in past few years, some interesting and rare plants have been collected which were pressed, dried and their herbarium sheets were prepared. Plant identification was done following standard literature (Haines, 1924; Duthie, 1952; Cooke, 1957; Maheshwari, 1963 and Bailey, 1966) Herbarium sheets are deposited in Botany department, Government P.G. College, Khargone for future record. Following is the list of the collected plants which are arranged alphabetically with their scientific names, synonyms, if any, local names, english names, if any, name of family and their distribution in the viscinity of Khargone.

***Adhatoda vasica* N.**

Local name: Adusa

Family: Acanthaceae

Distribution: It is found in wild condition on road sides at Khargone.

***Aristolochia bracteata* Retz.**

Local name: Girdhan

Family: Aristolochiaceae

Distribution: Previously it was frequently growing in cultivated fields but gradually disappearing from sight.

***Cadaba indica* Lamk.**

Local name: —

Family: Capparidaceae

Distribution: It is rarely seen on the hedges of cultivated fields.

***Clematis triloba* Heyne**

Local name: Bandarsethi

Family: Ranunculaceae

Distribution: It is found on slopy region near Kunda river on Sirwel hills.

***Cuscuta chinensis* Lamk**

Local name: Amarbel

Family: Convolvulaceae

Distribution: It was observed once as a parasite on *Solanum xanthocarpum*.

***Gloriosa superba* L.**

Local name: Kalihari

Family: Liliaceae

Distribution: It is frequently seen growing on hedges of cultivated fields in Bistan.

***Gynandropsis gynandra* (L.) Briq. (= *G. pentaphylla* DC.)**

Local name: Hurera

Family: Capparidaceae

Distribution: Previously it was growing wild but now it is less frequent in cultivated fields and along the road sides.

***Indigofera* Houer, Forsk.**

Local name:

Family: Fabaceae

Distribution: It was collected only once from stadium, area near the canal.

***Maerua arenaria* Cambess.**

Local name:

Family: Capparidaceae

Distribution: It is reported on the hedges of cultivated lands at Khargone.

***Passiflora foetida* L.**

Local name: Rakhi

Family: Passfloraceae

Distribution: It is a white flowered climber and is less common at Khargone.

***Psoralia corylifolia* L.**

Local name: Bawchi

Family: Fabaceae

Distribution: It is a medicinal plant growing wild in the viscinity of Khargone.

***Pterospermum acerifolium* (L.) W.**

Local name: Kanakchampa

Family: Sterculiaceae

Distribution: Only two plants have been observed growing at Khargone.

***Salvadora persica* L.**

Local name: Pilu

Family: Salvadoraceae

Distribution: It is an evergreen tree and generally seen at three places namely Balwant Hostel, Tehsil office and College Campus at Khargone.

***Spathodea companulata* B.**

English name: Fountain tree.

Family: Bignoniaceae

Distribution: There is only one tree which is found to be growing near J.N.A. Research station, Khargone.

***Heliconia caribaea* Lam.**

English name: Bird of paradise

Family: Musaceae

Distribution: It is found to be growing in private garden at Khargone.

***Striga asiatica* (L.) Kuntze. (= *S. lutea* Lour.)**

Local name: Agyo

Family: Scrophulariaceae

Distribution: It is a small root parasite which grows on maize and jowar.

***Trianthema crystallina* Vahl.**

Local name: Lonia

Family: Aizoaceae

Distribution: It has been observed near old temple and Kamal talai at Oon.

***Withania somnifera* (L.) Dun.**

Local name: Ashwgandha

Family: Solanaceae

Distribution: It is a medicinal plants which generally grows along road sides at Khargone.

***Zeuxine sulcata* Lindl.**

Local name:

Family: Orchidaceae

Distribution: It was only once collected from slopy region near the canal at Banihar dam.

Results and Discussion

Thus in the present survey in all 19 interesting and rare species belonging to 19 genera and 15 angiospermic families are reported. It is well known that BSI and ZSI have studied and documented 45,000 plants species and 75,000 animal species in our country respectively. Khargone district claims about 723 angiosperm species and 142 vertebrate animals, numerous insects and other microscopic invertebrate species.

Total area protected by the forest is only 107 hectares, which needs to be increased in the present context. In order to save our flora and fauna there is an urgent need to create public awareness and also to take strict action against those found to destroy natural vegetation and wild animals.

Acknowledgements

Authors are thankful to the Principal, Government P.G. College, Khargone for facilities and encouragement.

References

Bailey, L.H., 1966. *Manual of Cultivated Plants,* The Macmillan Company, New York.

Cooke, T., 1957. *Flora of the Presidency of Bombay,* Vols. I–II.

Duthie, J.F., 1952. *Flora of the Upper Gangetic Plain and of the Adjacent Siwalik and Sub-Himalayan Tracts,* 1903-22, Kolkata, 3 Vols., Delhi.

Haines, H.H., 1924. *The Botany of Bihar and Orissa,* Part VI.

Mahajan, S.K., 1984. A survey of climbers and parasites at Khargone, Madhya Pradesh. In: *54th Annual Sess., Nat. Acad. Sci., India,* Madurai (Bioi. Sect.) Abst. p. 34.

Mahajan, S.K. and Paliwal, P.R., 1985. Biological spectrum of the flora of Sirwel hills, Madhya Pradesh. *Geobios,* 12: 212–214.

Mahajan, S.K., 1987. Further additions to the flora of Khargone, Madhya Pradesh. In: *Proc. 74th Ind. Sci. Cong.* Part III (Bot. Sect.) Abst. p. 106.

Mahajan, S.K., 1990. A preliminary ethnobotanical survey in the Sirwel hills of Western M.P. In: *Natl. Seminar on Ethnobotany of Tribals of M.P.* (Sponsored by MAPCOST) organised by S.G.S. Government P.G. College, Sidhi, M.P. Abst. No. 14.

Mahajan, S.K., 2002. Studies in the seasonal aspects of wall vegetation of Khargone and its suburbs. *J.B.N.H.S* (In Press).

Mahajan, S.K. and Patel Pushpa, 2004. Study of lithontriptic plants used by the tribals of Khargone district of M.P. In: *Natl. Symposium on Medicinal Plants Farming, Science and Practice for Improving Financial Status of Indian Farmers Vision 21st Century and Herbal Trade Fair/Exhibition;* June 26-27. DDU Gorakhpur University, Gorakhpur, India.

Maheshwari, J.K., 1963. *The Flora of Delhi.* CSIR, Delhi.

Shastri, M.B., 1977. *Flora of Khargone, Madhya Pradesh: Recent Trends and Contacts between Cytogenetics, Embryology and Morphology,* p. 445–454.

Medicinal Plants: Conservation, Cultivation and Utilization (2007) *Pages 415–417*
Editors: **A.K. Chopra, D.R. Khanna, G. Prasad, D.S. Malik and R. Bhutiani**
Published by: **DAYA PUBLISHING HOUSE**

Chapter 54

Healthy Heart by Ayurvedic Herbs

V.K. Pandey[1] and Reena Pandey[2]
[1]Reader, Sharir Kriya, Government Ayurveda College and Hospital, Gurukul Kangri Haridwar (U.A.)
[2]Lecturer, CDM College of Ayurveda, Jagadhari, Distt. Yamuna Nagar (HR)

Introduction

In the present era, the life of man has become very mechanized due to fast moving technology. People are forgetting simple principle of healthy life due to competition in all aspect i.e. study, immediate gaining of money and fame. According to Ayurveda the concept of healthy person is not restricted only on physical or body level but the physical, mental and spiritual, all the three states must be in proper condition. It is the equilibrium state of a healthy person.

Heart disease is a global phenomenon. It is now becoming a major health problem in developed and developing countries causing much morbidity and mortality. Different Heart diseases can be classified under the five type of Haridroga described in Ayurveda. Ayurvedic scientists have classified all bodily constituents into three categories–*Doshas* (Humours), *Dhatus* (Tissues) and *Malas* (Waste Materials). Aggrivated doshas directly vitiate dhatus and changed their function. If this state continues for a long time, than pathogenesis takes place in that tissues.

Thus, the aggravated doshas vitiate to Rasa-Rakta dhatu (Blood) so the composition of blood becomes changed like hyper cholesterolemia etc. After some years permanent changes occur in arterial wall called atherosclerosis (Dhamani Kathinya). This state is responsible for the development of cardiac diseases *i.e.* angina; ischeamic heart disease, myocardial infarction, arrhythmia, heart failure etc.

In this respect father of surgery Acharya Sushruta says-

दूषयित्वा रसं दोषा विगुणा हृदय गता।
हृदि बाधां प्रकुर्वन्ति हृदरोग तं प्रचक्षते।। (Su.u. 43/4)

Table 54.1

Name of Drug	*Botanical Name*	*Part Used*	*Dose*	*Chemical Composition*	*Action on Digestive System*	*Action on Nervous System*	*Action on Cardiovascular System*
Rason	*Allium sativum*	Bulb, Oil	Paste: 3–6 g Oil: 1–3 drops	Volatile oil 0.06–01 per cent Allyle propyl Sulphate 6 per cent Diallyl disulphide 6 per cent and two other sulphur compounds	Liver stimulent, digestive, digestion promotive, pain reliever	Useful in paralysis, sciatica and all nervous diseases	Cholesterol level decreased, cardiac stimulant and edema remover
Arjun	*Terminalia Arjuna*	Bark	Powder: 3–6 g in Milk decoction: 5–10 ml	B-Cytosterol, Elegic acid, Arjunic acid, Arjunetin Feridilin, Ca, Mg and Tenin			Strengthening cardiac muscles, corrects the conducting system of heart, improved ardiac circulation
Tambul	*Piper betle*	Leaf	Juice: 5–10 ml	Ca, P, Fe, I, K, Vita B, C and A Eugenol Chavibetol, Hydroxychevicol	Appetite promotive and digestive, Removes anorexia, stomatitis, constipation		Cardiac stimulent and useful in bradycardia
Amlaki	*Emblica officinalis*	Fruit	Juice: 10–20 ml powder 3–6 g	Galic acid, Termic acid, Ca, P, Fe, Vit. C.	Appetizer, Digestive Hyperacidity, constipation, peptic ulcer and useful in liver disease	Brain and Sence Organs Tonic; Antioxidant	Useful in all type of cardiac diseases
Haritaki	*Terminalia chebula*	Fruit	Powder: 3–6 g	Chebulic acid, Chebulimic acid, corilegin	Appetizer and Liver stimulant, Mild Purgative and useful in digestive diseases	Brain and Nervine Tonic	Cardiac health promotive, improved circulation
Guduchi	*Tinospora cordifolia*	Stem	Powder: 3–6 g Decoction: 50–100 ml Satval: 2 g	Berberin, Giloin, Voletile oil	Liver stimulant		Cholesterol level decreased, cardiac stimulant, Gout and Rheumatoid arthritis
Brahmi	*Centella asiatica*	Leaves/ whole plant	Juice: 10–20 ml	Hydrocotyline, Asiaticocide, Brahmic acid and stigmasterol	Digestion Promotive, sprue	Brain Tonic, Neurons Function improved, epilepsy	Strengthening to heart and edema removes that developed by cardiac disorder

The most popular medical system *i.e.* allopathic system has comprehensive-treatment for heart disease but lacuna is that most of the treatment leads to another cardiac or extra cardiac diseases. Therefore, for the better personal and social health, we should adopt Ayurvedic system of medicine. Ayurveda is better alternate in this respect because of its holistic approach.

Common Cardiac Disorders

Atherosclerosis is a progressive inflammatory disorder of arterial wall that is characterized by the deposition of cholesterol and narrowing of lumen and loss of elasticity. The role of many risk factors for the development of atherosclerosis has been defined in many studies. The common risk factors are Age and gender, Family history, Obesity, smoking, Alcohol consumption, diabetes mellitus, physical inactivity, dietary factors and mental stress. Atherosclerotic disease may manifest as coronary heart disease *e.g.* angina, myocardial infarction and systemic hypertension.

Coronary heart disease is the most common form of heart disease and the single important cause of death. It is the most common cause of angina transient myocardial ischemia. Angina is characterized by central chest pain, discomfort or breathlessness that is precipitated by exertion or stress. Myocardial infraction is almost due to the formation of occlusive thrombus at the site of rupture or erosion of an atheromatous plaque in a coronary artery. Pain is the cardinal symptom of m.i. but breathlessness, vomiting and syncope are common features. Systemic blood pressure rises with the incidence of atherosclerosis, as it is most common risk factor for the hypertension.

Herbs and their Action in Cardiovascular Disorder

Various ayurvedic herbs are being used by Ayurvedic physician for protection and promotion of heart functions. On the basis of clinical study and chemical analysis, it has established that some ayurvedic herbs are very effective in prevention and treatment of cardiac disorders. The specific drugs are giving in Table 54.1.

Conclusion

The Ayurvedic system provides more effective and reliable treatment of cardiovascular diseases. In this regard various herbs have been described and presently in practiced. Different clinical studies and chemical analysis have been proved the efficacy of drugs in management of various heart disease as supportive add on therapy. These herbs promotes the functions as well as the capacity of cardiac muscles, conduction of impulses and circulation of blood. Some drugs (*Allium sativum* and *Tinospora cordifolia*) acts on lipids with decreasing the cholesterol level. These drugs (*Emblica officinalis, Terminalia chebula* and *Piper betle*) are correct the digestive system and cardiovascular system. The *Terminalia arjuna* gives strength to cardiac muscles and corrects the conducting system.

The *Centella asiatica* gives strength to nervous system and removed mental tension. If a healthy person takes these drugs (Herbs) in routine than he can prevent their heart from diseases because the atherosclerosis processs inhibit by mentioned drugs.

Medicinal Plants: Conservation, Cultivation and Utilization (2007) *Pages 419–424*
Editors: A.K. Chopra, D.R. Khanna, G. Prasad, D.S. Malik and R. Bhutiani
Published by: DAYA PUBLISHING HOUSE

Chapter 55

An Approach to Cure Paralysis and Arthiritis Using *Sida cordifolia* by Panchakarma

Harish Chauhan[1]*, D.R. Khanna[2] and R. Bhutiani[2]
[1]Ashtavaidyaratnam Vaidyasala Hospital and Research Centre, Shyampur Kangri, Haridwar
[2]Department of Zoology and Environment Science, Gurukul Kangri University Haridwar

ABSTRACT

In the present paper an approach has been made to cure paralysis and arthiritis through Panchakarma. The experiment was done on twenty patients of different age groups for required period or as per the condition of the patient. During the course of the study it was observed that patients to whom regular treatment was given get relief to about 15 per cent in first week, 25 per cent in second week and 30-35 per cent in the third week of treatment.

Introduction

Ayurveda literally means "the Science of life". Ayurveda in India and its neighbouring countries is in practice since time immemorial. According to ayurveda it does not mean only freedom from diseases but it also considers the equilibrium of mind, sense organs and the soul. Besides this ayurveda also consider the Healthy body i.e free from any kind of diseases. In ayurvedic system various therapeutic measures, both for patients and healthy persons are prescribed. One of the important aspect of ayurveda

* Corresponding Author: E-mail: vaidyasala@indiatimes.com.

is Panchakarma therapy, the present paper is an approach to cure paralysis and arthiritis using Sida cordifolia by Panchakarma.

Panchakarma

If one opens any chapter on the treatment of diseases in ayurvedic classics, the first point, which will strike his attention, is the description of the panchakarma measures for that ailment.

Panchakarma therapy primarily aims at cleaning the body of its accumulated impurities and nourishing the tissue. Once this is achieved, it becomes very easy to rejuvenate these tissues and prevent the process of ageing. The span of life is thus prolonged and the individual leads a disease free old age.

The term Panchakarma literally means five (Pancha) specialized therapies (Karma). The therapies, which are included under this collective term, are as follows:

Vamana Karma or Emetic therapy

Virechana Karma or Purgation therapy

Niruha vasti or Medicated anema containing decoction of drugs

Anuvasana vasti or anema containing medicated oil

Nasya Karma or inhalation therapy

Susruta includes rakta mokshana karma or bloodletting therapy in the place of Nasya karma or inhalation therapy.

Prior to the administration of these therapies, the body of the patient is to be suitably prepared and the therapeutic measures used for this purpose are called Purka Karma or prepatory therapies. These are two in number as follows:

1. Snehana karma or oleatic therapy
2. Swedana karma or formen testing therapy.

During the course of time some special massage therapies have been developed in ayurveda and are still in practice. These special massage therapies cause both oleation and fomentation of the body if used periodically; they prevent the ageing process while simultaneously preventing the manifestation of diseases.

These process which cause both oleation and fomentation of the body, is called Pinda Swedana. In Pinda swedana there is specialized process called sainti pinda swedana used very effectively a part of panchakarma for treatment of paralysis and arthiritis or other degeneration ailment.

The hindi name of *Sida cordifolia* is Bala found all over India and Ceylon and is growing wild along the roadside. All the parts *i.e.* Roots, Stems, Seeds and Leaves should be used for ailments. *Sida cordifolia* is used as cooling , astringent, stomachic and tonic aromatic bitter febrifuge, demulcent and diuretic. The seeds of *Sida cordifolia* are considered to be aphrodisiac.

Sida cordifolia is used in infusion in nervous and urinary diseases and disorders of the blood and bile. It is also used in bleeding piles, in strangury and haematuria gonorrhoea, cystitis, leucorrhoea, chronic dysentery, nervous diseases in asthma, paralysis, arthiritis etc.

Material and Methods

For therapy of Paralysis and Arthiritis by *Sida cordifolia* various equipments and instruments were used these includes:

1. Droni: 1
2. Stools: 5
3. Stove: 1
4. Big Vessels: 3
5. Cloth pieces: (18′ × 18″)

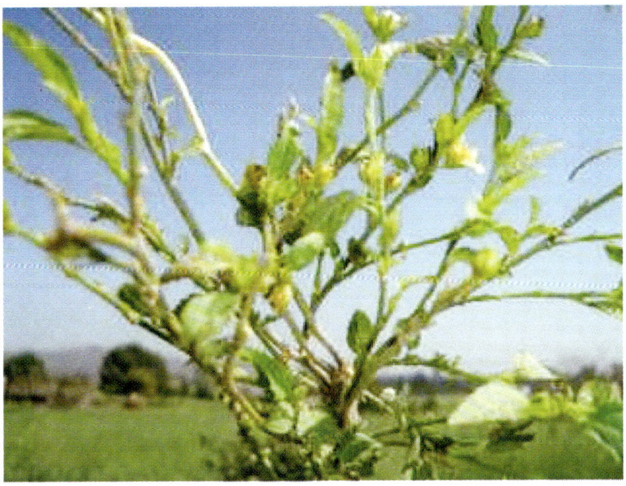

Figure 55.1: Showing Plant of *Sida cordifol*ia

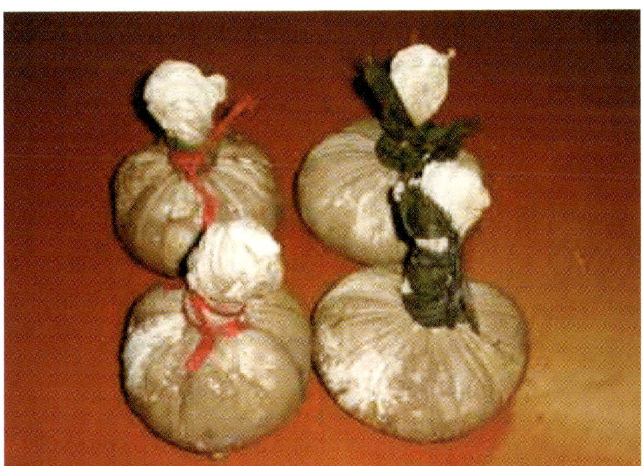

Figure 55.2: Showing Preparation of Bolus

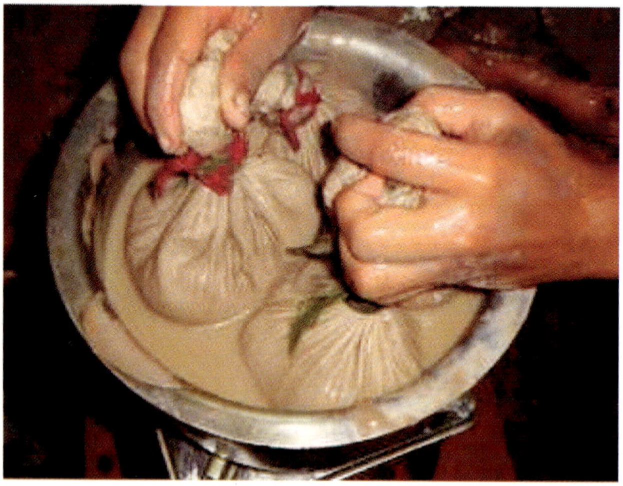

Figure 55.3: Showing Bolus Dipped in Decoction Milk

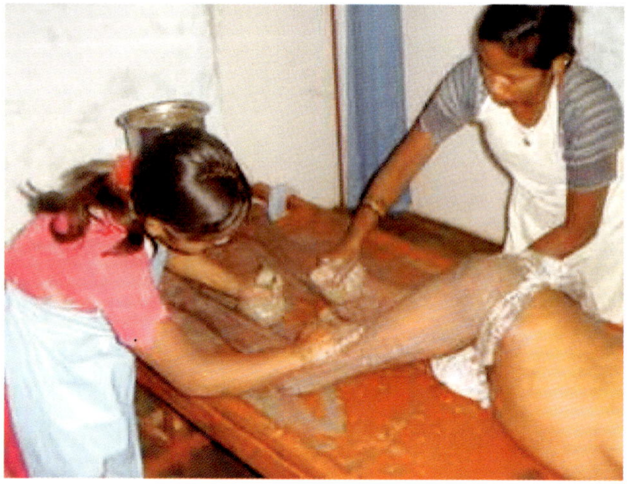

Figure 55.4: Showing Application of Bolus on Patient

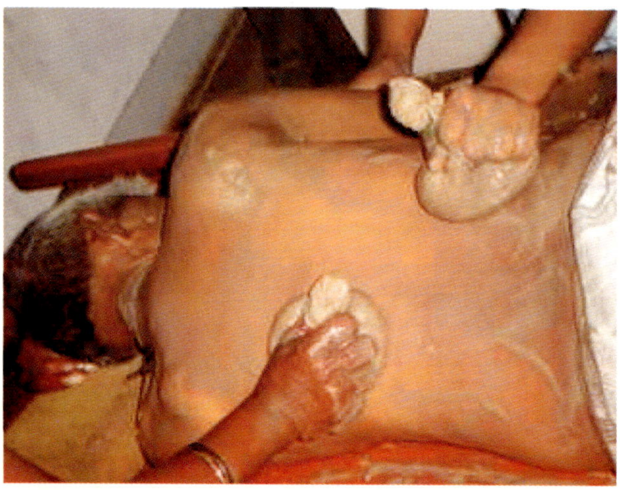

Figure 55.5: Showing Application of Bolus on Patient

Contents

1. Sasthi Rice: 600 gms
2. Bala Root: 500 gms
3. Milk: 2 litres
4. Water: 8 litres

Preparation of Milk Decoction

Mix 500 gms of Bala roots in 8 litres of water then boil the mixture till the quantity of water remains one fourth. Half of this decoction i.e approximately one litre is added with one litre of Cow's milk rest of the decoction i.e another one litre of decoction was kept for later stages.

Cooking of Red Rice

One litre of Milk was added to the above prepared one litre of decoction, to this add 600gms of Shasthi rice (Red rice) and cooked until it becomes semi-solid like pudding.

Preparation of Bolus

Four pieces of muslin cloth (about 18") width were taken and the above-prepared pudding was divided in to four equal parts and in this way four boluses were prepared.

Pinda Swedana

Pinda means bolus and Swedana means Heat. After performing the spiritual rites, Snehana or Oleation on body was done using suitable oil according to the need of the patient.The duration of Snehana was for about 15 minutes after Snehana the bolus was dipped in remaining two litres of milk decoction and rubbed vigorously over the entire body, focusing on the muscle tissue and joints. For severe conditions it is performed for about forty five minutes.The application of the Pinda Swedana improves the muscle tone, it nourishes Mamsa dhatu and vata. It is also beneficial treatment for hemiplegia and also helpful in multiple sclerosis and muscular atrophy. The therapy is used in conjunction with Panchakarma. The present Pinda Swedana was done to cure paralysis and arthiritis on several patients, which are described in table 1 and details, are given in results section.

Results

The present study was carried on twenty patients, ten patients for paralysis and ten for arthiritis of different age groups of 40-50 years, 51-60 years, 61-75 years. The treatment was given for three weeks during the course of study it was observed that patients to whom regular treatment was given get relief after one week but for those patients who did not get the regular treatment get little relief in the second week or third week of the treatment.

From the above study it was observed that in the first week of treatment about 15 per cent relief was observed in patients to whom regular Pinda Swedana was done besides this various types of ayurvedic medicines were also given to the patients time to time inspite of this certain changes in one's diet and daily routine was also done during the application period. In the second week of the treatment 25 per cent relief was observed for regular patients while the percentage for those patients who were not regular the relief observed was little less than regular patient's *i.e* 10 per cent in the first week and 18-20 per cent in the second week. The relief for regular patients in the third week goes up to 35 per cent while for irregular patients it goes up to 25 per cent only. Beside this it was observed that the patients enjoys a strong appetite digestion and feel light and energetic after Pinda Swedana. The patients feel happiness and experience satisfaction and enthusiasm for life.

Conclusion

From the present study it has been concluded that if proper guidelines would be followed from beginning of the procedure to the end, this Panchakarma therapy will be of great success in curing paralysis and arthiritis. At last we can say that Panchakarma is a very powerful therapy that provides a unique opportunity for the system to repair and rejuvenate and those undergoing this programme gain the maximum from it if they focus completely on the healing process taking place.

References

Charaka Samhita, 1982. Translated by Pundit Krishna Shastri and Dr. Garakhanath Chaturvedi, Vol. I & II. Chaukhambha Vishwabharati , Varanasi.

Dash, Bhagwan, 1991. *Materia Medica of Ayurveda based on Madanapala's Nighantu.* B. Jain Publisher, New Delhi.

Das, Vaidya Bhagwan, 1998. *Massage Therapy in Ayurveda.* Panchakarma Therapy of Ayurveda Series No. 1 . Concept Publishing Company, New Delhi, pp. 192.

Joshi, Sunil V., 1998. *Ayurveda and Panchakarma: The Science of Healing and Rejuvenation.* Motilal Banarsidas Publishers Pvt. Ltd., Delhi, pp. 1–309.

Sushruta Samhita, 1982. Translated by Kaviraj Ambika dutta Shastri, Vol. I & II. Chaukhambha Vishwabharati , Varanasi.

Medicinal Plants: Conservation, Cultivation and Utilization (2007) *Pages 425–426*
Editors: **A.K. Chopra, D.R. Khanna, G. Prasad, D.S. Malik and R. Bhutiani**
Published by: **DAYA PUBLISHING HOUSE**

Recommendations

During the sessions, there were five invited talks and a total of fifty papers were presented. The following important recommendations based on different technical sessions were made unanimously at the concluding session:

(1) The proper survey, identification and documentation of inventory of medicinal plants of Uttaranchal region including information on the list of species with local names, part(s) used and distribution range should be envisaged to documentation of inventories. The current status of medicinal plant resources of the state should be worked out.

(2) On priority, the strategy must address the conservation of wild medicinal plants, threatened with extinction and efforts should be made to prevent extinction through *ex-situ* & *in-situ* conservation practices.

(3) The traditional knowledge system needs to be studied, documented, preserved and used for the benefit of humankind. Uttaranchal is home to a variety of ethnic communities living in harmony with the rich and unique biodiversity elements. Among the tribes, Bhotia, Rajees, Tharus and Boxas live in Uttaranchal. They rely, to a large extent, on native plant species for obtaining various types of raw material which are thus of vital importance in traditional health care. This requires a holistic approach, involvement and participation of local inhabitants.

(4) Tribal knowledge databases should be taken up as a project by universities and a chapter on medicinal and veterinary plants should included in the textbooks at school levels also. The potentiality and role of medicinal plants in the state economy should be highlighted.

(5) At present, farming of medicinal plants is insignificant, scattered and largely informal. Keeping in view the increasing global population and consequent rise in demand for medicinal plants, one feasible option would be to regard medicinal plants as under-utilized

crops. This would promote farming of the species, which will help a great deal to offset pressure on natural wild types. Cultivation will also help in the production of uniform material for obtaining quality products, consistently. Cultivation should be a major part of the strategy.

(6) Contract farming of drug plants in this area and their marketing should be in proper way through farmer cooperative societies under guidance of Govt. to facilitate more funds and facilities like seeds, fertilizers, equipments etc. Organic farming certification, quality seed certification and patenting agencies should interact with farmers and NGOs to provide them these certificates for global marketing scopes.

(7) There is a need for in-depth and extensive investigation on the extent of availability and natural recruitment processes of high-value medicinal plants used extensively for the preparation of drugs in various systems of medicine. It will help in planning a strategy to offset the expected widening of gap between demand and supply (availability) of raw material.

(8) Scientific community should recommend authenticated formulations and not flair with the wave of misconception of farmers. There is great need for conscientious R & D for developing packages and their documentation. Since rural inhabitants possess incredible knowledge of a number of plant-based formulations, there help should be taken for experimentation and observations.

(9) Development of proper harvesting, post harvesting and storages practice should be promoted.

(10) Wastelands should be used for cultivation as alternatives to generate remuneration with proper reclamation and active ingredient testing.

(11) There is a need to inculcate greater mass awareness about the benefits of medicinal plants among different sections of the society.

(12) A collaborative work plan involving scientists, universities, government institutions and non-governmental organizations is suggested for preserving the traditional knowledge system and practices which will help in strengthening the conservation of medicinal plants and in the up-liftment of the rural economy of this mountain state.

Acknowledgements

The organizers are thankful to various funding agencies CSIR, UGC, NABARD and DST along with all the advertisers for providing us the partial financial assistance for organizing the National Seminar on "Medicinal Plants Conservation, Cultivation and Utilization" and making this event a grand success.

Index